Essential
Endocrinology
and Diabetes

FIFTH EDITION

Essential Endocrinology and Diabetes

Richard IG Holt

Reader of Endocrinology and Metabolism
School of Medicine
University of Southampton

Neil A Hanley

Professor of Endocrinology
School of Medicine
University of Southampton

Blackwell
Publishing

Published by Blackwell Publishing Ltd
Blackwell Publishing, Inc., 350 Main Street, Malden, Massachusetts
    02148-5020, USA
Blackwell Publishing Ltd, 9600 Garsington Road, Oxford OX4 2DQ, UK
Blackwell Publishing Asia Pty Ltd, 550 Swanston Street, Carlton, Victoria
    3053, Australia

First published 1983   Second edition 1988   Third edition 1996
Fouth edition 2001   Fifth edition 2007

2   2008

Library of Congress Cataloging-in-Publication Data

Holt, Richard I.G.
    Essential endocrinology and diabetes. – 5th ed. / Richard I.G. Holt,
    Neil A. Hanley.
        p. ; cm.
    Rev. ed. of: Essential endocrinology / Charles G.D. Brook, Nicholas
    J. Marshall. 4th ed. 2001.
    Includes bibliographical references and index.
    ISBN 978-1-4051-3648-8 (alk. paper)
        1.   Endocrinology–Case studies.   2.   Diabetes–Case studies.
    I. Hanley, Neil A.   II. Brook, C. G. D. (Charles Groves Darville). Essential
    endocrinology.   III. Title.
        [DNLM: 1.   Endocrine Glands–physiology–Case Reports.
    2.   Diabetes Mellitus–Case Reports.   3.   Endocrine System Diseases–Case
    Reports.   4.   Hormones–physiology–Case Reports.   WK 100 H758e
    2006]
    RC648.H65 2006
    616.4–dc22

2006008614

ISBN 978-1-4051-3648-8
A catalogue record for this title is available from the British Library

Set in 9 on 12 pt Palatino by SNP Best-set Typesetter Ltd., Hong Kong
Printed and bound in Singapore by Fabulous Printers Pte Ltd.

Commissioning Editor: Martin Sugden
Editorial Assistant: Eleanor Bonnet
Development Editor: Karen Moore
Production Controller: Kate Charman

For further information on Blackwell Publishing, visit our website:
http://www.blackwellpublishing.com

Contents

Preface

The fifth edition of this book has been extensively rewritten. We are grateful for the skilled help of Blackwell Publishing in bringing our work to fruition and also to our predecessors, Charles Brook and Nicholas Marshall, for their excellent starting point. Since the first edition of Essential Endocrinology by O'Riordan, Malan and Gould in 1982, medical education has changed; with the new design, layout and content of the book we have tried to keep up with this progression and, indeed, facilitate the widening access to medicine and the use of systems-based learning. There are now three clear sections to the text and even the title has changed to reflect the evolution of diabetes into its own specialty.

The first section focuses on basic principles. Recognizing that many students now come to medicine from nonscientific backgrounds, we have tried to limit assumptions on prior knowledge. For instance, the new chapter on biological principles explains meiosis, a prerequisite for grasping key aspects of reproductive endocrinology. Similarly, molecular genetics has advanced so much that new diagnostic tools are becoming standard practice. It is important that aspiring clinicians, as well as scientists, appreciate these laboratory methods and understand the language of molecular genetic investigation. The chapter on endocrine investigation has also been broadened to include an introduction to imaging techniques. Not everything has expanded. As molecular endocrinology advances, it becomes increasingly important to summarize the science that is salient to clinical practice without ever-expanding detail. As a result, the chapter on molecular endocrinology has actually been shortened. Taken together, the first four chapters should prepare the reader for the clinical

sections. Cross-references have been made where possible, including invitations to review the basic principle chapters at relevant points of the clinical sections.

The clinical endocrinology section retains an organ-based approach; however, the introductory basic science in these chapters has been condensed in favour of greater detail on clinical disorders and their management. The section on diabetes is entirely new and reflects the growth of this subject into a separate entity. The fact that diabetes is taught alongside endocrinology from undergraduate study until the completion of advanced training, presses for its inclusion in the same textbook. The combination of basic science and clinical information aims to bridge the gap from lecture theatre, through clinical training, to the knowledge required for the foundation years and specialist training. To this end, case scenarios are now included at relevant points of the text with detailed answers provided at the end of each clinical chapter. Clinical descriptions can be greatly enhanced by pictures and for this reason we have also included a series of clinical colour plates.

The text goes beyond core undergraduate medical education. Learning objectives, boxes, and concluding 'key points' aim to emphasize the major topics. The extra detail hopefully provides a 'refresher' where necessary for more advanced clinicians who, like the authors, enjoy trying to interpret clinical medicine scientifically, but for whom memory occasionally fails.

We have brought our clinical and research expertise together to create this book. While it has been a truly collaborative venture and the book is designed to read as a whole, inevitably one of us has taken a lead with each of the chapters depending on our own interests. As such, NAH was responsible for writing Part 1 and the chapters on the hypothalamus and pituitary, the adrenal gland, reproductive endocrinology and thyroid gland, while RIGH was responsible for Part 3 and the chapters on calcium and endocrine neoplasia.

R.I.G. Holt
N.A. Hanley
University of Southampton

The Authors

Richard Holt is Reader of Endocrinology and Metabolism at the University of Southampton and Honorary Consultant in Endocrinology at Southampton University Hospitals NHS Trust. His research interests are broadly focused around the pathogenesis of the insulin resistance syndrome and its interactions with the growth hormone axis.

Neil Hanley has a personal Chair at the University of Southampton and is an Honorary Consultant in Endocrinology at Southampton University Hospitals NHS Trust. His research interests are development of the human endocrine organs and stem cell biology.

Both authors play a role in the teaching of undergraduate medical students and doctors at the University of Southampton. RIGH is a member of the In-stitute of Learning and Teaching in Higher Education.

Further reading

The following major international textbooks make an excellent source of secondary reading:

Williams Textbook of Endocrinology, Reed Larsen, Henry Kronenberg, Shlomo Melmed and Kenneth Polonsky, 10th edition, Saunders, 2002.

Textbook of Diabetes, John Pickup and Gareth Williams, 3rd edition, Blackwell Publishing, 2002.

In addition, the following textbooks cover topics, relevant to some chapters, in greater detail:

Roitt's Essential Immunology, Peter J Delves, Seamus J. Martin, Dennis, R. Burton and Ivan M. Roitt, 11th edition, Blackwell Publishing, 2006.

Essential Reproduction, Martin Johnson and Barry Everitt, 5th edition, Blackwell Publishing, 2000.

Lehninger's Principles of Biochemistry, David Nelson and Michael Cox, Palgrave Macmillan, 2004.

List of Abbreviations

5-HIAA	5-hydroxyindoleacetic acid		FISH	fluorescence *in situ* hybridization
5-HT	5-hydroxytryptophan		FSH	follicle-stimulating hormone
αMSH	α-melanocyte stimulating hormone		fT_3	free triiodothyronine
ACTH	adrenocorticotrophic hormone		fT_4	free thyroxine
ADH	arginine vasopressin/antidiuretic hormone		GC	gas chromatography
			GDM	gestational diabetes
AFP	α-fetoprotein		GFR	glomerular filtration rate
AGE	advanced glycation end-product		GH	growth hormone (somatotrophin)
AGRP	Agouti-related protein		GHR	growth hormone receptor
AI	angiotensin I		GHRH	growth hormone releasing hormone
AII	angiotensin II		GI	glycaemic index
ALS	acid labile subunit		GIP	gastric inhibitory peptide
AMH	anti-Müllerian hormone		GLUT	glucose transporter
AR	androgen receptor		GnRH	gonadotrophin-releasing hormone
AVP	arginine vasopressin		GPCR	guanine-protein coupled receptor
CAH	congenital adrenal hyperplasia		GR	glucocorticoid receptor
cAMP	cyclic adenosine monophosphate		Grb2	type 2 growth factor receptor-bound protein
CBG	cortisol binding globulin			
cGMP	guanosine monophosphate		hCG	human chorionic gonadotrophin
CRE	cAMP response element		hMG	human menopausal gonadotrophin
CREB	cAMP response element-binding protein		HMGCoA	hydroxymethylglutaryl coenzyme A
			HNF	hepatocyte nuclear family
CNS	central nervous system		HPLC	high performance liquid chromatography
CRH	corticotrophin-releasing hormone			
CSF	cerebrospinal fluid		HRE	hormone response element
CT	computed tomography		HRT	hormone replacement therapy
CVD	cardiovascular disease		ICSI	intracytoplasmic sperm injection
DAG	diacylglycerol		IDDM	insulin-dependent diabetes mellitus
DEXA	dual energy X-ray absorptiometry			
DHEA	dehydroepiandrosterone		IFG	impaired fasting glycaemia
DHT	5α-dihydrotestosterone		IFMA	immunofluorometric assay
DI	diabetes insipidus		IGF	insulin-like growth factor
EGF	epidermal growth factor		IGFBP	IGF binding protein
EPO	erythropoietin		IGT	impaired glucose tolerance
FFA	free fatty acid		IP	inositol phosphate
FGF	fibroblast growth factor		IPF	insulin promoter factor
FIA	fluoroimmunoassay		IR	insulin receptor

IRMA	intraretinal microvascular abnormalities (Chapter 14)		PPAR	peroxisome proliferator-activated receptor
IRMA	immunoradiometric assay (Chapter 4)		PRL	prolactin
IRS	insulin receptor substrate		PTH	parathyroid hormone
IVF	*in vitro* fertilization		PTHrP	parathyroid hormone-related peptide
JAK	Janus-associated kinase		PTU	propylthiouracil
LDL	low-density lipoprotein		RER	rough endoplasmic reticulum
LH	luteinizing hormone		RIA	radioimmunoassay
MAO	monoamine oxidase		rT_3	reverse triiodothyronine
MAPK	mitogen-activated protein kinase		RXR	retinoid X receptor
MEN	multiple endocrine neoplasia		SERM	selective oestrogen receptor modulators
MIS	Müllerian inhibiting substance			
MODY	maturity onset diabetes of the young		SHBG	sex hormone binding globulin
MR	mineralocorticoid receptor		SIADH	syndrome of inappropriate antidiuretic hormone
MRI	magnetic resonance imaging			
MS	mass spectrometry		SoS	son of sevenless protein
MSH	melanocyte-stimulating hormone		SRE	serum response element
NEFA	nonesterified fatty acids		SS	somatostatin
NICTH	nonislet cell tumour hypoglycaemia		StAR	steroid acute regulatory protein
NIDDM	noninsulin dependent diabetes mellitus		STAT	signal transduction and activation of transcription protein
NPY	neuropeptide Y		T1DM	type 1 diabetes
NVD	new vessels at the disc		T2DM	type 2 diabetes
NVE	new vessels elsewhere		$T_{1/2}$	half-life
OGTT	oral glucose tolerance test		T_3	triiodothyronine
PCR	polymerase chain reaction		T_4	thyroxine
PDE	phosphodiesterase		TGFβ	transforming growth factorβ
PGE2	prostaglandin E2		TK	tyrosine kinase
PI	phosphatidylinositol		TPO	thyroid peroxidase
PIT1	pituitary-specific transcription factor 1		TR	thyroid hormone receptor
PKA	protein kinase A		TRE	thyroid hormone response element
PKC	protein kinase C		TRH	thyrotrophin-releasing hormone
PLC	phospholipase C		TSH	thyroid-stimulating hormone
PNMT	phenylethanolamine *N*-methyl transferase		UFC	urinary free cortisol
			VEGF	vascular endothelial growth factor
POMC	pro-opiomelanocortin		VIP	vasoactive intestinal peptide

PART 1

1 Principles of Endocrinology

LEARNING OBJECTIVES

- To be able to define endocrinology
- To understand the underlying principles of endocrinology as a basic science and a clinical specialty
- To appreciate the history of endocrinology

- To understand the classification of hormones into peptides, steroids and amino acid derivatives
- To understand the principle of feedback mechanisms that regulate hormone secretion

This chapter introduces the background and basic principles that underlie endocrinology and diabetes

Introduction

An organism comprised of a single or a few cells analyses and responds to its external environment with ease. No cell is more than a short diffusion distance from the outside world or its neighbours, allowing a constancy of internal environment ('homeostasis'). This simplicity has been lost with the evolution of more complex, larger, multicellular organisms. Simple diffusion has become inadequate in larger animal species where functions are localized to specific organs. In humans, there are $\sim10^{14}$ cells of 200 or more different types. With this compartmentalized division of purpose comes the need for effective communication to disseminate information throughout the whole organism—only a few cells face the outside world, yet all respond to it. Welcome to the world of communication systems and, in particular, the endocrine and nervous systems (Box 1.1).

The specialized ductless glands and tissues of the endocrine system release chemical messengers—hormones—into the extracellular space, from where they enter the bloodstream. It is this blood-borne transit that defines endocrinology; however, the principles are similar for hormone action on a neighbouring cell ('*paracrinology*') or, indeed, itself ('*auto* or *intra*crinology') (Fig. 1.1).

The nervous and endocrine systems interact. Many endocrine glands are under both nervous and hormonal control, while the central nervous system is affected by multiple hormonal stimuli—features reflected by the composite science of neuroendocrinology (Fig. 1.1).

The term 'hormone', derived from the Greek word 'hormaein' meaning 'to arouse' or 'excite', was first used in 1905 by Sir Ernest Starling in his Croonian Lecture to the Royal College of Physicians. Endocrinologists have recently held centenary celebrations of this landmark; however, the specialty is built on

BOX 1.1 The endocrine and nervous systems constitute the two main communication systems

The functions of the endocrine and nervous systems are to:
- allow appropriate adaptive changes
- monitor internal and external environments } maintain homeostasis
- communicate via chemical messengers

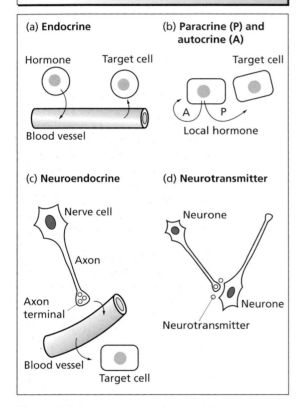

(a) Endocrine

Hormone Target cell

Blood vessel

(b) Paracrine (P) and autocrine (A)

Target cell

A P

Local hormone

(c) Neuroendocrine

Nerve cell

Axon

Axon terminal

Blood vessel

Target cell

(d) Neurotransmitter

Neurone

Neurone

Neurotransmitter

Figure 1.1 Cells that secrete regulatory substances to 'communicate' with their target cells and organs. (a) Endocrine. Cells secrete hormone into the blood vessel, where it is carried, potentially for large distances, to its target cell. (b) Paracrine (P). Cells secrete hormone that acts on nearby cells (e.g. glucagon and somatostatin act on adjacent β-cells within the pancreatic islet to influence insulin secretion). Autocrine (A). Insulin-like growth factors can act on the cell that produces them, representing autocrine control. (c) Stimulated neuroendocrine cells secrete hormone (e.g. epinephrine) from axonic terminals into the bloodstream. (d) Neurotransmitter cells secrete substances from axonic terminals to activate adjacent neurones.

foundations that are far older. Aristotle described the pituitary, while the associated condition, gigantism, was referred to in the Old Testament, two millennia or so before the 19th century recognition of the gland's anterior and posterior components by Rathke, and Pierre Marie's connection of pituitary tumours to acromegaly. Diabetes was recognized by the ancient Egyptians before Areteus described the disorder in the second century AD as 'a melting down of flesh and limbs into urine'—diabetes comes from the Greek word meaning siphon. The disorder was only narrowed to the pancreas relatively recently by realizing that the organ's removal in dogs mimicked the human condition (Minkowski, 1889).

The roots of reproductive endocrinology are equally long. The Bible refers to eunuchs and Hippocrates recognized that mumps could result in sterility. Oophorectomy in sows and camels was used to increase strength and growth in ancient Egypt. However, it was only in the 17th century that it gained microscopic understanding with the visualization of spermatozoa by Leeuwenhoek and later, in the 19th century, when the mammalian ovum was discovered in the Graafian follicle.

During the last 500 years, other endocrine organs and axes have been identified and characterized. In 1564, Bartolommeo Eustacio noted the presence of the adrenal glands. Almost 300 hundred years later (1855), Thomas Addison, one of the forefathers of clinical endocrinology, described the consequences of their inadequacy. Catecholamines were identified at the turn of the last century, in parallel with Oliver and Schaffer's discovery that these adrenomedullary substances raise blood pressure. This followed shortly after the clinical features of myxoedema were linked to the thyroid gland, when, in 1891, physicians in Newcastle treated hypothyroidism with sheep thyroid extract. This was an important landmark, but long after the ancient Chinese recognized that seaweed, as a source of iodine, held valuable properties in treating goitre.

Early clinical endocrinology tended to recognize and describe the features of endocrine syndromes. Since then, our understanding has advanced due to: the successful quantification of circulating hormones; the pathophysiological identification of endocrine dysfunction; and the molecular unravelling of complex hormone action. Some of the landmarks from the last 100 years are shown in Box 1.2.

Traditionally, endocrinology has studied specialized hormone-secreting organs (Fig. 1.2), largely built on the 'endocrine postulates' of Edward Doisy (Box 1.3). While the focus of this textbook remains with these organs, many tissues display hitherto unappreciated degrees of hormone biosynthesis, and, perhaps more importantly, modulate hormone action. All will become increasingly important for a complete appreciation of endocrinology and its significance.

The role of hormones

Hormones are synthesized by specialized cells (Table 1.1), which may exist as distinct endocrine glands or be located as single cells within other organs, such as the gastrointestinal tract. Classically, all are defined by the secretion of hormones into the bloodstream; however, autocrine or paracrine actions may also be prevalent and, indeed, modulate the function of the original endocrine cell type.

Hormones act by binding to specific receptors, either on the surface or within the target cell, to

---

BOX 1.2 Some landmarks in endocrinology over the last 100 years

1905	First use of the term 'hormone' by Starling in the Croonian Lecture at the Royal College of Physicians
1909	Cushing removed part of pituitary and saw improvement in acromegaly
1914	Kendall isolated iodine-containing substance from thyroid
1921	Banting and Best extracted insulin from islet cells of dog pancreas and used it to lower blood sugar
Early 1930s	Pitt-Rivers and Harrington determined the structure of the thyroid hormone, thyroxine
1935	Crystallization of testosterone
~1940	Identification of oestrogen and progesterone
1940s	Harris recognizes the relationship between the hypothalamus and anterior pituitary in the 'portal-vessel chemotransmitter hypothesis'
1952	Gross and Pitt-Rivers identified triiodothyronine in human serum
1955	The Schally and Guillemin laboratories showed that extracts of hypothalamus stimulated ACTH release
1956	Doniach, Roitt and Campbell associated antithyroid antibodies with some forms of hypothyroidism – the first description of an autoimmune phenomenon
1950s	Adams and Purves identified the stimulatory substances that proved to be thyroid stimulatory autoantibodies
1950s	Landmark experiments by Jost discovered the role of testosterone in rabbit sexual development
1955	Sanger reported the primary structure of insulin, for which he won the Nobel Prize in Medicine
1957	Growth hormone first used to treat short stature in patients
1969	Hodgkin reported the three dimensional crystallographic structure of insulin
1969–71	Discovery of TRH and GnRH by Schally's and Guillemin's groups
1973	Discovery of somatostatin by the group of Guillemin
1977	The sequential discovery of hypothalamic releasing factors was recognized by the award of the Nobel Prize in Medicine to Schally and Guillemin
1981–2	Discovery of CRH and GHRH by Wylie Vale's group
1994	Identification of leptin by Friedman and colleagues
1999	Discovery of Ghrelin by Kangawa and colleagues
1999	Sequencing the human genome – publication of the DNA code for the first chromosome, chromosome 22
2000	Establishment of the 'Edmonton protocol' by Shapiro and colleagues, revitalizing efforts to cure type 1 diabetes by transplantation

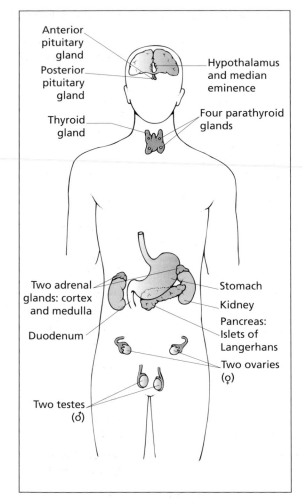

Figure 1.2 The sites of the principal endocrine glands. The stomach, kidneys and duodenum are also shown.

initiate a cascade of intracellular reactions, which frequently amplifies the original stimulus and generates a final response. These responses are altered in hormone deficiency and excess and it is these phenomena that marry basic science and clinical endocrinology. For instance, growth hormone (GH) underproduction leads to short stature in children, while excess causes overgrowth (either gigantism or acromegaly; Chapter 5).

Thyroid hormone acts on many, if not all, of the 200 cell-types in the body. The basal metabolic rate increases if it is present in excess and declines if there is a deficiency (Chapter 8). Similarly, insulin acts on most tissues, implying its receptors are widespread.

Its importance is also underlined by its role in the maintenance of many cell types in laboratory culture. In contrast, other hormones may act only on one tissue. Thyroid-stimulating hormone (TSH), adrenocorticotrophin (ACTH) and the gonadotrophins are secreted by the anterior pituitary and have specific target tissues—the thyroid gland, the adrenal cortex and the gonads, respectively.

Classification of hormones

There are three major groups of hormones according to biochemical structure and method of synthesis (Box 1.4). The biosynthesis of peptide hormones is similar to that of any cellular protein. The production of amino acid-derived and steroid hormones is a biochemical cascade catalyzed by a series of intracellular enzymes. Such cascades are central to all eukaryotic cells—it is subtle adaptation that co-opts them to endocrine duty and the biosynthesis of a hormone rather than another endpoint.

Peptide hormones

The majority of hormones are peptides and range in size from very small, only three amino acids (TRH), to small proteins of over 200 amino acids, such as TSH or luteinizing hormone (LH). Some peptide hormones are secreted directly, but most are stored in granules, the release of which becomes a major

Table 1.1 The endocrine organs and their hormones. The distinction between peptide and protein is somewhat arbitrary. Shorter than 50 amino acids is termed a peptide in this table

Gland	Hormone	Molecular characteristics
Hypothalamus/median eminence	*Releasing and inhibiting hormones*:	
	Thyrotrophin-releasing hormone (TRH)	Peptide
	Somatostatin (SS)	Peptide
	Gonadotrophin releasing hormone (GnRH)	Peptide
	Corticotrophin releasing hormone (CRH)	Peptide
	Growth hormone releasing hormone (GHRH)	Peptide
	Dopamine (Prolactin inhibiting factor)	Tyrosine derivative
Anterior pituitary	Thyrotrophin or thyroid-stimulating hormone (TSH)	Glycoprotein
	Luteinizing hormone (LH)	Glycoprotein
	Follicle-stimulating hormone (FSH)	Glycoprotein
	Growth hormone (GH) (also called somatotrophin)	Protein
	Prolactin (PRL)	Protein
	Adrenocorticotrophin (ACTH)	Peptide
Posterior pituitary	Arginine vasopressin/antidiuretic hormone (ADH)	Peptide
	Oxytocin	Peptide
Thyroid	Thyroxine (T_4) and triiodothyronine (T_3)	Tyrosine derivatives
	Calcitonin	Peptide
Parathyroid	Parathyroid hormone (PTH)	Peptide
Adrenal cortex	Aldosterone	Steroid
	Cortisol	Steroid
	Androstenedione	Steroid
	Dehydroepiandrosterone (DHEA)	Steroid
Adrenal medulla	Epinephrine (adrenaline)	Tyrosine derivative
	Norepinephrine (noradrenaline)	Tyrosine derivative
Stomach	Gastrin	Peptide
Pancreas (islets of Langerhans)	Insulin	Protein
	Glucagon	Protein
	Somatostatin (SS)	Protein
Duodenum and jejunum	Secretin	Protein
	Cholecystokinin	Protein
Liver	Insulin-like growth factor 1 (IGF1)	Protein
Ovary	Oestrogens	Steroid
	Progesterone	Steroid
Testis	Testosterone	Steroid

BOX 1.4 Major hormone groups

- Peptides and proteins
- Amino acid derivatives
- Steroids

control mechanism regulated potentially by another hormone, as part of a cascade, or by innervation.

Some peptide hormones have complex tertiary structures or are comprised of more than one peptide chain. Oxytocin and arginine vasopressin (AVP), the two posterior pituitary hormones, have ring structures linked by disulphide bridges. Despite being remarkably similar in structure, they have very different physiological roles (Fig. 1.3). Insulin consists of α- and β-chains linked by disulphide bonds. Like several hormones, it is synthesized as an inactive precursor that requires modification prior to release and activity. This model protects the synthesizing cell from a deluge of its own hormone action. The gonadotrophins, follicle-stimulating hormone (FSH) and LH, TSH and human chorionic gonadotrophin (hCG) also have two chains. However, these α- and β-subunits are synthesized quite separately, from separate genes. The α-subunit of each is shared; it is the distinctive β-subunit of each that confers biological specificity.

Amino acid derivatives

These hormones are small water-soluble compounds. Melatonin is derived from tryptophan, whereas the tyrosine derivatives include the thyroid hormones, the catecholamines, and dopamine from the hypothalamic–anterior pituitary unit and the central nervous system. The catecholamines of the adrenal medulla, epinephrine and norepinephrine, are identical to the sympathetic neurotransmitters, emphasizing the close relationship between the nervous and endocrine systems (Fig. 1.2). Like peptide hormones, they are stored in secretory granules prior to release.

Steroid hormones

Steroid hormones are lipid-soluble molecules derived from cholesterol, which is itself a basic constituent of the cell membrane. Produced by the adrenal cortex and gonad, steroid hormones are insoluble in water so need to circulate bound to plasma proteins.

Organization of the endocrine system

The synthesis and release of hormones is regulated by control systems, similar to those used in engineering. These mechanisms ensure that hormone signals can be limited in amplitude and duration. At the centre of regulation for many endocrine organs is the anterior pituitary gland, which, in turn, is controlled by a number of hormones released from specialized hypothalamic neurones. Thus, major endocrine axes are formed (hypothalamic–anterior pituitary–end organ), where the end organ might be adrenal cortex, thyroid, testis or ovary.

Mechanisms that regulate endocrine signalling

An appreciation of control is crucial to endocrinology, as it underpins not only the functions of many endocrine systems but also their clinical investigation.

Simple control

An elementary control system is one in which the signal itself is limited, either in magnitude or duration, so as to induce only a transient response. Certain neural impulses are of this type. Refinement allows discrimination of a positive signal from background 'noise' to ensure that the target cell cannot or does not respond below a certain threshold level. An example of this is the pulsatile release of gonadotrophin-releasing hormone from the hypothalamus.

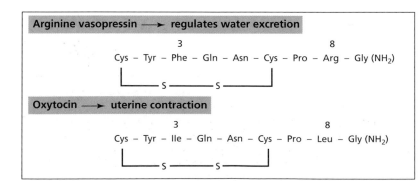

Figure 1.3 The structures of arginine vasopressin and oxytocin are remarkably similar, yet the physiological effects of the two hormones differ profoundly.

Negative feedback

Negative feedback is the commonest form of regulation used by many biological systems. For example, in enzymatic reactions, the product of a reaction frequently inhibits its own generation. In endocrinology, the hormone may act on its target cell to stimulate a substance (often another hormone) that then inhibits production of the first hormone (Fig. 1.4a). An extension of this scenario exists for many of the hypothalamic-anterior pituitary-end organ axes (Fig. 1.4b). The hypothalamic hormone (e.g. CRH) stimulates the release of anterior pituitary hormone (in this case ACTH) to increase peripheral hormone production (cortisol), which then feeds back on the anterior pituitary and hypothalamus to reduce the original secretions.

Hormone secretion may also be regulated by meta-bolic processes. For instance, the β-cell makes insulin in response to high blood glucose concentrations. The effect is to lower glucose, which, in turn, inhibits further insulin release.

Positive feedback

Under certain, more unusual, circumstances, hormones feedback to the pituitary gland to enhance, rather than inhibit, secretion of the primary hormone —called positive feedback (Fig. 1.4). In engineering, this is intrinsically unstable. However, in some biological systems it can be beneficial: for instance, the action of oestrogen on the pituitary gland to induce the ovulatory surge of LH and FSH (Chapter 7); or during childbirth, stretch receptors in the distended vagina send neurological signals to the brain, which stimulate oxytocin release. This hormone

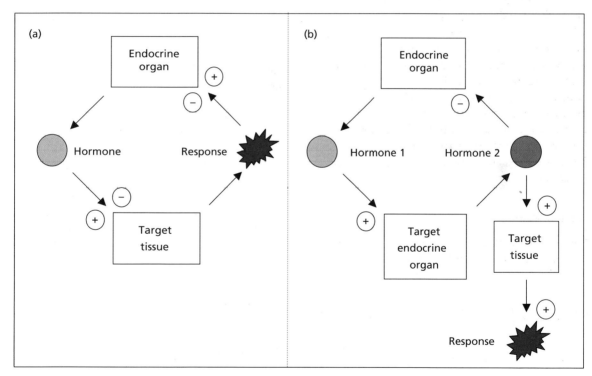

Figure 1.4 Two simplified models of hormone synthesis, action and feedback. (a) The endocrine organ releases a hormone, which acts on the target tissue to stimulate (+) or inhibit (−) a response. The response may feedback either to inhibit or stimulate the endocrine organ to decrease or increase supply of the hormone, respectively. (b) The endocrine organ produces hormone 1, which acts on a second endocrine gland to release hormone 2. In turn, hormone 2 acts dually on the target tissue to induce a response and feeds back negatively onto the original endocrine organ to regulate release of hormone 1. This model is illustrative of the axes between the anterior pituitary and its peripheral endocrine targets.

causes the uterus to contract, further activating the stretch receptors to establish positive feedback that is only terminated by delivery of the baby. The role of oxytocin in the suckling-milk ejection reflex is similar—a positive feedback loop that is only broken by the cessation of the baby's feeding.

Inhibitory control

The secretion of some hormones is under inhibitory as well as stimulatory control. Somatostatin, a hypothalamic hormone, prevents the secretion of GH, such that when somatostatin secretion is diminished, GH secretion is facilitated. A similar scenario controls prolactin release, which is under tonic inhibition from dopamine. This complexity from dual inhibitory and stimulatory control allows more precise regulation of hormone secretion.

Endocrine rhythms

Many of the body's activities show periodic or cyclical changes (Box 1.5). Control of these rhythms commonly arises from the nervous system, for instance the hypothalamic nuclei. Some appear independent of the environment, whereas others are co-ordinated and 'entrained' by external cues (e.g. the 24-hour light/dark cycle that becomes temporarily disrupted in 'jetlag').

Cortisol secretion is maximal between 0400 h and 0800 h as we awaken and minimal as we retire to bed. In contrast, GH and prolactin are secreted maximally ~1 hour after falling asleep. Clinically, knowledge of endocrine rhythms is important, as serum analysis of a hormone must take into account hour-by-hour and day-to-day variability. Otherwise, such measurements may not be useful, or indeed, they may be misleading.

BOX 1.5 Endocrine cycles

Circadian = 24-hour cycle
- circa = about, dies = day

Ultradian < 24-hour cycle
- e.g. GnRH release

Infradian > 24-hour cycle
- e.g. menstrual cycle

Endocrine disorders

Abnormalities of the endocrine axes largely present through *disordered, over*production or *under*production of hormone. Some clinical features occur because of compensatory overproduction of other hormones. For example, Addison's disease is a deficiency of cortisol from the adrenal cortex, which reduces negative feedback on ACTH production at the anterior pituitary. The gene that encodes ACTH also includes another hormone, melanocyte-stimulating hormone (MSH). This unavoidable, concomitant rise in MSH stimulates melanocytes to increase skin pigmentation—a cardinal sign of Addison's disease.

Imbalanced hormone production may occur when a particular enzyme is missing because of a genetic defect. For example, in congenital adrenal hyperplasia, the lack of 21-hydroxylase results in a failure to synthesize downstream cortisol. Other pathways remain intact leading to an excess production of sex steroids that can masculinize aspects of the female body. Endocrine disorders may also arise from abnormalities in hormone receptors or hormone-induced signalling pathways. The commonest example is type 2 diabetes, which frequently arises, in large part, from resistance to insulin action in target tissues.

For those endocrine glands under regulation of the hypothalamus and anterior pituitary, disorders can also be categorized according to site. Disease directly in the end organ is termed 'primary'. When the end organ is affected because of a problem in the anterior pituitary (either underactivity or overactivity) it is secondary, while in tertiary disease, the pathology resides in the hypothalamus.

Laboratory diagnosis and assessment of endocrine disorders

The ability to measure hormones in the circulation has transformed our understanding of endocrine disorders as well as dramatically altered our ability to care for patients. The methods for the determination of hormone concentrations are usually referred to as 'assays' (Chapter 4). Most commonly, these depend on antibodies that bind to specific antigenic sites on the hormone (immunoassays). Immunoassays are now a matter of routine biochemical testing and are carried out on a large scale in chemical pathology laboratories. They are sufficiently sensitive, precise and hormone-specific to meet the analytical challenges presented by the endocrine systems.

Principles of static and dynamic testing

The introduction to rhythmical or pulsatile hormone secretion and feedback highlights some problems and opportunities for the assessment of endocrine disorders. Pulsatile secretion, for instance of GH, renders the interpretation of single random samples impossible. GH can be examined, however, as a 'day series' of six to eight values over a number of hours. Alternatively, dynamic testing measures the response of a particular hormone within a defined time period following the administration of a stimulus. This might be a metabolic stimulus, such as hypoglycaemia, to study the response of GH and cortisol. Alternatively, it might be hormonal; for instance, hypothalamic hormones can be injected to stimulate

and assess secretion from the anterior pituitary (e.g. the response of TSH to TRH administration).

These provocative tests interrogate suspected hypofunction. In contrast, suppression testing takes advantage of negative feedback and investigates potential overactivity (Box 1.6). For instance, dexamethasone, a potent synthetic glucocorticoid, should 'switch off' ACTH production from the anterior pituitary according to the normal rules of negative feedback. However, in Cushing disease, ACTH secretion persists due to the autonomous function of a corticotroph adenoma. Examples of these different clinical tests will be discovered throughout Parts 2 and 3.

BOX 1.6 The principles of dynamic investigation in endocrinology

If underactivity is suspected: try to stimulate it
If overactivity is suspected: try to suppress it

KEY POINTS

- Endocrinology is the study of hormones and constitutes one of the body's major communication systems
- A hormone is a chemical messenger, classically distributed via the circulation, that elicits specific effects in target cells
- The three major types of hormones are peptides and the derivatives of amino acids and cholesterol
- Negative and positive feedback mechanisms operate to regulate hormone production
- Hormone secretion may be cyclical
- Clinical endocrine disorders most commonly arise due to hormone over or underactivity
- Clinical investigation of hormone secretion is commonly static but may require dynamic testing

CHAPTER 2

2

The biological principles of endocrinology

LEARNING OBJECTIVES

- To appreciate the organization, structure and function of DNA
- To understand protein synthesis and the cell biology that allows peptide hormone production
- To understand the function of enzymes and how enzyme cascades generate steroid and amino acid-derived hormones

This chapter aims to introduce some of the basic principles that are needed to understand later chapters

Introduction

The human genome is made up of deoxyribonucleic acid (DNA), assembled into 46 chromosomes, and resides in the nucleus (Box 2.1). The DNA contains the 'blueprints' for synthesizing proteins. These are the genes, of which humans possess ~30 000. Each gene serves as the template for generating many copies of messenger ribonucleic acid (mRNA), which is a means of amplifying the information contained in a single gene into the building blocks for many replica proteins. Specific proteins define the phenotype of a particular cell-type (e.g. a cell synthesizing peptide hormone); more commonplace proteins carry out basic functions, for instance the metabolic processes common to all cells. Proteins on the cell surface act as receptors that initiate intracellular signalling, which in turn is reliant on proteins that function as enzymes. Eventually, signalling information reaches the nucleus and the proteins within it called transcription factors. These latter proteins bind or release themselves from areas of DNA near genes to determine whether a gene is switched on ('expressed', when mRNA is transcribed) or silenced.

Chromosomes, DNA and protein synthesis

Genomic DNA in most human cells is packaged into chromosomes by being wrapped around proteins called histones. There are 22 pairs of 'autosomes' and two sex chromosomes—two X's in females, one X and a Y in males. This composition makes females 46,XX and males 46,XY. Distinct chromosomes are only apparent when they are lined up in double quantities in preparation for cell division, either 'mitosis' or 'meiosis' (Fig. 2.1). Mitosis generates two daughter cells, each with a full complement of 46 chromosomes and occurs ~10^{17} times during human life. Meiosis creates the gametes (i.e. spermatozoan

---

BOX 2.1 The structure of DNA

- A molecule of deoxyribose (a 5-carbon sugar) is linked covalently to one of two types of nitrogenous bases:
  - purine—adenine (A) or guanine (G)
  - pyrimidine—thymine (T) or cytosine (C)
  - the base plus the sugar is termed a 'nucleoside', e.g. adenosine
- The addition of a phosphate group to a nucleoside creates a nucleotide, e.g. adenosine mono-, di- or triphosphate (according to how many phosphate groups have been added)
- Phosphodiester bonds polymerize the nucleotides into a single strand of DNA
- Two strands, running in opposite directions, 5 prime (5'; upstream) to 3' (downstream) assemble as a double helix
  - Hydrogen bonds form between the strands, between the base pairs A–T and G–C
- ~3 billion base pairs comprise the human genome

---

or ovum) with 23 chromosomes so that full diploid status is only reconstituted at fertilization.

Several chromosomal abnormalities can result in endocrinopathy. During meiosis, if a chromosome fails to separate properly from its partner or if migration is delayed, a gamete might result that lacks a chromosome or has too many. Thus, it is easy to appreciate Turner syndrome (45,XO), where one sex chromosome is missing; or Klinefelter syndrome (47,XXY), where there is an extra one. Similarly, breaks and rejoining across or within chromosomes produce unusual 'derivative' chromosomes or ones with duplicated or deleted regions (see Fig. 4.4). If such events occur close to genes, function can be disrupted; for example, congenital loss of a hormone. Duplication can be equally significant; on the X chromosome, double dose of a region that includes the gene for DAX1 causes female development in a 46,XY fetus.

Gene transcription

The production of mRNA from a gene is called transcription. Within most genes, the stretches of DNA that encode protein, called exons, are separated by variable lengths of noncoding DNA called introns (Fig. 2.2). Upstream of the first exon is the 5' flanking region of the gene, which contains multiple 'promoter' elements, usually within a few hundred base pairs. Transcription factors bind to these elements to either promote (i.e. turn on) or repress (i.e. turn off) the production of mRNA by RNA polymerase, the enzyme that 'reads' the DNA code. Commonly, the signal that recruits RNA polymerase to the DNA occurs at a 'TATA' box, a short run of adenosines and thymidines, ~30 base pairs upstream of exon 1 (Fig. 2.2).

Superimposed on this, gene expression can be further increased or diminished by more specific transcription factors potentially binding to more distant stretches of DNA (either 'enhancer' or 'repressor' elements). For instance, the transcription factor, steroidogenic factor-1 (SF1) turns on many genes specific to the adrenal cortex and gonad; when SF1 is absent, both organs fail to form.

RNA contains ribose sugar moieties rather than deoxyribose. RNA polymerase 'sticks' ribonucleotides together to generate a single strand of mRNA that correlates to the DNA code of the gene, except that in place of thymidine, a very similar nucleoside, uridine, is incorporated. The initial mRNA strand (pre-mRNA) is processed so that intronic gene regions are excluded and only the exonic sequences are 'spliced' together. Not all exonic regions encode protein, stretches at either end constitute the 5' and 3' untranslated regions (UTR) (Fig. 2.2). Within the 3' UTR, mRNA transcription is terminated by a specific purine-rich motif, the polyadenylation signal, ~20 base pairs upstream of where the mRNA gains a stretch of adenosine residues. This poly-A tail provides stability as the mRNA is moved from the nucleus to the cytoplasm for translation into protein.

Translation into protein

The mRNA is transported to the ribosomes, where protein synthesis occurs by 'translation' (Fig. 2.3a). The ribosomes are attached to the outside of the endoplasmic reticulum (ER), leading to the description of 'rough' ER.

The ribosome is an RNA–protein complex that 'reads' the mRNA sequence. On the first occasion

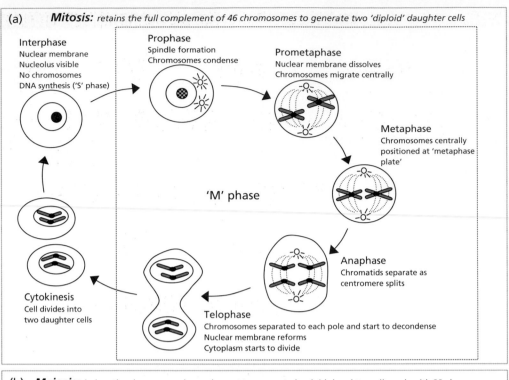

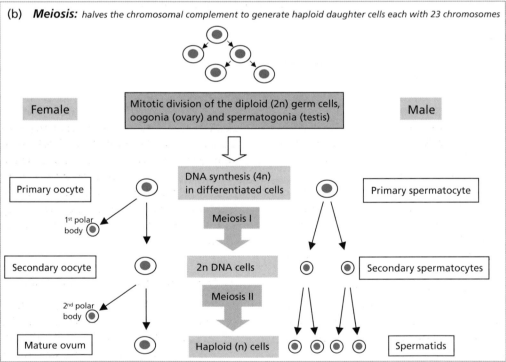

Figure 2.1 Cell division. Prior to mitosis and meiosis the cell undergoes a period of DNA synthesis ('S' phase) so that the normal diploid status of DNA (2n) temporarily becomes 4n. (a) The stages of mitosis result in each daughter cell containing diploid 2n quantities of DNA. (b) Meiosis is split into two stages, each of which comprises prophase, prometaphase, metaphase, anaphase and telophase. During prophase of meiosis I the maternally and paternally derived chromosomes align to allow crossing over ('recombination'), a critical aspect of genetic diversity. The two sister chromatids do not separate, so that the secondary oocyte and spermatocytes each contain '2n' quantities of DNA. During the second stage of meiosis, separation of the chromatids results in haploid cells (n). In males, meiosis is an equal process resulting in four spermatids. In contrast, in females, only one ovum is produced from a primary oocyte, smaller polar bodies being extruded at both stages of meiosis.

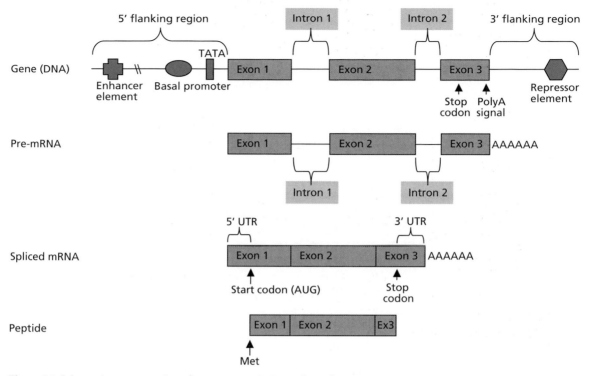

Figure 2.2 Schematic representation of a gene, transcription and translation.

that sequential A–U–G nucleotides are encountered (corresponding to ATG in the genomic DNA), translation starts (Fig. 2.2). From this point, every three nucleotides represent an amino acid. This nucleotide triplet is called a codon, AUG being a start codon that specifies the amino acid, methionine. Similarly, translation continues until a 'stop' codon is encountered (UAA, UGA or UAG).

By understanding these normal events of gene transcription and protein translation, it becomes possible to appreciate how mutations (sequence errors) in the genomic DNA lead to miscoded, and consequently malfunctional, protein (Box 2.2). An entire gene may be missing ('deleted') or duplicated. An erroneous base pair in the promoter region may impair a critical transcription factor from binding. A similar error in exonic coding sequence might translate a different amino acid or even create a premature stop codon. Small deletions or insertions of one or two base pairs throw the whole triplet code out of frame. A mutation at the boundary between an intron and an exon can prevent splicing so that the intron becomes included in the mature mRNA. All of these events affect endocrinology either as congenital defects (i.e. during early development so that the fault is present in the genome of many cells) or as acquired abnormalities later in life, potentially predisposing to the formation of an endocrine tumour (see Chapter 10).

Post-translational modification of peptides

Some polypeptides can function as hormones with simple removal of the start methionine (e.g. thyrotrophin releasing hormone (TRH), which is only three amino acids). Others undergo further modification or potentially fold together as different subunits of a hormone (e.g. luteinizing hormone (LH)). Peptides with any degree of complexity fold into three-dimensional structures, which may contain helical or pleated domains. These shapes provide stability and affect how one protein interacts

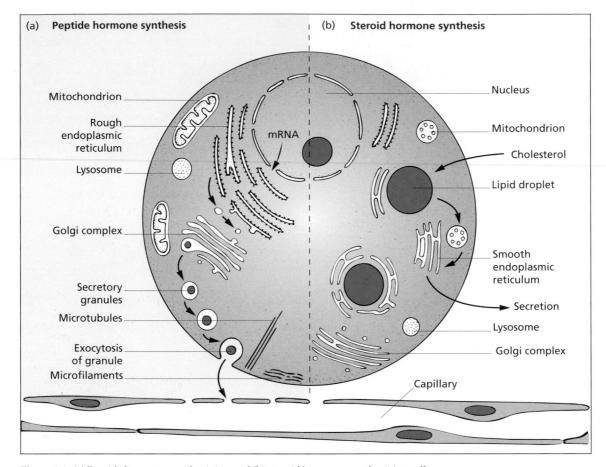

(a) Peptide hormone synthesis

- Mitochondrion
- Rough endoplasmic reticulum
- Lysosome
- mRNA
- Golgi complex
- Secretory granules
- Microtubules
- Exocytosis of granule
- Microfilaments

(b) Steroid hormone synthesis

- Nucleus
- Mitochondrion
- Cholesterol
- Lipid droplet
- Smooth endoplasmic reticulum
- Secretion
- Lysosome
- Golgi complex
- Capillary

Figure 2.3 (a) Peptide hormone-synthesizing and (b) steroid hormone-synthesizing cells.

BOX 2.2 Genetic and genomic abnormalities that can result in endocrinopathy

Abnormalities in DNA
- Base substitution — swapping different nucleotides
- Insertion or deletion — alters frame if exonic and not a multiple of three

Chromosomal abnormalities
- Numerical — three copies as in Down syndrome (trisomy 21)
- Structural
  - inversions — region of a chromosome is turned upside down
  - translocations — regions swapped between chromosomes
  - duplications — region of a chromsome is present twice
  - deletions — region of a chromosome is excised and lost

---

with another (e.g. how a hormone might bind to its receptor).

For hormones that require secretion out of the cell, additional modifications are common and important (Fig. 2.4). The precursor peptide, called a preprohormone, carries a lipophilic signal peptide at the amino terminus. This sequence is recognized by channel proteins so that the immature peptide can cross the ER membrane. Once inside the ER, the signal peptide is excised in preparation for other post-translational changes (Fig. 2.4a–d).

Disulphide bridges are formed in certain proteins (e.g. growth hormone or insulin; Fig. 2.4a and c). Certain carbohydrates may be added to form glycoproteins (Fig. 2.4d). Some prohormones need processing to give rise to several final products (e.g. pro-opiomelanocortin and glucagon), whereas others are assembled as a combination of distinct

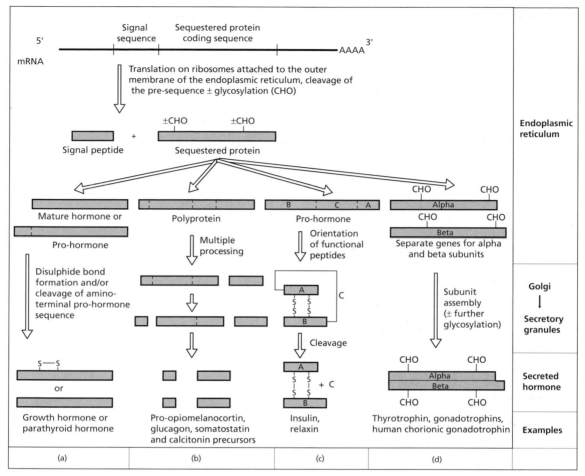

Figure 2.4 Post-translational modifications of peptide hormones. Four types are shown. (a) Simple changes such as removal of the amino terminal 'pro-' extension prior to secretion (e.g. parathyroid hormone) or the addition of intra-chain disulphide bonds (e.g. growth hormone). (b) Multiple processing of a 'polyprotein' into a number of different peptide hormones (e.g. pro-opiomelanocortin can give rise to adrenocorticotrophin plus melanocyte-stimulating hormone and β-endorphin). (c) Synthesis of insulin requires folding of the peptide and the formation of disulphide bonds. The active molecule is created by hydrolytic removal of a connecting (C-) peptide, i.e. proinsulin gives rise to insulin plus C-peptide in equimolar proportion. (d) Synthesis of larger protein hormones (e.g. TSH, LH, follicle-stimulating hormone and human chorionic gonadotrophin) from two separate peptides that complex together. The four hormones share the same α-subunit with a hormone-specific β-subunit.

peptide chains, each synthesized from different genes (e.g. thyroid-stimulating hormone, TSH).

The completed protein is then packaged into membrane-bound vesicles, which may contain specific 'endopeptidases'. These enzymes are responsible for final hormone activation—cleaving the 'pro-' portion of the protein chain, as occurs with the release of C-peptide and insulin (Fig. 2.4c). Post-translational modifications are essential stages in hormone synthesis (Box 2.3).

Endocrine cell biology and biochemistry

Storage and secretion of peptide hormones

Endocrine cells usually store newly synthesized

peptide hormone in small vesicles or secretory granules. Movement of these vesicles to a position near the cell membrane is influenced by two types of filamentous structure: microtubules and microfilaments (Fig. 2.3a). Secretion of the stored hormone only occurs after appropriate stimulation of the cell. Whether this is hormonal, neuronal or nutritional, it usually involves a change in cell permeability to calcium ions. These divalent metal ions are required for interaction between the vesicle and plasma membrane and for the activation of enzymes, microfilaments and microtubules. The secretory process is called exocytosis (Fig. 2.3a). The membrane of the storage granule fuses with the cell membrane at the same time as vesicular endopeptidases are activated so that active hormone is expelled into the extracellular space from where it enters the blood vessels. The vesicle membrane is then recycled within the cell.

Enzymatic action and cascades

Enzymes can be divided into classes according to the reactions that they catalyse (Table 2.1). They frequently operate in cascades where the product of one reaction serves as the substrate for the next. Most simplistically, enzyme action is achieved by protein–protein interaction between the substrate and the enzyme at the latter's 'active site'. Other macromolecules bind elsewhere to the enzyme and function as 'cofactors', adding more complex regulation to the biochemical reaction.

Patients can present with many endocrine syndromes due to loss of enzyme function. For instance, a mutation in the corresponding gene might lead to substitution of an amino acid at a key position of an enzyme's active site. The three-dimensional structure might be affected so significantly that the substrate is no longer converted to the product. In the

---

BOX 2.3 Role of post-translational modifications

Post-translational modifications are important so that:
- active hormone is saved for its intended site of action
- the synthesizing cell is protected from a barrage of its own hormone action

---

Table 2.1 Definition and classification of enzymes

Definition

An enzyme is a biological macromolecule—most frequently a protein—that catalyses a biochemical reaction
Catalysis increases the rate of reaction, e.g. the disappearance of substrate and generation of product
Enzyme action is critical for the synthesis of hormones derived from amino acids and cholesterol

Classification

Enzyme	Catalytic function	Example
Oxidoreductase	Oxidation and reduction	11β-hydroxysteroid dehydrogenase isoforms (HSD11B)
Hydrolases	Cleavage of a bond by the addition of water	Cytochrome P450 11A/cholesterol side-chain cleavage (CYP11A)
Transferases	Transfer of a molecular group from substrate to product	Phenol ethanolamine N-methyl transferase (PNMT)
Lyases	Removal of a group to form a double bond or addition of a group to a double bond	Cytochrome P450 17α-hydroxylase/17-20 lyase (CYP17)
Isomerases	Intramolecular rearrangments	3β-hydroxysteroid dehydrogenase/Delta 4,5 isomerase isoforms (HSD3B)
Ligases or synthases	Join two molecules together	Thyroid peroxidase (TPO)

enzyme cascade to cortisol biosynthesis, this causes congenital adrenal hyperplasia (CAH) (see Chapter 6). Understanding the biochemistry allows accurate diagnosis as the substrate builds up in the circulation and its excess can be measured by immunoassay.

Cholesterol and steroidogenesis

The biosynthesis of steroid hormones centres on enzyme cascades that modify the four-carbon ring structure of cholesterol (Fig. 2.5). The precise complement of enzymes determines which steroids are generated as the final product (Box 2.4).

In addition to making steroid hormones, cholesterol is a critical building block of all mammalian cell membranes and the starting point for vitamin D synthesis, arguably also a hormone (see Chapter 9). It is acquired in approximately equal measure either from the diet or *de novo* synthesis (mostly in the liver; Box 2.4). From the diet, cholesterol is delivered to cells as a complex with low-density lipoprotein (LDL-cholesterol). Intracellular uptake is via the cell surface LDL receptor and endocytosis (Fig. 2.3b). *De novo* biosynthesis commences with acetate and proceeds via hydroxymethylglutaryl coenzyme A (HMGCoA) and mevalonic acid. The rate-limiting step is the reduction of HMGCoA by the enzyme HMGCoA reductase. Pharmacological inhibition of this enzyme in attempts to combat cardiovascular disease has spawned the most widely prescribed drug family in the world (the 'statins').

In steroidogenic cells, cholesterol is largely deposited as esters in large lipid-filled vesicles (Fig. 2.3b). Upon stimulation, cholesterol is released from its stores and transported into the mitochondria, a process that is facilitated by the steroid acute regulatory (StAR) protein in the adrenal and gonad and by the related protein, start domain containing 3 (STARD3), in the placenta. The first step in the synthesis of a steroid hormone is the conversion of cholesterol to pregnenolone. This step is rate limiting. Pregnenolone then undergoes a range of further enzymatic modifications in either the mitochondria or the ER to make active steroid hormones.

Nomenclature of steroidogenic pathways

Figure 2.5 shows a generic representation of human steroid hormone biosynthesis. Many of the enzymes are encoded by the cytochrome P450 (*CYP*) family of related genes that is also critical for hepatic detoxification of drugs. Some of the enzymes are important in both the adrenal cortex and gonad (e.g. CYP11A), whereas others are restricted and thus create the distinct steroid profiles of the different organs (e.g. CYP21, needed for cortisol and aldosterone biosynthesis, is only in the adrenal cortex).

Historically, the enzymes have been labelled according to their enzymatic action (e.g. hydroxylation) at a specific carbon atom, with a Greek letter indicating orientation above or below the four-carbon ring structure (e.g. 17α–hydroxylase attaches a hydroxyl group in the alpha position to carbon 17; Fig. 2.5).

The common names used for steroids also adhere to a loose convention. The suffix -ol indicates an important hydroxyl group, as in cholester*ol* or cortis*ol*, whereas the suffix -one indicates an important ketone group (testoster*one*). The extra presence of -di, as in -diol (oestra*diol*) or -dione (androstene*dione*), reflects two of these groups, respectively; '-ene' (androst*ene*dione) within the name indicates a significant double bond in the steroid nucleus.

It is tempting to dismiss this nomenclature as excessive, however familiarity with these features underpins the understanding of steroid endocrinology and its associated disorders. Furthermore, many of the more old-fashioned names remain in common usage.

Storage of steroid hormones

Unlike cells making peptide hormones, most steroid-secreting cells do not store hormones but synthesize them as required. A consequence of this is a slower

---

BOX 2.4 Hormones derived from cholesterol

Cholesterol sources:
- diet
- *de novo* synthesis

Major steroid hormone products:
- adrenal cortex: aldosterone, cortisol and sex steroid precursors
- testis: testosterone
- ovary and placenta: oestrogens and progesterone

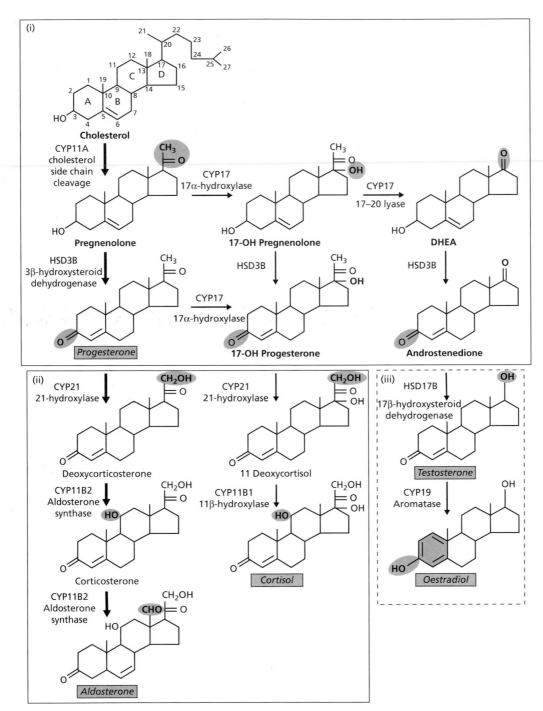

Figure 2.5 The structure of cholesterol and overview of the major steroidogenic pathways. Shading indicates the enzymatic change since the last step. The enzymes are shown by proper name and the common name according to their action. Note some enzymes perform two reactions (e.g. CYP17 acts as both hydroxylase and lyase). The simplified pathways are grouped into three blocks: (i) common to both the adrenal cortex and the gonad; (ii) adrenocortical steroidogenesis; and (iii) pathways largely restricted to the gonads. OH, hydroxy; DHEA, dehydroepiandrosterone.

onset of action for steroid hormones following the initial stimulus to the relevant endocrine organ.

Hormone transport

Most peptide hormones are hydrophilic, so they generally circulate free in the bloodstream with little or no association with serum proteins. In contrast, steroid hormones circulate bound to proteins because their cholesterol origin makes them hydrophobic. There are specific transport proteins for many of the steroid hormones (e.g. cortisol-binding globulin and sex hormone-binding globulin) as well as for thyroid hormone (thyroxine-binding globulin). Many hormones also loosely associate with other circulating proteins, especially albumin.

The equilibrium of whether a hormone is protein-bound or unbound ('free') determines activity, as free hormone diffuses into tissues much more readily. This is relevant to hormone assays where only total hormone is measured as results may be markedly altered by changes in the concentration of binding protein. However, the change in free hormone concentration may be very small and biological activity remains unaltered. This is particularly relevant to circulating testosterone (Chapter 7) and thyroid hormone (Chapter 8).

KEY POINTS

- Genes are stretches of DNA responsible for the encoding of protein

- Common mechanisms govern basal transcription; specific factors orchestrate cell-restricted gene expression

- Meiosis is central to reproductive endocrinology

- Mutations in DNA and chromosomal errors cause congenital and sporadic endocrine disease

- Synthesis as a pro-hormone requiring post-translational modification saves peptide hormones for their intended site of action and protects the synthesizing cell from a deluge of their effects

- Enzyme cascades biosynthesize hormones derived from amino acids and cholesterol

- Unlike peptide hormones, steroid hormones are not stored in cells but made 'on demand'

- Many peptide hormones are free in the circulation compared to steroid or thyroid hormones, which associate with binding proteins

CHAPTER 3

3

The molecular basis of endocrinology

LEARNING OBJECTIVES

- To understand the basic principles of hormone–receptor interaction
- To know the different families of hormone receptors and understand the biology of:
  - tyrosine kinase receptors and associated signalling pathways
  - G-protein coupled receptors and associated signalling pathways
  - nuclear receptors and the associated influence on gene expression
- To appreciate the role of endocrine transcription factors
- To appreciate how abnormalities in hormone receptors or their downstream signalling can cause endocrinopathy

This chapter describes the key events that occur within the cell following stimulation by hormone

Introduction

There are two superfamilies of hormone receptors, which display characteristic features (Fig. 3.1 and Box 3.1).

Cell surface receptors

Cell surface receptors are comprised of three components, each with characteristic structural features, which reflect its location and function (Fig. 3.2).

Stage 1: binding of hormone to receptor (Box 3.2)

Hormone–receptor interactions have been charac-
terized using radiolabelled hormones and isolated preparations of receptors to define two properties:
1. The hormone–receptor interaction is saturable (Fig. 3.3).
2. The hormone–receptor interaction is reversible (Fig. 3.4)

Using methodology similar to that of immunoassays (see Chapter 4), constant amounts of labelled hormone and receptor preparations can be incubated with increasing, known amounts of unlabelled hormone for a specified time. Separating and measuring the receptor-bound labelled fraction allows curves to be plotted and mathematical modelling of the hormone (H)–receptor (R) interaction; for instance, whether it is conforms to the equation $H + R \rightleftharpoons HR$.

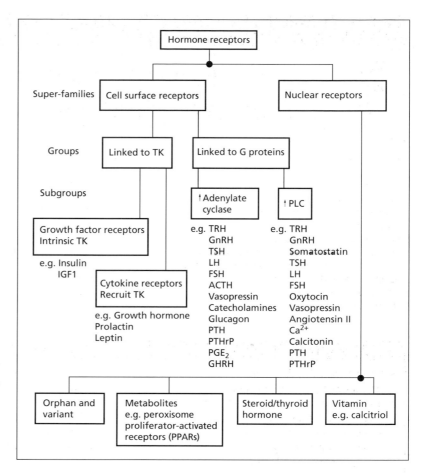

Figure 3.1 The different classes of hormone receptor. Some hormone receptors (e.g. the PTH receptor) can link to different G-proteins, which couple to either adenylate cyclase or phospholipase C (PLC). TK = tyrosine kinase.

BOX 3.1   Basic principles of hormone receptors

- Tissue distribution of hormone receptor determines the scope of hormone action
  - thyroid-stimulating hormone (TSH) receptor limited to thyroid, therefore TSH action also restricted to the thyroid
  - thyroid hormone receptor is widespread, therefore thyroid hormone action is diverse
- Binding of hormone induces a conformational change in its receptor that initiates downstream effects
- Downstream effects differ in different cell-types according to which intracellular pathways are present
- Control is exerted through the constant synthesis and degradation of hormone receptors—most target cells have 2000–100 000 receptors for a particular hormone

Hormone superfamilies
- Water-soluble hormones (e.g. peptide hormones)
  - plasma membrane is impenetrable
  - cell surface receptors transduce signal through membrane
  - activate intracellular signalling pathways
  - fast responses (seconds) as well as slow ones
- Lipid-soluble hormones (e.g. steroid and thyroid hormones)
  - pass through plasma membrane
  - receptors function as transcription factors in the nucleus
  - activate or repress gene expression
  - tend to be relatively slow responses (hours–days)

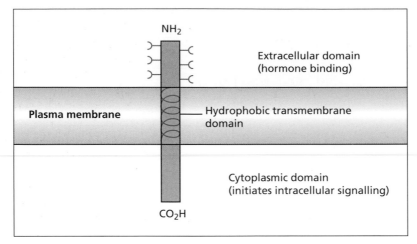

Figure 3.2 A membrane-spanning cell surface receptor. The hormone acts as a ligand. The ligand-binding pocket in the extracellular domain is comparatively rich in cysteine residues that form internal disulphide bonds and repeated loops to ensure correct folding. For some hormones (e.g. GH), this extracellular domain can also be identified in the circulation as a binding protein. Circulating fragments of the TSH receptor may be an immunogenic source for antibody formation in autoimmune thyroid disease. The α-helical membrane-spanning domain is rich in hydrophobic and uncharged amino acids. The C-terminal cytoplasmic domain either contains, or links to, separate catalytic systems, which initiate the intracellular signals after hormone binding.

BOX 3.2 Binding characteristics of hormone receptors

- High affinity: hormones circulate at low concentrations—receptors are like 'capture systems'
- Reversible binding: allows the transient nature of endocrine responses
- Specificity: receptors distinguish between closely related molecular structures

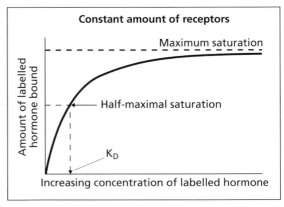

Figure 3.3 Hormone–receptor systems are saturable. Increasing amounts of labelled hormone are incubated with a constant amount of receptors. The amount of bound labelled hormone increases as more is added until the system is saturated. At this point, further addition fails to increase the amount bound to receptors. The concentration of hormone that is required for half-maximal saturation of the receptors is equal to the dissociation constant (K_D) of the hormone–receptor interaction.

Ultimately, these types of experiment can allow estimation of the number of hormone receptors present per target cell.

Stage 2: signal transduction

When a hormone binds to a cell surface receptor, the cascade of cytoplasmic responses is mediated

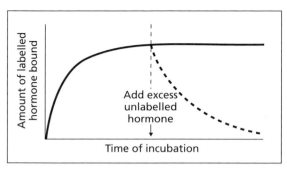

Figure 3.4 Hormone–receptor interactions are reversible. Constant amounts of labelled hormone and receptors are incubated together for different times. The bound label increases with time until it reaches a plateau, when the bound and free hormone have reached a dynamic equilibrium. In a dynamic equilibrium, hormone continually associates and dissociates from its receptor. By adding excess unlabelled hormone, competition with the label is established for access to the receptors. Consequently, the amount of bound labelled hormone decreases with extended incubation (broken line).

BOX 3.3 Categories of cell surface receptors

G-protein coupled receptors
- Activate or inhibit adenylate cyclase and/or phospholipase C (PLC)
- Second messengers: cyclic adenosine monophosphate (cAMP), inositol triphosphate (IP$_3$), diacylglycerol (DAG) and intracellular calcium
- Phosphorylation of serine and threonine amino acids

Tyrosine kinase receptors
- Phosphorylation of the amino acid, tyrosine

---

through protein phosphorylation or the generation of 'second messengers'. This process amplifies the hormone response as many second messenger molecules are produced for each hormone–receptor complex. The cell surface receptors are classified into two groups, G-protein coupled and tyrosine kinase receptors, according to the second messenger and signalling cascades that are stimulated (Fig. 3.1 and Box 3.3).

Protein phosphorylation is a key molecular switch. Approximately 10% of proteins are phosphorylated at any given time in a mammalian cell. The phosphate group is donated from ATP and the reaction catalysed by a 'kinase' enzyme. It is accepted by the polar hydroxyl group of serine, threonine or tyrosine (Fig. 3.5a) and causes a conformational change in the three-dimensional shape of the protein (Fig. 3.5b). In many signalling pathways, the phosphorylated protein can also act as a kinase and phosphorylate the next protein in the sequence. In this way, a phosphorylation cascade is generated, which relays and amplifies the intracellular signal generated by the hormone binding to its receptor (Fig. 3.5c).

Tyrosine kinase receptors

Phosphorylation of tyrosine kinase (TK) receptors can occur through: (i) intrinsic TK activity located in the cytosolic domain of the receptor; or (ii) separate TKs recruited after receptor activation (Fig. 3.1). By either mechanism, conformational change induced by phosphorylation creates 'docking' sites for other proteins. Frequently, this occurs via conserved motifs within the target protein known as 'SH2' or 'SH3' domains. These domains may be involved in the activation of downstream kinases or they may play a more passive role, stabilizing signalling proteins within a phosphorylation cascade.

Receptors with intrinsic tyrosine kinase activity

Intrinsic TK receptors autophosphorylate upon binding of the appropriate hormone. The group includes the receptor for insulin and those for ligands such as epidermal growth factor (EGF), fibroblast growth factor (FGF) and insulin-like growth factor 1 (IGF1). The EGF and FGF receptors exist as monomers that dimerize upon hormone binding to activate tyrosine phosphorylation: those for insulin and IGF1 exist in their unoccupied state as preformed dimers. The signalling pathways for all these receptors are heavily involved in cell growth and proliferation.

Insulin signalling pathways
The dimerized insulin receptor (IR) is composed of

(a)

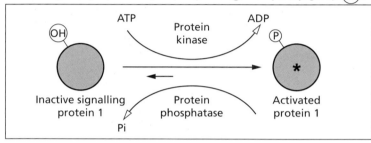

(b) Phosphorylation of protein 1 induces an activating conformational change due to the energetically favourable phosphorylation ℗ of a hydroxyl group (OH).

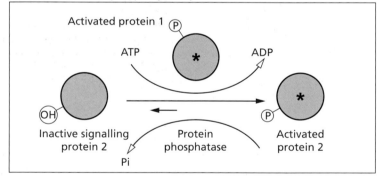

(c) The initiation of a phosphorylation cascade. Phosphorylated protein 1 acts as a kinase and phosphorylates protein 2.

Figure 3.5 Intracellular signalling via phosphorylation. (a) Amino acids serine, threonine and tyrosine carry polar hydroxyl groups that can be phosphorylated. Over 99% of all protein phosphorylation occurs on serine and threonine residues, however phosphorylation of tyrosine, the only amino acid with a phenolic ring, generates particularly distinctive intracellular signalling pathways. (b) Protein 1 is inactive until its hydroxyl group is phosphorylated by the action of a kinase enzyme. This induces a conformational change, resulting in an activated phosphorylated protein. Energy for the transfer of the phosphate group comes from the hydrolysis of ATP to ADP. The reverse reaction, from active to inactive Protein 1, is catalysed by a phosphatase. (c) The initiation of a signalling cascade. Activated, phosphorylated Protein 1 itself acts as a kinase and catalyses the phosphorylation of Protein 2. Amino acid specificity means that serine/threonine kinases usually show no cross-reactivity with tyrosine residues and *vice versa*.

two α- and two β-subunits linked by a series of disulphide bridges (Fig. 3.6; see Chapter 11). The earliest response to insulin binding is autophosphorylation of the cytosolic domains of the β-subunit. The activated receptor then phosphorylates a key intermediary, insulin receptor substrate (IRS) 1 or 2, which is thought to be essential for almost all biological actions of insulin. IRS1 has many potential tyrosine phosphorylation sites, at least eight of which are phosphorylated by the activated IR.

Multiple phosphorylation of IRS1 or 2 leads to the docking of several proteins with SH2 domains, and the activation of divergent intracellular signalling. For example, docking of phosphatidylinositol-3-kinase (PI3-kinase) leads to deployment of the glucose transporter (GLUT) family members. In the target organs of adipose tissue and muscle, this leads to the translocation of GLUT4 from intracellular vesicles to the cell membrane and glucose uptake into the cell. The mitogenic effects of insulin are mediated via a

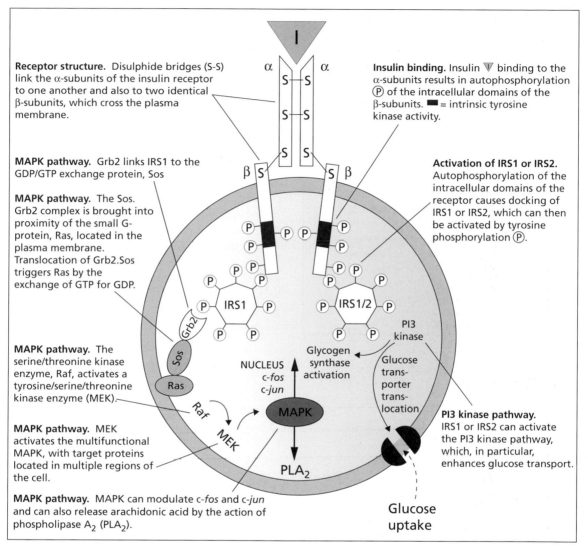

Receptor structure. Disulphide bridges (S-S) link the α-subunits of the insulin receptor to one another and also to two identical β-subunits, which cross the plasma membrane.

Insulin binding. Insulin ▽ binding to the α-subunits results in autophosphorylation Ⓟ of the intracellular domains of the β-subunits. ■ = intrinsic tyrosine kinase activity.

MAPK pathway. Grb2 links IRS1 to the GDP/GTP exchange protein, Sos

MAPK pathway. The Sos. Grb2 complex is brought into proximity of the small G-protein, Ras, located in the plasma membrane. Translocation of Grb2.Sos triggers Ras by the exchange of GTP for GDP.

Activation of IRS1 or IRS2. Autophosphorylation of the intracellular domains of the receptor causes docking of IRS1 or IRS2, which can then be activated by tyrosine phosphorylation Ⓟ.

MAPK pathway. The serine/threonine kinase enzyme, Raf, activates a tyrosine/serine/threonine kinase enzyme (MEK).

MAPK pathway. MEK activates the multifunctional MAPK, with target proteins located in multiple regions of the cell.

PI3 kinase pathway. IRS1 or IRS2 can activate the PI3 kinase pathway, which, in particular, enhances glucose transport.

MAPK pathway. MAPK can modulate c-*fos* and c-*jun* and can also release arachidonic acid by the action of phospholipase A₂ (PLA₂).

Figure 3.6 The insulin receptor and some of its signalling pathways. The number of insulin receptors on target cells varies, commonly from 100 to 200 000, with adipocytes and hepatocytes expressing the highest numbers. Not all insulin-signalling pathways are shown (e.g. Grb2 can be stimulated independently of IRS1). Phosphatidylinositol-3-kinase, PI3-kinase.

different intracellular pathway. Activated IRS1 docks with the SH2/SH3 domains of the type 2 growth factor receptor-bound (Grb2) protein. This adaptor protein links IRS1 to the son of sevenless (SoS) protein and, ultimately, to activation of the mitogen-activated protein kinase (MAPK) pathway leading to gene expression that promotes mitosis and growth.

These molecular events lie at the heart of insulin's clinical action (see Part 3). Defects in the insulin signalling pathway can result in rare syndromes of resistance to insulin action as well as a considerable, if somewhat ill-defined, component of Type 2 diabetes (see Chapter 13 and Box 3.4).

Receptors which recruit tyrosine kinase activity

The subfamily of receptors that bind growth hormone (GH), prolactin (PRL) and leptin includes
those for numerous cytokines and erythropoietin
(EPO). The basic receptor composition, with major
homology between family members in the extracellular domain, is shown in Fig. 3.2.

GH and PRL signalling pathways — the Janus family of tyrosine kinases

Similar mechanisms govern GH and PRL receptor
binding and signal transduction. Two different sites
on the hormone are each capable of binding receptors. The hormone–receptor interaction of the first
leads to the binding of the second to another receptor
molecule. The close proximity of the two receptor
molecules leads to dimerization of their cytoplasmic
regions and signal transduction. Discovery of this
phenomenon has been utilized in drug design to
combat excessive GH action in acromegaly (Fig. 3.7).

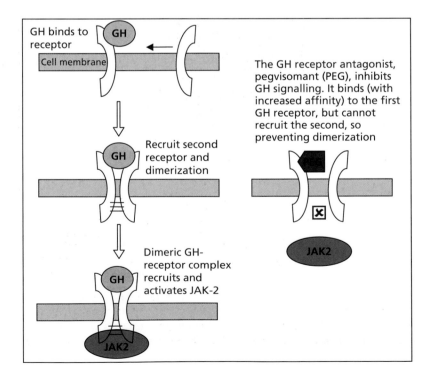

GH binds to receptor

Cell membrane

The GH receptor antagonist, pegvisomant (PEG), inhibits GH signalling. It binds (with increased affinity) to the first GH receptor, but cannot recruit the second, so preventing dimerization

Recruit second receptor and dimerization

Dimeric GH-receptor complex recruits and activates JAK-2

Figure 3.7 GH signalling and its antagonism. GH binds to its cell surface receptors and, via the formation of receptor dimers, recruits JAK2. This model led to the design of the growth hormone receptor antagonist, pegvisomant.

With the exception of the receptor for EPO, other cytokine receptors tend to form heterodimers with diverse partner proteins.

Activation of the hormone receptor rapidly recruits members of the Janus family of TKs (Fig. 3.8). The four members of the family contain distinctive, tandem kinase domains at their carboxy terminals leading to their name 'Janus associated kinase' (JAK1–4) after the two-faced Roman deity, Janus. GH, PRL and EPO receptors tend to associate with JAK2 and it is probable that their dimerization brings together two JAK2 molecules that cross-phosphorylate each other. The major downstream substrates of JAK are the STAT family of proteins (hence the term 'JAK-STAT' signalling; Fig. 3.8). The name STAT comes from dual function: (i) *s*ignal *t*ransduction, located in the cytoplasm, and (ii) nuclear *a*ctivation of *t*ranscription. Both activities rely on phosphorylation by JAK, facilitated by SH2-mediated docking onto the hormone receptor (Fig. 3.8). Phosphorylated STAT proteins dissociate from the occupied receptor/kinase complex and, themselves, dimerize to gain access to the nucleus. There, they activate genes regulating proliferation or the differentiation status of the target cell. One of the major targets is IGF1 (Box 3.5). JAK signalling does not focus exclusively on STAT. GH receptor (GHR) occupancy also stimulates MAPK and PI3-kinase pathways. This

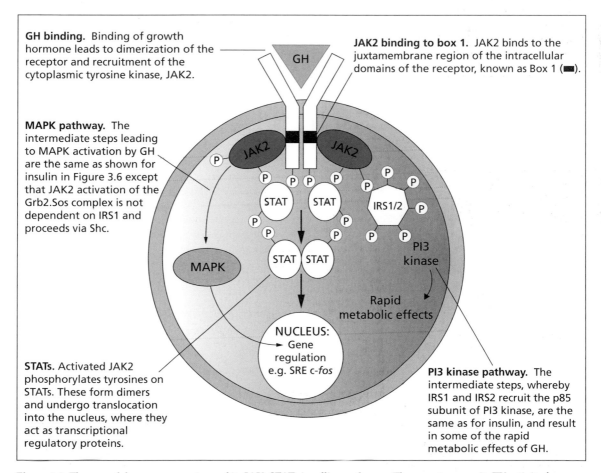

GH binding. Binding of growth hormone leads to dimerization of the receptor and recruitment of the cytoplasmic tyrosine kinase, JAK2.

JAK2 binding to box 1. JAK2 binds to the juxtamembrane region of the intracellular domains of the receptor, known as Box 1 (■).

MAPK pathway. The intermediate steps leading to MAPK activation by GH are the same as shown for insulin in Figure 3.6 except that JAK2 activation of the Grb2.Sos complex is not dependent on IRS1 and proceeds via Shc.

STATs. Activated JAK2 phosphorylates tyrosines on STATs. These form dimers and undergo translocation into the nucleus, where they act as transcriptional regulatory proteins.

PI3 kinase pathway. The intermediate steps, whereby IRS1 and IRS2 recruit the p85 subunit of PI3 kinase, are the same as for insulin, and result in some of the rapid metabolic effects of GH.

Figure 3.8 The growth hormone receptor and its JAK–STAT signalling pathways. The receptor recruits TK activity from JAK2. SREs (serum response elements) are MAPK-responsive promoter and enhancer elements that mediate the induction of target genes, such as c-*fos*.

BOX 3.5 One of the major targets of GH signalling is the *IGF1* gene

- Measuring serum IGF1 is a useful measure of GH activity in the body

BOX 3.6 Defects in the GH signalling pathways and GH resistance syndromes

Severe resistance to GH, mainly due to mutations in the GH receptor that commonly affect the hormone-binding domain, is characterized by grossly impaired growth and is termed Laron syndrome after his first report in 1966 (Fig. 3.9). It is an autosomal recessive disorder with a variable phenotype typified by normal or raised circulating GH and low levels of serum IGF1.

For some patients, no *GHR* mutations can be identified, implicating genes that encode downstream components of GH signalling. For instance, defects in the *IGF1* gene have been associated with severe intrauterine growth retardation, mild mental retardation, sensorineural deafness and postnatal growth failure.

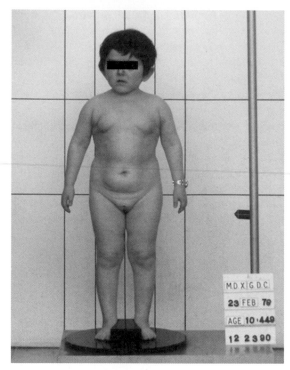

Figure 3.9 Laron syndrome. This boy presented aged 10.4 years but with a height of 95 cm—equivalent to that of a 3-year old. There is a prominent forehead, depressed nasal bridge, underdevelopment of the mandible, truncal obesity and a very small penis. These features could represent severe GH deficiency. However, serum GH levels were elevated with undetectable IGF1. These findings diagnose growth hormone resistance. Laron syndrome was due to an inactivating mutation of the gene encoding the GH receptor.

overlap may account for some of the rapid metabolic effects of GH (Fig. 3.8).

Defects in the GH signalling pathway can result in rare syndromes of resistance to GH action (Box 3.6 and Fig. 3.9)

G-protein coupled receptors

Receptor structure

The commonest subset of cell surface receptors (>140 members) couple to guanine (G)-proteins at the inner surface of the cell membrane. This leads to the generation of intracellular second messengers such as cAMP, DAG and IP$_3$—the latter two arising from phosphatidylinositol (PI) metabolism (Fig. 3.10). In addition to hormones, G-protein coupled receptors (GPCRs) also exist for glutamate, thrombin, odourants and the visual transduction of light. The most striking structural feature of all these receptors lies in the transmembrane domain, comprised of hy-

drophobic helices, which cross the lipid bilayer of the plasma membrane seven times (Fig. 3.11).

G-protein coupling

G-proteins mediate GPCR signalling by their ability to hydrolyze GTP to GDP. In their resting state, the G-proteins exist in the cell membrane as heterotrimeric complexes with α, β and γ subunits. In practice, the β and γ subunits associate with such affinity that the functional units are Gα and Gβ/γ (Fig. 3.11). Hormone occupancy results in conformational change of receptor structure. In turn, this causes a conforma-

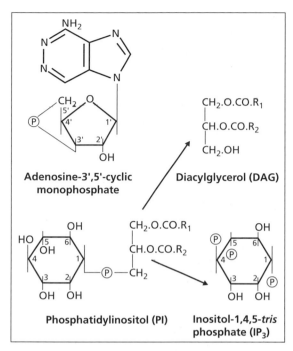

Figure 3.10 Second messengers involved in signalling from G-protein-coupled receptors. The symbol P is the abbreviation for a phosphate group. Carbon atoms are numbered in their ring position. R_1 and R_2 represent fatty acid chains.

tional change in the α-subunit leading to an exchange of GDP for GTP. The acquisition of GTP causes the α-subunit to dissociate from the heterotrimeric complex and bind to a downstream catalytic unit, either adenylate cyclase in the generation of cAMP or phospholipase C (PLC) for DAG/IP_3. The energy to activate these targets comes from the cleavage of phosphate from GTP. This regenerates Gα-GDP, which no longer associates with adenylate cyclase or PLC, thus switching off the cascade and recycling the Gα-GDP back to the start.

G Subunits

There are over 20 isoforms of the Gα subunit that may be grouped into four major subfamilies (Box 3.7). These are used differentially by the various hormone receptor signalling pathways (Table 3.1).

More than half of GPCRs can interact with different Gα subunits and thus modulate contrasting, and

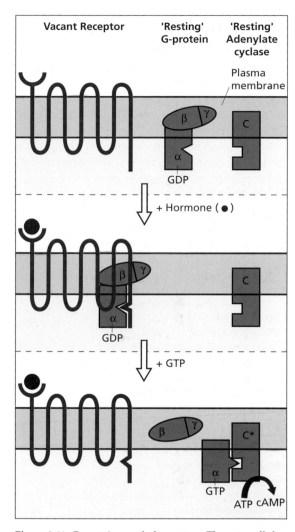

Figure 3.11 G-protein coupled receptors. The extracellular domain is ligand-specific and, hence, less conserved across family members (e.g. only 35–45% for the TSH, LH/hCG and FSH receptors). The transmembrane domain has a characteristic heptahelical structure, most of which is embedded in the cell membrane and provides a hydrophobic core. Conserved cysteine residues can form a disulphide bridge between the second and third extracellular loops. The cytoplasmic domain links the receptor to the signal-transducing G-proteins and, in this example, is linked to membrane-bound adenylate cyclase. The activation of adenylate cyclase is shown as C to C*.

sometimes apparently conflicting, intracellular second messenger systems (Fig. 3.12). In part, this promiscuity can be attributed to the degree of hormonal stimulation or activation of different receptor subtypes. For instance, at low concentrations, TSH, calcitonin and LH receptors associate with $G_s\alpha$ to activate adenylate cyclase, whereas higher concentrations recruit $G_q\alpha$ to activate PLC. Calcitonin receptor subtypes are differentially expressed according to the stage of the cell cycle. Defects in the G protein signalling pathways can result in many endocrine disorders (Box 3.8 and Figs 3.13 and 3.14).

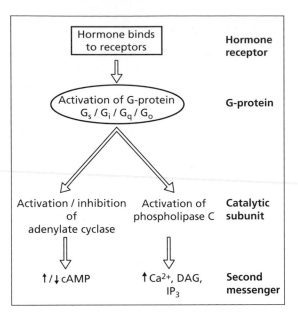

Figure 3.12 Hormonal activation of G-protein-coupled receptors can link to different second messenger pathways. The two alternative pathways are not mutually exclusive and may, in fact, interact.

BOX 3.7 Subfamilies of G protein subunits

- $G_s\alpha$: activates adenylate cyclase
- $G_i\alpha$: inhibits adenylate cyclase
- $G_q\alpha$: activates PLC
- $G_o\alpha$: activates ion channels

Hormone	Dominant G-protein α-subunit(s)
Thyrotrophin-releasing hormone (TRH)	$G_q\alpha$
Corticotrophin-releasing hormone (CRH)	$G_s\alpha$
Gonadotrophin-releasing hormone (GnRH)	$G_q\alpha$
Somatostatin (SS)	$G_i\alpha/G_q\alpha$
Thyroid-stimulating hormone (TSH)	$G_s\alpha/G_q\alpha$
Luteinizing hormone (LH)/human chorionic gonadotrophin (hCG)	$G_s\alpha/G_q\alpha$
Follicle-stimulating hormone (FSH)	$G_s\alpha/G_q\alpha$
Adrenocorticotrophic hormone (ACTH)	$G_s\alpha$
Oxytocin	$G_q\alpha$
Arginine vasopressin (AVP)	$G_s\alpha/G_q\alpha$
Catecholamines (β-adrenergic)	$G_s\alpha$
Angiotensin II (AII)	$G_i\alpha/G_q\alpha$
Glucagon	$G_s\alpha$
Calcium	$G_q\alpha/G_i\alpha$
Calcitonin	$G_s\alpha/G_i\alpha/G_q\alpha$
Parathyroid hormone (PTH)/PTH-related peptide (PTHrP)	$G_s\alpha/G_q\alpha$
Prostaglandin E2	$G_s\alpha$

Table 3.1 Use of different Gα subunits by various hormone signalling pathways

For SS, AVP, AII, calcitonin and PTH/PTHrP different receptor subtypes, potentially in different tissues, determine α-subunit specificity. This provides opportunities for selective antagonist therapies.

Second messenger pathways

Cyclic adenosine monophosphate

Activation of membrane-bound adenylate cyclase catalyses the conversion of ATP to the potent second messenger cAMP (Fig. 3.11). cAMP interacts with protein kinase A (PKA) to unmask its catalytic site, which phosphorylates serine and threonine residues on a transcription factor called CREB (*c*AMP *r*esponse *e*lement *b*inding protein) (Fig. 3.15). CREB then translocates to the nucleus where it binds to a short palindromic sequence in the promoter regions of cAMP-regulated genes. This signalling pathway regulates major metabolic pathways, including those for lipolysis, glycogenolysis and steroidogenesis.

The cAMP response is terminated by a large family of phosphodiesterases (PDEs), which can be activated by a variety of systems including phosphorylation by PKA in a negative feedback loop. PDEs rapidly hydrolyse cAMP to the inactive 5′AMP. In addition, activated PKA can phosphorylate serine and threonine residues of the GPCR to cause receptor desensitization.

BOX 3.8 Defects in the GPCR/G-protein signalling pathways

Several endocrinopathies occur due to activating or inactivating mutations of GPCRs or the G-proteins coupled to them. Activating mutations cause constitutive overactivity; inactivating mutations cause hormone resistance syndromes characterized by high circulating hormone levels but diminished hormone action.

- Gain of function
  - LH receptor: male precocious puberty (Fig. 3.13)
  - TSH receptor: toxic thyroid adenomas
  - $G_s\alpha$: McCune–Albright syndrome (Fig. 3.14), some cases of acromegaly and some autonomous thyroid nodules
- Loss of function
  - V2 receptor: nephrogenic diabetes insipidus (high AVP)
  - TSH receptor: resistance to TSH
  - $G_s\alpha$: pseudohypoparathyroidism (Fig. 9.9) and Albright's hereditary osteodystrophy

---

Diacylglycerol and Ca^{2+}

Signalling from hormones, such as TRH, GnRH and oxytocin, recruits G-protein complexes containing the $G_q\alpha$ subunit. This activates membrane-associated PLC, which catalyses the conversion of PI 4,5-bisphosphate (PIP$_2$) to DAG and IP$_3$ (Fig. 3.16). IP$_3$ stimulates the transient release of calcium from the endoplasmic reticulum to activate several calcium-sensitive enzymes, including the protein kinase, calmodulin, and some isoforms of protein kinase C

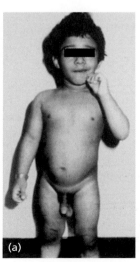

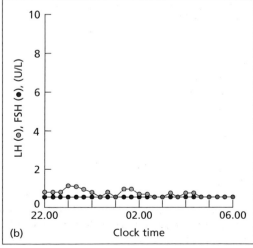

Figure 3.13 Familial male precocious puberty ('testotoxicosis'). This 2-year old presented with signs of precocious puberty. He was the size of a 4-year old. His overnight gonadotrophins (LH and FSH) were undetectable as the testosterone was arising from autonomous Leydig cell function.

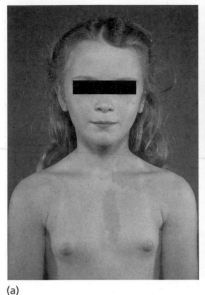
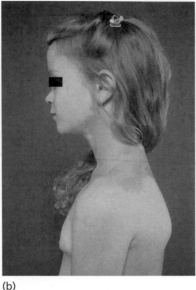

(a)   (b)

Figure 3.14 McCune–Albright syndrome. At 6 years of age, this girl presented with breast development and vaginal bleeding in the absence of gonadotrophins. An activating mutation in $G_s\alpha$ had created independence from MSH causing skin pigmentation ('café-au-lait' spots) and similar constitutive activation in the ovary (i.e. independence from gonadotrophins) giving rise to premature breast development. In some cases, constitutive overactivity can manifest in bones (causing 'fibrous dysplasia'), the adrenal cortex (Cushing syndrome) and the thyroid (thyrotoxicosis).

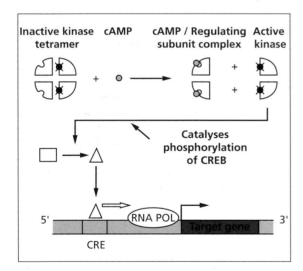

Figure 3.15 The activation of protein kinase A, a cAMP-dependent protein kinase. The four-subunit complex is inactive. When cAMP binds to the regulatory subunits, dissociation occurs so that the active kinase subunits are released to catalyse the phosphorylation of the cAMP response element-binding protein (CREB). This activates CREB so that it can bind to its DNA target, the cAMP response element (CRE) to switch on transcription of cAMP-inducible genes.

(PKC). Calcium ions also activate cytosolic guanylate cyclase, an enzyme that catalyses the formation of cyclic guanosine monophosphate (cGMP). The effects of atrial natriuretic peptide are mediated by receptors linked to guanylate cyclase.

The major target of DAG signalling is PKC, which activates phospholipase A_2 to liberate arachidonate from phospholipids and generate potent eicosanoids, including thromboxanes, leucotrienes, lipoxins and prostaglandins (Fig. 3.17). The latter are well-recognized paracrine and autocrine mediators capable of amplifying or prolonging a response to a hormonal stimulus.

Nuclear receptors

Classification and structure of nuclear receptors

The nuclear receptors are classified by their ligands, which are small lipophilic molecules that diffuse across the plasma membrane of target cells. The receptors, encoded by a single gene, typically bind DNA and function as transcription factors (Fig. 3.18). Distinct polypeptide-encoding regions can be identified (Fig. 3.19), for which evolutionary conservation can be as high as 60 to 90%.

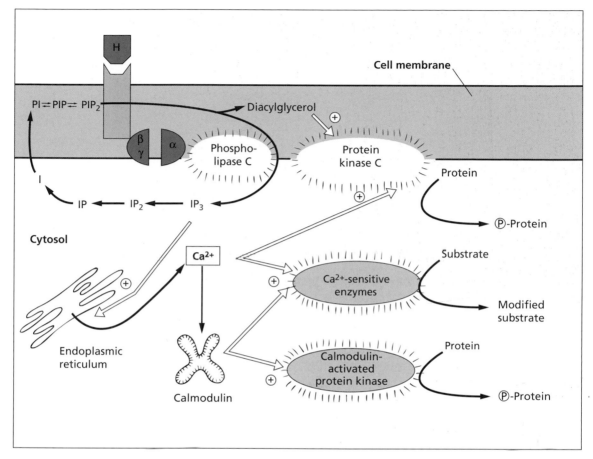

Figure 3.16 Hormonal stimulation of phospholipid turnover and calcium metabolism within the cell. PI metabolism includes the membrane intermediaries, PI monophosphate (PIP) and PI bisphosphate (PIP_2). Hormone action stimulates phospholipase C, which hydrolyses PIP_2 to DAG and IP_3. IP_3 mobilizes calcium, particularly from the endoplasmic reticulum. DAG activates protein kinase C and increases the enzyme's affinity for calcium ions, which further enhances activation. Collectively, these events stimulate phosphorylation cascades of proteins and enzymes to alter intracellular metabolism.

Many nuclear receptors exist for which no endogenous ligand has been identified and are termed 'orphan' nuclear receptors. In addition, some variant receptors have atypical DNA-binding domains and potentially function via indirect interaction with the genome. All the different types are associated with endocrinopathies.

The receptor family predominantly resides in the nucleus, although increasingly nuclear import and export appears to be an important regulatory mechanism, as has been long recognized for the glucocorticoid receptor (GR). The receptors are structurally related (Fig. 3.19) and control the expression of specific target genes. This need for transcription and translation to elicit an effect means that biological responses are relatively slow compared to cell surface receptor signalling.

Target cell conversion of hormones and vitamins destined for nuclear receptors

A further characteristic of several nuclear hormone receptors includes enzymatic modification of the

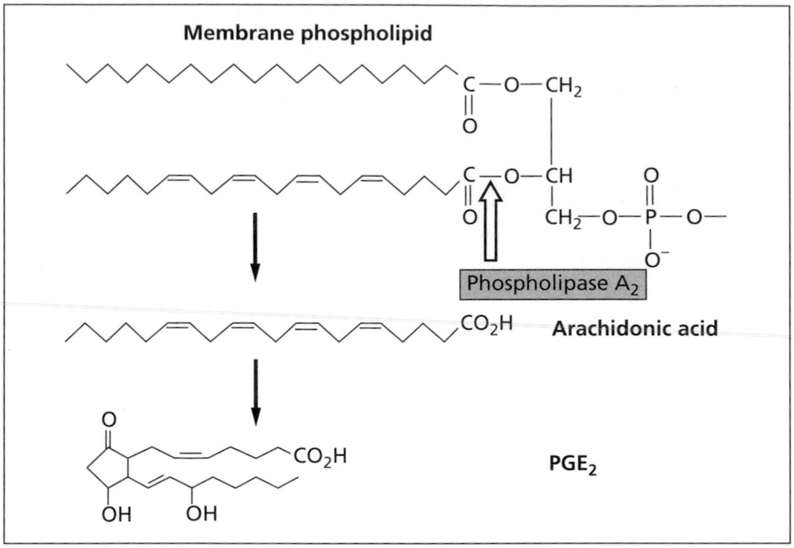

Figure 3.17 Eicosanoid signalling. Arachidonic acid, released by phospholipase A$_2$, is the rate-limiting precursor for generating eicosanoid signalling molecules by cyclooxygenase and lipoxygenase pathways. The example shown produces prostaglandin E$_2$ (PGE$_2$). There are at least 16 prostaglandins—structurally related, 20- carbon, fatty acid derivatives. They are released from many cell types and exert paracrine and autocrine actions (e.g. the inflammatory response and contraction of uterine smooth muscle). Their circulating half-life is short (~3–10 min). Aspirin inhibits prostaglandin production at sites of inflammation.

ligand within the target cell. This converts the circulating hormone into a more, or less, potent metabolite prior to receptor binding (Table 3.2).

The inactivation of cortisol to cortisone by type 2 11β-hydroxysteroid dehydrogenase (HSD11B2) in kidney tubular cells is interesting. It functions, not to affect the GR, but to preserve aldosterone action at the mineralocorticoid receptor (MR). Without this, cortisol, present in the circulation at much higher concentrations than aldosterone, would swamp the MR causing inappropriate overactivity. Impaired function of HSD11B2 leads to hypertension and hypokalaemia in the syndrome of apparent mineralocorticoid excess.

Nuclear localization, DNA binding and transcriptional activation

In their resting state, unbound steroid hormone receptors associate with heat-shock proteins, which obscure the DNA-binding domain, so that they cannot bind the genome. Steroid binding causes conformational change and dissociation of the heat-shock protein. This reveals two polypeptide loops stabilized by zinc ions, known as zinc fingers. Once two steroid receptors have dimerized, these motifs bind to target DNA at the specific hormone response element (HRE) (Fig. 3.20).

Interestingly, the thyroid hormone receptor (TR) is located exclusively in the nucleus bound to DNA at the thyroid hormone response element (TRE). In the absence of hormone, the TR dimerizes with the retinoid X receptor and tends to recruit nuclear proteins that inhibit transcription (corepressors). The binding of thyroid hormone leads to dissociation of these factors and the recruitment of transcriptional coactivators. These effects take place either in gene promoters or in more distant enhancer/repressor regions. In the case of transcriptional activation, this leads to the recruitment of DNA-dependent RNA polymerase (Fig. 3.20).

The principles of nuclear hormone resistance syndromes are similar to those for cell surface receptors—inactivating mutations in the receptor prohibit the hormone's effect on the target cell. Mutations have been identified which lead to

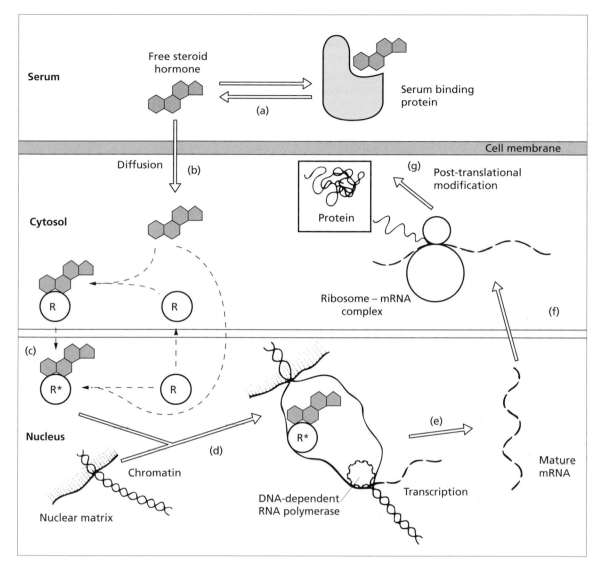

Figure 3.18 Steroid hormone action. Free steroid, in equilibrium with that bound to protein (a), diffuses across the target cell membrane (b). Binding to its receptor ® may occur in the cell cytoplasm (e.g. the glucocorticoid receptor) or in the cell nucleus (e.g. other steroid hormone receptors). The activated hormone–receptor complex ®*, now present in the nucleus (c), binds to the hormone- response element (HRE) of its target genes (d). This interaction promotes DNA-dependent RNA polymerase to start transcription (e) of mRNA. Post-transcriptional modification and splicing sees the mRNA exit the nucleus (f) for translation into protein on ribosomes. Post-translational modification provides the final protein (g).

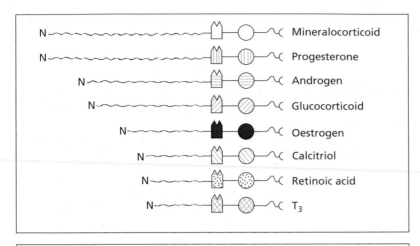

Highly conserved, DNA-binding domain, comprised of two zinc fingers

Specific hormone-binding domain, which forms a hydrophobic pocket

C-terminus 'AF2' region, which recruits the nuclear components for transcriptional activation

Variable N-terminal domain

Figure 3.19 The nuclear hormone receptor superfamily. The receptors range in size from 395 to 984 amino acids. Ligands are shown to the right.

Table 3.2 Potential modifications to nuclear hormones

Modification that increases activity	Modification that decreases activity
Deiodination of T_4 to T_3 by selenodeiodinases (Fig. 8.3)	Inactivation of cortisol to cortisone by Type 2 11β-hydroxysteroid dehydrogenase (HSD11B2) (Chapter 6)
Reduction of testosterone to DHT by 5α-reductase (Fig. 7.7) Conversion of 25-OH vitamin D to 1,25-OH vitamin D (calcitriol) by 1α-hydroxylase (Fig. 9.4)	

Biological importance of these examples is underlined by rare mutations presenting with endocrine overactivity or underactivity.

reduced hormone binding, impaired receptor dimerization and decreased DNA binding to the HRE (Table 3.3).

Orphan nuclear receptors and variant nuclear receptors

Some orphan and variant receptors play very important roles in endocrinology. Steroidogenic factor 1 (SF1), for which the ligand has recently been discovered, is a critical mediator of endocrine organ forma-tion. Without it, the anterior pituitary gonadotrophs, the adrenal gland and the gonad fail to develop. It is also critical for the on going expression of many important genes within these cell types (e.g. the enzymes that orchestrate steroidogenesis). A variant receptor with a similar expression profile is DAX1, mutation of which causes congenital adrenal hypoplasia (i.e. underdevelopment). As mentioned before, duplication of the region that includes the gene encoding DAX1 causes male-to-female sex reversal (see Chapters 6 and 7).

(a) Steroid receptors form homodimers

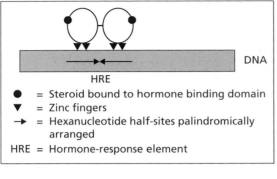

DNA

HRE

● = Steroid bound to hormone binding domain
▼ = Zinc fingers
→ = Hexanucleotide half-sites palindromically arranged
HRE = Hormone-response element

(b) The thyroid hormone receptor forms heterodimers

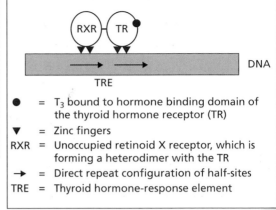

DNA

TRE

● = T_3 bound to hormone binding domain of the thyroid hormone receptor (TR)
▼ = Zinc fingers
RXR = Unoccupied retinoid X receptor, which is forming a heterodimer with the TR
→ = Direct repeat configuration of half-sites
TRE = Thyroid hormone-response element

(c)

● = T_3 bound to the TR
▼ = Zinc fingers
RXR = Retinoid X receptor
TIC = Transcription initiation complex
RNA POL = RNA polymerase
TRE = Thyroid hormone-response element

Figure 3.20 Nuclear hormone receptor–DNA interactions. (a) Steroid hormone receptors form homodimers on palindromic hexanucleotide target DNA sequences. (b) The TR, similar to receptors for retinoic acid and calcitriol, forms heterodimers with the retinoid X receptor. (c) Once occupied by T_3, the TR bound to DNA recruits coactivator proteins which, in turn, bridge to, activate and stabilize the multiple components of the transcription initiation complex at the basal promoter of the target gene.

Other critical endocrine transcription factors

Although distinct from the nuclear receptor super-family, other transcription factors play critical roles in the endocrine system.

The pituitary gland

In the pituitary, pituitary-specific transcription factor 1 (PIT1) regulates the expression of genes encoding GH, PRL and the β-subunit of TSH. Patients with inactivating mutations in PIT1 show reduced, or absent, levels of these hormones causing short stature and, potentially, a congenital form of secondary hypothyroidism with severe learning disability.

The endocrine pancreas

The development of the pancreas and, in particular, the specification and on going function of β-cells relies on several transcription factors. Insulin promoter factor 1 (IPF1) and several members of the hepatocyte nuclear family (HNF) are critical in this regard; inactivating mutations have been identified, which cause type 2-like diabetes at an early age, called maturity onset diabetes of the young (MODY) (see Table 13.3). Potentially, these patients never accrue a normal number of β-cells, which also fail to function properly.

Table 3.3 Defects in nuclear hormone signalling

Mutations in receptor for	Clinical effects
Androgen (AR)	Partial or complete androgen insensitivity syndromes
Glucocorticoid (GR)	Generalized inherited glucocorticoid resistance
Oestrogen (ER)	Oestrogen resistance
Thyroid hormone (TR)	Thyroid hormone resistance
Vitamin D (VDR)	Vitamin D (Calcitriol)-resistant rickets

KEY POINTS

- Hormone action is mediated by binding to receptors and triggering intracellular responses

- The tissue distribution of the receptor determines where a hormone will exert its effect

- The two major subdivisions of hormone receptors are either cell surface or intracellular (usually nuclear)

- Peptide hormones and catecholamines act on cell surface receptors

- Activation of cell surface receptors can generate fast responses in seconds or minutes

- Steroid and thyroid hormones act on intracellular, usually nuclear, receptors

- Activation of intracellular/nuclear receptors generates slower responses due to the need to produce protein from the expression of target genes

- Mutations in genes encoding any part of the cascade from hormone receptor to action can result in either underactive or overactive endocrinopathy and potentially include tumour formation

CHAPTER 4

4 Investigations in endocrinology

LEARNING OBJECTIVES

- To understand how circulating hormones are measured by a range of different immunoassays
- To understand the principles of bioassay and receptor assays
- To develop awareness of other laboratory investigations that can be applied to clinical endocrinology
- To appreciate the molecular biology that now provides genetic diagnoses in endocrinology
- To appreciate the options that are available to image endocrine disease

This chapter details the basic principles by which clinical endocrinology is investigated

Clinical endocrinology and diabetes have been advanced by methodology to aid diagnosis and to monitor and assess treatment. Laboratory investigation, largely measuring serum hormone concentrations, is heavily centred in clinical biochemistry. There is an increasing contribution from molecular biology as patient-specific genetic diagnoses become possible for some disorders. Clinical investigation of the endocrine system draws upon expertise from the specialties of radiology and nuclear medicine.

The measurement of circulating hormones

Precise diagnosis largely depends on an ability to measure the appropriate hormones in the circulation. Immunoassays, introduced in the 1960s, have been developed that are sufficiently sensitive, precise and hormone-specific to meet the high through-put analytical challenge. Bioassays, the measurement of physiological responses induced by a stimulus, are less suited to the demands of routine chemical pathology and are now more restricted to research and development. All assays rely on a comparison between the response of the patient sample and those produced by different known concentrations of a reference compound. For immunoassays and bioassays, a calibration curve is generated with the reference preparation from which the unknown concentration of the hormone in the patient sample can be deduced.

Immunoassays

'Immunoassay' is a broad term for one of two different techniques: true 'immunoassay', as in radioimmunoassay (RIA); and 'immunometric' assay, as encountered in immunoradiometric assay (IRMA). Both RIAs and IRMAs employ a radioactive isotope as a 'label' or 'tracer', such as iodine-125 (I^{125}), which generates the quantitative signal for the assay; however, alternative nonisotopic labelling systems are increasingly used. Assays that employ these other labelling systems, such as fluorescence, have been given similar names, for example fluoroimmunoassays (FIAs) and immunofluorometric assays (IFMAs).

Principles of immunoassays

Both forms of immunoassay are based on the hormone to be measured acting as an antigen, which is bound by a specific laboratory antibody. Using the example of growth hormone (GH), anti-GH antibodies bind the hormone to form an antibody–antigen complex (Fig. 4.1). This reaction is reversible with the antigen and its antibody continuously associating and dissociating. To set up a calibration or standard curve for the immunoassay, a constant amount of antibody is added to a series of tubes with increasing, known amounts of a GH reference preparation. After incubation, the reaction reaches equilibrium and the tubes with the greater amount of GH generate more bound complex. Measuring the amount of this bound complex can thus be related to the quantity of GH that was originally added. This allows a calibration curve to be plotted, against which the same process can now determine the GH concentration in a patient sample.

Immunometric assays: the sandwich assays

The principle of an immunometric assay for GH is shown in Fig. 4.2. A constant amount of anti-GH antibody is added to each tube with increasing, known amounts of the GH reference preparation. After incubation, the amount of GH bound to the antibody is detected by adding, to all the tubes, an excess amount of a second labelled anti-GH antibody. The second antibody is directed against a different antigenic site on GH from the first antibody. Thus, a triple complex is formed, with the GH sandwiched between the two antibodies. The unbound fraction of the second antibody is removed, leaving the amount of triple complex to be determined by quantifying the bound label, for example by measuring the radioactivity or fluorescence emitted. This emission is plotted against the increasing, known amount of GH standard to generate a calibration curve (Fig. 4.2). To determine the standard curve with precision, against which patient samples can be interpolated, usually between five and eight different concentrations of hormone are used.

The immunometric assay is suitable only when the hormone to be measured is large enough to permit the discrete binding of two antibodies. This would not be suitable for hormones such as thyroxine (T_4) or triiodothyronine (T_3), for which the competitive-binding immunoassay system must be used.

Immunoassays: the competitive-binding assays

The principle underlying this alternative immunoassay system is shown in Fig. 4.3, which illustrates how a two-point calibration curve can be generated. Constant amounts of antibody and labelled antigen are

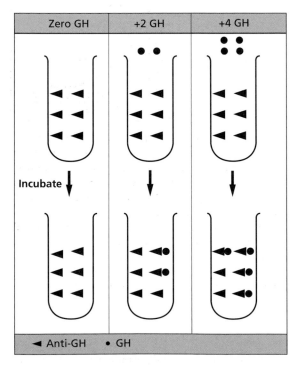

Figure 4.1 Representation of the basic immunoassay system for human growth hormone (GH). For the sake of clarity, in Figs 4.1–4.3 only small numbers of hormone molecules and antibodies are shown. In practice, the numbers of molecules of a given reagent will be in the order of 10^8–10^{13}.

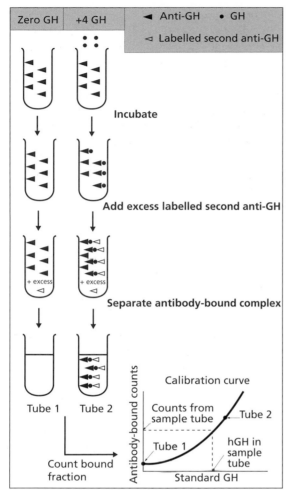

Figure 4.2 Diagram illustrating a two-point calibration curve for an immunometric assay for GH. In practice, the incubation steps for the first and second antibodies are usually held simultaneously. Because the hormone is bound between the two antibodies in the triple complex (◀•◁), this type of immunoassay is sometimes referred to as a sandwich assay. Separation of the complex from the excess labelled second antibody is usually achieved physically, for instance by precipitation and centrifugation, such that the supernatant contains the unbound labelled second antibody and can be discarded. This leaves the bound labelled second antibody to be quantified by counting radioactivity or measuring fluorescence emitted by the pellet. The low measurement from the 'zero' tube, Tube 1, and the higher value from tube 2 are plotted on the calibration curve. Tube 1 is not zero because of a small amount of nonspecific antibody binding. The calibration line is also curved, rather than straight, due to the reversible nature of the interaction between antibodies and their antigens.

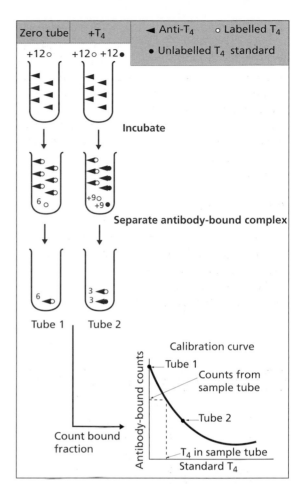

Figure 4.3 Diagram of a two-point calibration curve for an immunoassay for thyroxine. As in Fig. 4.1, in practice large numbers of molecules are present for each reagent. Under the conditions shown, the competition between labelled and unlabelled thyroxine (T_4) in tube 2 will be such that 'on average', 50% of the antibody binding sites will be occupied by labelled T_4 when it is competing with an equal amount of unlabelled T_4. Because of this competition between the labelled and unlabelled hormone for a limited amount of antibody, this type of immunoassay is sometimes called a 'competitive-binding' assay.

added to each tube. In the example shown for T_4, a 'zero' tube is set up that only contains labelled T_4, as well as a tube that includes a known amount of unlabelled standard T_4. A suitable incubation period allows the antigen–antibody complex to form. Since tube 1 contains twice as much labelled T_4 as anti-T_4

antibody, half of the labelled hormone will be bound and the other half will be free ('in excess'). In tube 2, the unlabelled and the labelled T_4 compete for the limited opportunity to bind to the antibody. The total antibody-bound T_4 is separated (e.g. by precipitation) and the label measured by radioactive or fluorescence emission (depending on the method employed). Less signal will be measured from tube 2 due to the competition from the unlabelled T_4. The decrease is a function of the amount of unlabelled T_4 that was added, that is the signal decreases as the amount of unlabelled T_4 increases, allowing the construction of a calibration curve (Fig. 4.3).

To measure T_4 clinically, the standard T_4 is replaced by the patient sample, while keeping all other assay conditions identical. The T_4 present in the sample can then be interpolated from the calibration curve.

Reference ranges

A typical adult reference range is listed for a number of hormones, as determined by immunoassays (Table 4.1). Whenever possible, hormones are measured in molar units (e.g. pmol/L) or mass units (e.g. ng/L). However, this is not possible for complex hormones such as the glycoproteins thyroid-stimulating hormone (TSH), luteinizing hormone (LH) and follicle-stimulating hormone (FSH), because they circulate in a variety of slightly different forms. In this scenario, an international reference preparation for a given hormone is agreed, which has a potency expressed in 'units' (U) and subdivisions thereof, e.g. milliunits (mU). This potency is assigned after large collaborative trials involving many laboratories worldwide using a range of bioassays and immunoassays, together with physical analytical techniques. Patient results are then expressed relative to this reference preparation.

Bioassay

At least theoretically, bioassays offer a valuable alternative to immunoassay. Biological efficacy of more complex hormones, such as TSH, may not entirely match immunoassay detection, which takes no account of functional response. In practice, the antibodies currently used in immunoassays minimize this issue (e.g. the TSH immunoassay is clinically sound and used on a large scale). There are two forms of endocrine bioassay (Table 4.2). *In vivo* bioassays investigate the biological potency of a hormone following its administration to an animal and quantification of a specific response. *In vitro* bioassays measure biological effects when hormone is added to an isolated laboratory preparation of the target tissue.

In vivo bioassays are typically used in animal experiments in conjunction with other assay techniques to establish the potency of new preparations of complex polypeptide hormones, now produced by recombinant technology. The potency may then be assigned in terms of 'units' of bioactivity. *In vivo* bioassays are also used to analyse the consequences of site-directed mutagenesis on the potency of recombinant products—a research approach that can map the bioactive site of a hormone. *In vivo* bioassays also uniquely reflect both the efficacy of the hormone preparation on its target receptor and the *in vivo* clearance rate or metabolism. For example, by *in vivo* assay, a serum binding protein may increase the potency of a hormone by prolonging its circulating half-life even though, when tested *in vitro*, the binding protein may appear to inhibit hormone action.

Receptor assay

Receptors can replace antibodies as hormone-binding agents in assays. Principles and designs are similar to immunoassays, the hormone–receptor complex replacing the hormone–antibody complex. Generally, the competitive binding system is used where the hormone is labelled (as in Fig. 4.3). Receptors may be either in solubilized form or, in the case of cell surface receptors, used while still part of isolated cell membranes. The hormone receptors, and hence the assays derived from them, have high affinity and hormone specificity, often generating favourable sensitivity, precision and sample capacity. By definition, they are based on direct interaction with the bioactive site and therefore bridge the gap between bioassays and immunoassays.

Other analytical methods

There are still situations for which satisfactorily specific and sensitive immunoassays have not been developed, commonly due to antibodies lacking

Table 4.1 Hormone reference ranges

Adult reference hormone	Range	Units
Adrenocorticotrophic hormone (ACTH, 9 AM)	0–40	ng/L
Aldosterone		
recumbent	20–190	ng/L
after 4 h standing (ambulant)	30–340	ng/L
Cortisol (9 AM)	140–700	nmol/L
Follicle-stimulating hormone (FSH)		
males	1.0–8.0	U/L
females: early follicular phase	1.0–11.0	U/L
postmenopausal	>20	U/L
Glucagon (fasting)	<50	pmol/L
Gastrin (fasting)	<40	pmol/L
Growth hormone		
after a glucose load	<2	mU/L
stress-induced	>20	mU/L
Insulin		
fasting	<10	mU/L
during hypoglycaemia (glucose <2.5 mmol/L)	<5	mU/L
during hypoglycaemia (glucose <1.5 mmol/L)	<2	mU/L
Luteinizing hormone (LH)		
males	0.5–9.0	U/L
females: early follicular phase	0.5–14.5	U/L
postmenopausal	>20	U/L
Oestradiol		
males	37–130	pmol/L
females: early follicular phase	100–500	pmol/L
mid-cycle	700–1900	pmol/L
luteal phase	300–1250	pmol/L
Parathyroid hormone (PTH)	<4.4	pmol/L
Prolactin	80–500	mU/L
Progesterone (day 21, luteal phase)	>30	nmol/L (indicates ovulation)
Renin		
recumbent	2–30	mU/L
ambulant	3–40	mU/L
Testosterone		
male	8–30	nmol/L
female	0.5–2.5	nmol/L
Thyroid-stimulating hormone (TSH)	0.3–5.0	mU/L
Thyroxine, free (fT_4)	11–24	pmol/L
Triiodothyronine, free (fT_3)	3.5–8.2	pmol/L
Vitamin D (25-OH-cholecalciferol)	4–40	µg/L
Vitamin D (1,25-OH-cholecalciferol)	48–110	pmol/L

Ranges vary slightly between laboratories due to differences in the methods employed. These examples are only intended to be illustrative. The data were kindly provided by Dr Peter Wood and Miss Catherine Noyce, Southampton General Hospital.

Table 4.2 Bioassays

Hormone	Experimental system	Response measured
In vivo bioassays		
Growth hormone	Hypophysectomized rats or hypopituitary strain of dwarf mice	Body weight gain or increase in the width of tibial epiphyseal cartilage
Prolactin	Pigeon crop sac	Increased in crop weight or thickening
Parathyroid hormone	Parathyroidectomized rats	Increase in serum calcium
Insulin	Rabbits and mice	Lowering blood glucose
FSH	Hypophysectomized female rats	Increase in ovarian weight
LH	Hypophysectomized male rats	Increase in prostate weight
TSH	Mice: thyroids prelabelled with I^{131}	Discharge of I^{131} into the circulation
In vitro bioassays		
Growth hormone	Nb2 rat lymphoma cell line	Increase in cell number and metabolic activity
Prolactin	As for growth hormone	As for growth hormone
Parathyroid hormone	Renal plasma membranes	Increase in adenylate cyclase activity
Insulin	Rat diaphragm muscle	Increase in glucose uptake and glycogen synthesis
FSH	Cultured ovarian granulosa cells or CHO cells that express the human FSH receptor	Increase in aromatase (CYP19) activity
LH	Cultured Leydig cells	Increase in testosterone production
TSH	Immortalized rat thyroid cells (FRTL-5 cells) or CHO cells that express the human TSH receptor	Increase in adenylate cyclase activity or, for instance, I^{131} uptake

sufficient specificity. For some steroid hormones or intermediaries from their biosynthetic pathway, other techniques, such as high performance liquid chromatography (HPLC) or gas chromatography coupled to mass spectrometry (GC/MS), are becoming increasingly helpful. These approaches provide definitive identification of the relevant hormone or compound from its physical characteristics. They have proved helpful in combating the use of performance enhancing agents in professional sport.

Molecular biology approaches to endocrine diagnosis

Karyotype and fluorescence *in situ* hybridization

Karyotype refers to the complement of chromosomes within an individual's cells—normal karyotype for females being 46,XX and for males 46,XY. The term is also commonly used to describe metaphase chromosomes on glass slide (although more correctly, this is the 'karyogram') (see Fig. 2.1). More detail comes from Giemsa (G) staining of metaphase chromosomes, where each chromosome can be identified by its particular staining pattern, called 'G-banding'.

Ascertaining the karyotype can be useful in paediatric cases of genital ambiguity (i.e. is it 46,XX or 46,XY?), or when there is concern over Turner syndrome (45,XO) or Klinefelter syndrome (47,XXY) (see Chapter 7). G-banding allows experienced cytogeneticists to identify deletions, duplications or translocations of chromosomes, the limit of resolution being in the order of a few megabases.

When a syndrome is suspected, for which the causative gene or genomic position ('locus') is known, fluorescence *in situ* hybridization (FISH) allows assessment of duplications and deletions on a smaller scale. For instance, a locus for congenital hypoparathyroidism, as part of DiGeorge syndrome,

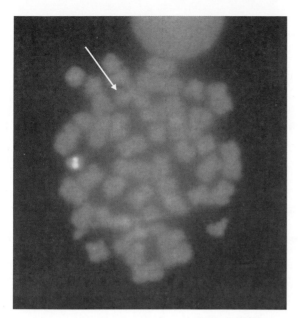

Figure 4.4 FISH in a case of DiGeorge syndrome with congenital hypoparathyroidism. Human metaphase chromosomes from a patient with hypocalcaemia and congenital heart disease were hybridized with a fluorescent probe from chromosome 22q11. The two bright dots indicate hybridization on the sister chromatids of the normal chromosome 22. The arrow points to the other chromosome 22 that lacks signal, indicating a deletion. Images provided by Professor David Wilson, University of Southampton.

exists on the long arm of chromosome 22 (22q). FISH utilizes the principle that complementary DNA sequences hybridize together. Stretches of DNA from the region of interest are fluorescently labelled and hybridized to the patient's DNA. The fluorescence is visible as a dot on each sister chromatid of each relevant chromosome (Fig. 4.4). Therefore, normal autosomal copy number is viewed as two pairs of two dots; one pair indicates a deletion; and three pairs indicate either duplication or potentially a translocation breakpoint (where the probe detects sequence either side of the breakpoint on different chromosomes).

New technology using the principles of FISH for comparative genomic hybridization (CGH) on a genome-wide microarray format is called array CGH and offers much increased resolution down to several kilobases. It examines the entire genome for microdeletions and duplications in one experiment and is entering clinical diagnostic service.

Mutation detection by PCR-based methodology and sequencing

With the advance of molecular genetics and the discovery of a vast number of disease-associated genes, very precise genetic testing is rapidly moving into clinical endocrinology. In time, it will offer increasingly precise genotype–phenotype correlations *and predictions*. For instance, in type 2 multiple endocrine neoplasia (MEN2; see Chapter 10), certain mutations in the *RET* proto-oncogene have never been associated with phaeochromocytoma, normally one of the commonest features of the syndrome. As such, defining molecular genetics will begin to inform clinical management rather than just confirm a diagnosis.

Polymerase chain reaction (PCR) is used to identify a mutation in a specific gene (Fig. 4.5). This method amplifies the exons of a gene of interest in DNA isolated from the patient's white blood cells. The enzymatic reaction utilizes bacterial DNA polymerases that are capable of withstanding high temperature (up to the mid-90s °C). These enzymes originated from the microorganisms that live in hot springs. A second, modified PCR reaction provides the base pair sequence of the DNA demonstrating whether or not the gene is mutated.

Imaging in endocrinology

Ultrasound

Ultrasound travels as sound waves beyond the range of human hearing and, according to the surface encountered, is reflected back towards the emitting source (the ultrasound probe). Different tissues have different reflective properties. By knowing the speed of the waves and the time between emission and detection, the distance between the reflective surfaces and the source can be calculated. These data allow a two-dimensional image to be generated (Fig. 4.6). The major advantage of ultrasound is its simplicity and noninvasiveness. Machines are portable. It is helpful as an initial imaging investigation of many endocrine organs. For instance, the thyroid has a characteristic appearance in Graves disease due its

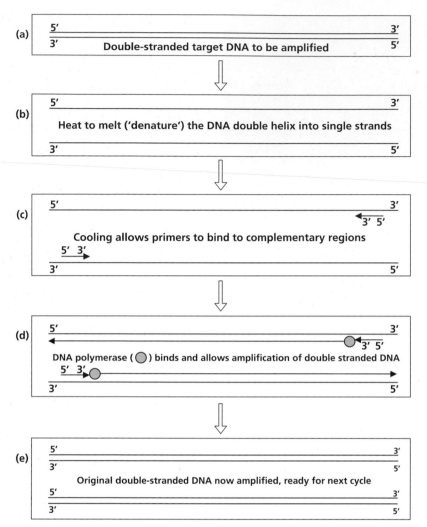

Figure 4.5 The basic principles of polymerase chain reaction. Polymerase chain reaction (PCR) allows the amplification of a user-defined stretch of genomic DNA (the 'target' DNA in (a)). In diagnostic molecular genetics, this is commonly the exonic sequence of a gene, mutation of which is suspected to underlie the patient's phenotype. (a) The starting DNA. (b) The double helix is separated into two single strands by heating to mid 90's °C. (c) Cooling from this high temperature allows the binding of user-designed short stretches of DNA ('primers') that are complementary to the opposite strands at each end of the region to be amplified. The binding takes place specifically at the complementary base pairs of the target DNA. (d) DNA polymerase catalyses the addition of new deoxynucleotide residues based on the complementary base pairs of the template strand. (e) Once complete, two double-stranded sequences are generated from the original target DNA. Another cycle then recommences at (a), only this time with twice as much template, i.e. the increase in target DNA is exponential. Having amplified large amounts of the desired DNA sequence, a modified PCR reaction and analysis determines the precise sequence of the DNA to discover the presence or absence of a mutation.

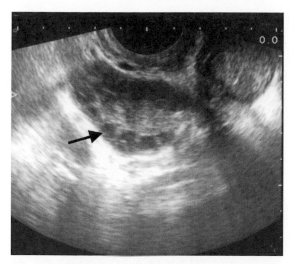

Figure 4.6 Ultrasound of a polycystic ovary. Although controversial, the presence of multiple small cysts (see arrow) is consistent with, but not required for, the diagnosis of polycystic ovarian syndrome. Ultrasound does, however, help to exclude an androgen-secreting tumour (see Chapter 7). Image kindly provided by Dr Sue Ingamells, University of Southampton.

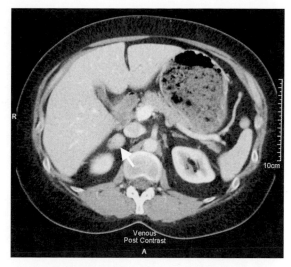

Figure 4.7 Abdominal CT with contrast demonstrating a right adrenal mass. This patient presented with Cushing syndrome. The mass (see arrow) on CT was a hypersecreting adrenocortical adenoma.

increased vascularity. The ovaries can be delineated transabdominally, or with specific consent, trans-vaginally, when the shorter distance between probe and ovary and fewer reflective surfaces create higher resolution images (Fig. 4.6).

Computed tomography and magnetic resonance imaging

Computed tomography (CT) and, more latterly, magnetic resonance imaging (MRI) provide excellent depiction of the body's internal organs and tissues. The principle of CT is the same as that for X-ray imaging. X-rays pass differently through the various organs and tissues of the body. For instance, bone is not penetrated very well so a plain X-ray image is obtained as if the skeleton has cast a shadow. In CT scanning, the patient lies on a table that slides through a motorized ring, which rotates and emits X-rays. Data are acquired on penetration from different angles, which are then constructed by computer into a single transverse 'slice' through the body (Fig. 4.7).

The skull is a bony casing, hence imaging the brain by CT is limited.

In comparison to CT, MRI does not rely on X-rays and is particularly useful at imaging intracranial structures, such as the anterior pituitary (Fig. 4.8). The key components of MRI are magnets. At their centre is a hollow tube, into which the patient passes on a horizontal table. Once inside the tube, the patient is in a very strong magnetic field (the reason why MRI is dangerous in patients with metallic implants such as pacemakers or aneurysm clips). Within the magnetic field, some of the body's hydrogen atoms resonate after absorbing energy from a pulse of radio frequency waves. Once the pulse ends, the resonating atoms give up energy as they return to their original state. These emission data are collected. They differ slightly for different tissues allowing the construction of high definition images.

Contrast agents are very useful for both CT and MRI scanning (Fig. 4.7). In MRI, agents such as gadolinium can subtly alter the data acquired, for instance allowing the identification of an adenoma within normal anterior pituitary tissue.

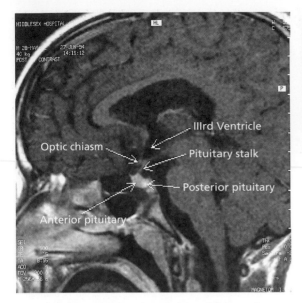 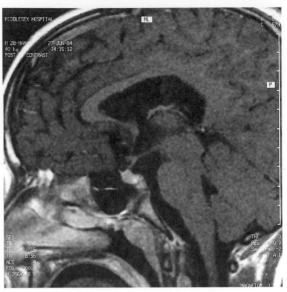

Figure 4.8 Sagittal (side-on) MRI of the adult central nervous system. Because of its composition, the posterior pituitary characteristically appears bright under particular MRI settings. Loss of the 'posterior pituitary bright spot' indicates altered tissue composition and may indicate pathology.

Nuclear medicine and uptake markers

Simple X-rays, CT and MRI depict the body's tissues and organs but provide limited insight into the cells that compose these structures or their function. In later life, many organs develop benign tumours of little or no significance. For instance, adrenal 'incidentalomas' can affect ~5% of the population after ~40 years. In a patient with hypertension, it would be important to distinguish these from a phaeochromocytoma that could be the curable cause of the elevated blood pressure (see Chapter 6). The uptake of markers (or 'tracers') specific to a particular cell-type can provide valuable clues. For instance, meta-iodobenzylguanidine (mIBG) acts as an analogue of norepinephrine and is taken up by adrenal medulla cells. When labelled with radioactive I^{123} it can be used to distinguish a phaeochromocytoma from other tumours (Plate 4.1, facing p. 246). At higher doses, it can even be used as targeted therapy, when instead of marking cells it kills them. Technetium-99m pertechnetate can be used to distinguish different causes of hyperthyroidism (see Chapter 8). It is taken up by the thyroid gland like iodide. In Graves disease, the uptake is homogeneous; with a solitary 'toxic' adenoma, the uptake is restricted to the relevant nodule.

KEY POINTS

- Diagnosing or excluding endocrine disorders relies on an ability to measure serum hormone levels

- Immunoassays provide accurate, reliable laboratory measurement of serum hormone concentrations

- Molecular biology is applied increasingly to provide patient-specific diagnoses of congenital disorders or endocrine neoplasia syndromes; the information

can predict and influence patient outcome and management

- Imaging investigations are key to localizing endocrine disorders and assist surgical intervention, however:

- 'Incidentalomas' are common and conscientious effort is needed to correlate a biochemical endocrine abnormality to a tumour identified on imaging

PART 2

2 Clinical Endocrinology

5 The hypothalamus and pituitary gland

LEARNING OBJECTIVES

- To appreciate the nature of the various hypothalamic–anterior pituitary axes and their end organ interactions
- To understand the clinical disorders that arise from *over* and *under*secretion of the anterior pituitary hormones
- To acquire familiarity with the hormones of the posterior pituitary and the associated clinical conditions
- To understand the nature of tumours within the pituitary gland and their clinical consequences

This chapter integrates the basic biology of the hypothalamus and the pituitary gland with important clinical conditions

Parts of the hypothalamus and pituitary gland act co-ordinately as several organs in one, regulating a number of distinct hormone axes, each with their own clinical disorders relating to *over* and *under*production. Rather than providing sequential basic science and clinical sections, clinical details are given for each hormone axis as it is encountered. Similarly, the destructive consequences of pituitary tumours follow on from the description of pituitary anatomy and surrounding landmarks. As underactivity of the pituitary commonly involves many of the hormone axes, the concluding section of the chapter ties these features together.

Embryology, anatomy and vasculature

The anterior and the posterior pituitary develop as two independent organs from very different starting points (Fig. 5.1). The anterior pituitary (also known as the adenohypophysis) is derived from the epithelial lining of the roof of the mouth prior to closure of the bony palate. This invasion of proliferating epithelial cells (Rathke's pouch) detaches from the oral lining and moves upwards. At the same time, central nervous system cells proliferate in the floor of the third ventricle (a region called the infundibulum) and migrate downwards to form the posterior pituitary (also known as the neurohypophysis). The downward movement creates the stalk of the pituitary, below which the anterior and posterior components become apposed within the bony casing of the pituitary fossa (also called the sella turcica, part of the sphenoid bone) (Fig. 5.2). Sometimes, incomplete fusion of Rathke's pouch can result in fluid-filled cysts that, like pituitary tumours, cause detrimental effects from local pressure (see the clinical

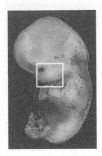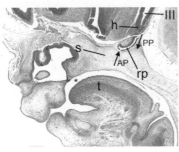

Figure 5.1 The human pituitary gland forms at ~8 weeks of development. The boxed region is enlarged to the right. The arrows show the respective migration of the cells that form the anterior (AP) and posterior pituitary (PP). III, third ventricle; h, hypothalamus; rp, Rathke's pouch; s, sphenoid bone; t, tongue; *, oral cavity.

consequences of anatomy, below). Above the pituitary, clusters of neurosecretory cells form the various hypothalamic nuclei (Fig. 5.2), which can be divided both anatomically and functionally into two components (Table 5.1).

Hormone-containing granules are continually transported down the neurones to the posterior pituitary at a rate of 8 mm/h. Upon stimulation, these hormones are released from the nerve terminals into the adjacent fenestrated capillaries. In essence, the posterior pituitary functions largely as a store. As some of the arginine vasopressin (AVP) fibres terminate in the median eminence of the hypothalamus (Fig. 5.2), a patient with destruction of the posterior pituitary can commonly recover AVP function.

The adult pituitary weighs ~0.5 g, three-quarters of which is anterior pituitary; however, this can double during puberty or pregnancy. Hypothalamic hormones released into the capillary plexus at the median eminence flow down the portal veins to the anterior pituitary (Fig. 5.2). In turn, this stimulates the specific cell types of the anterior pituitary to secrete their own hormones from storage granules.

Pituitary tumours — clinical consequences of anatomy

The commonest space-occupying lesion of the pituitary fossa is a benign adenoma. If these tumours arise from endocrine cell types, the patient may present with features of hormone excess. These are dealt with in the following sections and case reports. Here, we consider the physical consequences of the pituitary, lying in a bony case surrounded by important structures (Box 5.1).

Nonfunctioning adenomas

The commonest pituitary tumour does not secrete known active hormones and is termed a 'nonfunctioning' adenoma. On post-mortem analysis, foci of pituitary adenoma are recognized in up to 20% of individuals. The reason for this incredibly high rate of benign tumour formation is contentious; attention has fallen on the pituitary's unusual location where it receives privileged access to high concentrations of hormones and growth factors directly from the hypothalamus. Molecular genetics has also advanced understanding. For instance, ~40% of GH-secreting adenomas contain a mutation in $G_s\alpha$ (review Chapter 3). Pituitary carcinoma is exceptionally rare.

The distinction between microadenoma and macroadenoma (a diameter smaller or larger than 1 cm) is arbitrary and reflects historical resolution of imaging techniques. Magnetic resonance imaging (MRI) is now the investigation of choice for visualizing the pituitary gland and is capable of resolving tumours a few millimetres in diameter (see Fig. 4.8).

Tumours restricted to the pituitary fossa may compress nearby cells and cause various forms of 'hypopituitarism' (i.e. deficiency of pituitary hormone, described later). Pituitary adenomas can also expand beyond the pituitary fossa, eroding the sella turcica, and bulge in all directions (Box 5.1). Upward growth can compress the optic chiasm where the optic nerves cross, relaying information from the eye to the visual cortex. This creates a characteristic defect, where the fibres first affected are those from the inner portions of the retina. This leads to loss of peripheral vision, termed 'bitemporal hemianopia'. It progresses insidiously and patients may present with profound visual loss. A classical description is a road traffic accident where cars or pedestrians coming from either side were unappreciated.

Lateral extension into the cavernous sinus can cause ophthalmoplegia (paralysis of eye movement) due to pressure on any of the three cranial nerves that innervate the extraocular muscles of the eye

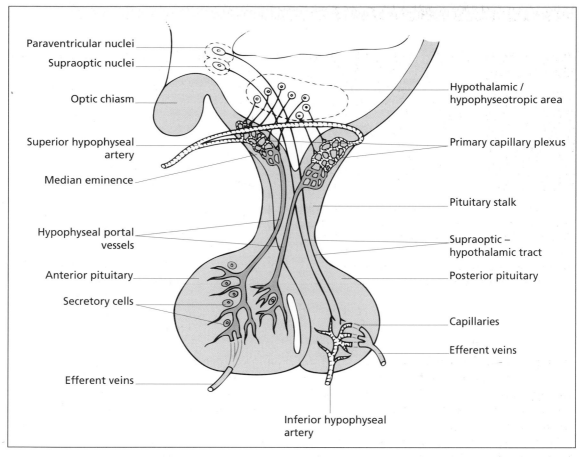

Figure 5.2 The structure of the hypothalamus and its neural and vascular connections with the pituitary. The superior hypophyseal artery branches to form the primary capillary plexus in the median eminence and the upper part of the pituitary stalk. From the plexus arise the hypophyseal portal vessels, which terminate in the anterior pituitary to form a secondary plexus of sinusoidal capillaries and supply the hormone-secreting anterior pituitary cell types. Efferent veins drain from the anterior pituitary into dural sinuses. The axons from the hypothalamic–hypophyseotrophic area terminate close to the primary capillary plexus. The posterior pituitary is supplied by the inferior hypophyseal artery. The axons of the supraoptic and paraventricular nuclei run down the pituitary stalk and terminate close to the capillaries supplying the posterior pituitary. The entire pituitary gland is encased in the bony sella turcica.

Table 5.1 Anatomical and functional aspects of the hypothalamic nuclei

Nuclei	Anatomy and function
Supraoptic and paraventricular nuclei	Influence posterior pituitary function
	Paired structures in the anterior hypothalamus
	Large neurones pass through the pituitary stalk as the 'supraoptic–hypothalamic tract' to the posterior pituitary
	Oxytocin and arginine vasopressin secreted into the circulation from storage granules at the nerve terminals
Hypothalamic–hypophyseotropic nuclei	Influence anterior pituitary function
	Lie in the lateral wall of the third ventricle
	Small neurones pass to the median eminence where hormones are stored as small vesicles
	Hormones released into capillary network and carried to the anterior pituitary
	Individual hypothalamic hormones regulate specific anterior pituitary cell types

(Table 5.2). Involvement of each nerve can give rise to characteristic forms of diplopia (double vision), exacerbated by looking away from the action of the paralysed muscle. Laterally, tumour can also envel-op the internal carotid artery in the cavernous sinus. Restricted access and the dangers of operating around major vessels makes curative surgery impossible once tumours have extended in this direction.

Other more generalized symptoms of pituitary masses include headache (especially frontal/retro-orbital) from stretching of the meninges or obstruction to cerebrospinal fluid (CSF) drainage. Very rarely, tumours extend anteriorly through the sphenoid sinus to cause CSF leakage through the nose ('CSF rhinorrhoea').

Not all pituitary masses are adenomas. The differential diagnosis includes metastasis, meningioma, lymphoma, sarcoid, histiocytosis, or an unusual tumour that more commonly presents to the paediatric endocrinologist called a craniopharyngioma. Histologically, this tumour is benign but it still invades. It most likely arises from the epithelial cells that lined Rathke's pouch and can cause coincident diabetes insipidus (deficiency of AVP, see later).

Treating pituitary tumours

Pharmacological treatment is available for some hormone-secreting tumours (see later sections). For all others, there are essentially three choices (Box 5.2).

Compression of the optic chiasm is a neurosurgical emergency. Profound visual loss can be restored quickly by relieving pressure on the chiasm. This is an example where surgery is advantageous over radiotherapy, which is less invasive, but can take up to 10 years for its complete effect and frequently results

---

> **BOX 5.1 The consequences of pituitary tumours**
>
> The consequences of pituitary tumours are twofold:
> - Potential hormone excess from the tumourous cell type (see later sections)
> - Local pressure from the space-occupying lesion on other pituitary cell types and external structures
>   - >1 cm diameter = 'macroadenoma'
>   - <1 cm diameter = 'microadenoma'
>
> The anterior pituitary is bordered by a number of very important structures that can be affected by expanding pituitary tumours:
> - Superiorly—optic chiasm
>   - compression causes loss of vision (classically, a bitemporal hemianopia)
> - Anteriorly—sphenoid sinus
>   - the surgical route for transsphenoidal removal of pituitary tumours
> - Laterally—cavernous sinuses
>   - contain cranial nerves III, IV and VI, which can be compressed, and the internal carotid artery, which can be encased
>   - veins, into which anterior pituitary hormones drain, that can be accessed under radiological guidance ('inferior petrosal sinus sampling')

Table 5.2 Cranial nerves in the cavernous sinus

Cranial nerve	Function	Consequences of compression
Oculomotor nerve (III)	Innervation of suprapalpebral muscles	Ptosis is the most obvious feature
	Associated with parasympathetic nerve fibres from the Edinger–Westphal nucleus	Fixed, dilated pupil and loss of accommodation
	Innervation of all extraocular muscles except those supplied by IV and VI	Down and outward-looking vision (unopposed actions of superior oblique and lateral rectus)
		Double vision if eye lid is raised
Trochlear nerve (IV)	Innervation of the superior oblique muscle	Weak downward and inward gaze
		Double vision on walking down stairs
Abducent nerve (VI)	Innervation of the lateral rectus muscle	Inward (medial)-looking gaze.
		Double vision most pronounced on looking to affected side

in hypopituitarism due to death of the other hormone-secreting cell types.

The hypothalamic–anterior pituitary hormone axes

There is a special relationship between an anterior

BOX 5.2 Summary of nonpharmacological treatment of pituitary tumours

Observe — repeat MRI scan and monitor anterior pituitary hormone function
- Increasingly common as 'incidentalomas' are discovered with the use of MRI to investigate headaches
- An option for tumours that are not compressing the optic chiasm

Transsphenoidal surgery
- Conducted from behind the upper lip or through the nose. The sphenoid sinus is entered, crossed and the pituitary encountered through the sella turcica
- Used in an emergency to treat compression of the optic chiasm (except for prolactinomas — see later)

Transfrontal surgery is less commonly used now, but can be considered for particularly large tumours

Radiotherapy
- Radiation is delivered to the tumour region, while taking great care to avoid the optic chiasm

---

pituitary cell type, its hypothalamic regulator and its secreted hormone, which in several instances goes on to regulate major endocrine end organs (Table 5.3). The adrenal gland, testis, ovary and thyroid are *Essential Endocrinology* chapters in their own right; here, details relating to their basic and clinical science will be kept brief.

As they are mostly small peptides, hypothalamic hormones have short circulating half-lives and their release is generally pulsatile. Therefore, action on the pituitary is of limited duration. Clinically, they are rarely measured, but their action may be monitored by the relevant anterior pituitary hormone (e.g. a rise in TSH concentration in response to intravenous TRH). *In vivo* action is very fast by virtue of specific anterior pituitary cell-surface receptors linked to characteristic second messenger pathways (see Chapter 3) and the release of stored hormone granules. How the inhibitory hormones somatostatin and dopamine act is less well understood.

Generic regulation of hypothalamic–anterior pituitary hormone secretion

Regulation of anterior pituitary hormone release is complex and where axis-specific processes occur (e.g. for the adrenal cortex, testis, ovary and thyroid), these are discussed in the relevant 'end organ' chapter. Nevertheless, there is a basic model (Fig. 5.3). 'Closed loop' feedback, most commonly negative, can act on the transcription and translation of

---

Table 5.3 Hormone-secreting cell types of the anterior pituitary

Anterior pituitary cell type	Hormone secreted	Size (amino acids)	Target organ	Hypothalamic regulator (+ or − effect)
Somatotroph	Growth hormone (GH)	191	Diverse	GH-releasing hormone (GHRH, +) and somatostatin (SS, −)
Lactotroph	Prolactin (PRL)	199	Breast	Dopamine (−) and thyrotrophin-releasing hormone (TRH, +)
Corticotroph	Adrenocorticotrophin (ACTH)	39	Adrenal cortex	Corticotrophin-releasing hormone (CRH, +)
Thyrotroph	Thyroid-stimulating hormone (TSH)	204	Thyroid	TRH (+)
Gonadotroph	Follicle-stimulating hormone (FSH) and luteinizing hormone (LH)	Both 204	Ovary or testis	Gonadotrophin-releasing hormone (GnRH, +)

particular hormone-encoding genes as well as the release of hormone stores and the number of cell-surface receptors available to mediate hormone action. For example, increased thyroid hormone reduces the number of TRH receptors on anterior pituitary thyrotrophs.

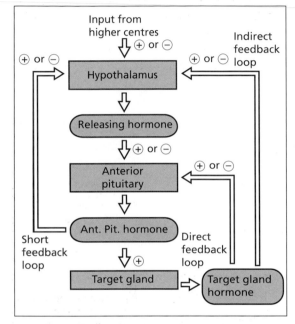

Figure 5.3 Endocrine feedback circuits. The diagram shows interactions between higher centres, the hypothalamus, the anterior pituitary and peripheral endocrine glands. The controlling factors can be stimulatory (+) or inhibitory (−).

Pulsatility of hypothalamic hormone release can also impact on target cell responsiveness. Constant GnRH 'switches off' the gonadotroph, and, consequently, 'shuts down' the testis or ovary. Thus, continuous intravenous supply can be used as a contraceptive or a means of pharmacological castration (e.g. in hormone-dependent prostrate or breast cancer). In contrast, pulses of GnRH every 90 min can be used to restore fertility in patients with hypothalamic dysfunction.

In addition to autonomous regulation, transient 'open loop' neural inputs from higher centres modulate the system at the hypothalamus (Table 5.4). Several endocrine responses to environmental changes, such as psychological stress, exercise and temperature, are mediated in this way. Several anterior pituitary hormones exhibit a circadian rhythm, the regulation of which remains poorly understood but probably involves the pineal gland. In mammals, this gland appears to transduce neural information on the day–night light cycle from the retina into a circadian rhythm of melatonin secretion.

Growth hormone

Growth hormone (GH) is the most abundant hormone of the adult anterior pituitary, accounting for up to 10% of its dry weight. The major form of human GH is a protein with 191 amino acids, two disulphide bridges and a molecular weight of 22 kDa, although there are some minor variants. The structure of GH is species-specific. Human GH differs markedly from that of nonprimates. This is thought to reflect the dramatic evolution of the GH/PRL gene family

Table 5.4 The hypothalamus controls vital functions and its regulation is very complex

Autonomous regulation	Nonautonomous regulation
Demonstrated by surgical disconnection when: Basal secretion of GH, FSH and LH remain largely unchanged Insulin-induced hypoglycaemia or stress release of ACTH is unaffected	Input from within the hypothalamus itself or from other parts of the brain (e.g. hippocampus, anterior thalamus, amygdala, pyriform cortex and midbrain)

Norepinephrine, epinephrine, dopamine, serotonin and acetylcholine influence hypothalamic neurosecretory cells
Monoamine-secreting neurones synapse on hypothalamic neurones and their axons
Peptide neurotransmitters (e.g. opioid peptides and substance P) modulate hypothalamic hormone secretion

with the appearance of primates. One practical consequence is the obligatory use of human GH, now produced recombinantly, to treat children and adults with GH deficiency.

Effects of growth hormone

Growth hormone has both metabolic and anabolic actions (Fig. 5.4). The latter are mediated largely through the generation of the mitogenic polypeptide insulin-like growth factor 1 (IGF1). IGF1 is produced in many tissues, including large amounts from the liver. In turn, the endocrine action of IGF1 is regulated by a family of at least six highly specific IGF binding proteins (IGFBPs). Most (>95%) serum IGF1 is bound in a complex with IGFBP3 and a protein called acid labile subunit (ALS). The production of IGFBP3 and ALS is also increased by GH.

Metabolic actions

Intermediate metabolism. The direct metabolic effects of GH tend to synergize with cortisol and generally antagonize insulin, giving rise to the 'diabetogenic' properties of excess GH. GH leads to a stimulation of lipolysis and increases fasting free fatty acid (FFA) concentrations. During times of fasting or energy restriction, this lipolytic effect of GH is enhanced, while the effect is suppressed by coadministration of

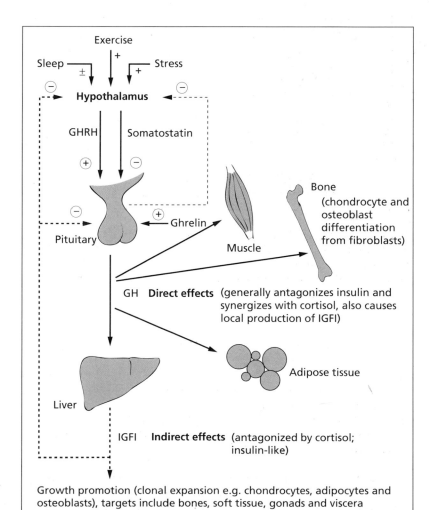

Figure 5.4 Summary of the regulation and effects of growth hormone. Glucagon and free fatty acids increase somatostatin release.

food or glucose. In the long term, and important clinically, GH leads to a reduction in fat mass.

GH and IGF1 both have roles in normal glucose homeostasis. GH increases fasting hepatic glucose output, by increasing hepatic gluconeogenesis and glycogenolysis, and decreases peripheral glucose utilization through the inhibition of glycogen synthesis and glucose oxidation. These effects are antagonistic to those of insulin and acute reductions in GH secretion are associated with enhanced insulin sensitivity. Longer-term reductions in GH are associated with the development of insulin resistance in association with changes in body composition. In contrast to GH, IGF1, as suggested by its name, acts like insulin to lower blood glucose by stimulating peripheral glucose uptake, glycolysis and glycogen synthesis while having a minimal effect on hepatic glucose production.

Sodium and water homeostasis. The mechanisms enabling the body to regulate sodium and water homeostasis are complex. Although incompletely understood, there is evidence that GH induces sodium and fluid retention, possibly by increasing glomerular filtration rate. The main clinical implication of this phenomenon is the side-effect of swollen hands or feet or pitting oedema reported by adults receiving GH replacement therapy.

Energy expenditure. GH causes an increase in basal metabolic rate through a number of mechanisms including an increase in lean body mass, increased FFA oxidation and enhanced peripheral tri-iodothyronine production (see Chapter 8).

Anabolic actions

GH output increases with size to sustain growth during childhood. A person destined to become tall secretes GH at rather higher circulating concentrations than his or her smaller peers. The consequence is that he or she grows rather faster than average and, year-by-year, gains height. There is a marked rise in GH concentration at puberty.

The anabolic effects of GH on protein metabolism are mainly mediated by IGF1. This promotes growth of long bones at the epiphyseal plates, where there are actively proliferating cartilage cells. This 'growth spurt' ceases once the epiphyses of the long bones

fuse at the end of adolescence—the reason why too much GH after this time leads to the progressively dysmorphic growth of acromegaly. GH also has profound effects on bone turnover. Again it is likely that these effects are largely indirect, as IGF1 concentrations correlate well with estimates of bone mineral density. In addition, GH and IGF1 may modify intestinal calcium absorption and serum concentrations of active vitamin D (see Chapter 9).

Acute administration of GH modestly stimulates muscle and whole body protein synthesis leading to nitrogen retention and increased lean body mass. The converse effects are seen with the decline in GH secretion with ageing; features, which can be partially reversed by GH administration. As well as GH, IGF1 concentrations also decline with advancing age. The latter is particularly important, as age and sex-matched normal ranges are necessary for the appropriate interpretation of serum IGF1 assays. Without them, there is a risk of incorrectly diagnosing overactivity or underactivity of the GH–IGF1 axis.

Mechanism of action of GH and IGFs

GH signals within the cell via the JAK–STAT pathway (review Figs 3.7 and 3.8). GH receptors have been detected within the first year of life in all of the known target tissues. The number of receptors in a target tissue (e.g. the liver) can be changed both by peripheral factors, such as sex hormones, and also by GH itself, which induces downregulation. As suggested by the name, the indirect effects of GH via IGF1 are often 'insulin-like'. They can be antagonized by cortisol and are mediated intracellularly by pathways very similar to those described for insulin signalling (review Chapter 3 and Fig. 3.6).

Growth hormone regulation

Dual input from higher centres

GH secretion is stimulated by sleep and exercise and is inhibited by food ingestion. During deep sleep, bursts of secretion occur every 1 to 2 h (Fig. 5.5). Stress (e.g. excitement, cold, anaesthesia, surgery or haemorrhage) also produces a rapid increase in serum GH. The regulation of GH production comes from dynamic, opposing interplay between GHRH and somatostatin (Fig. 5.4). GHRH and somatostatin are released by the hypothalamus and their dual input

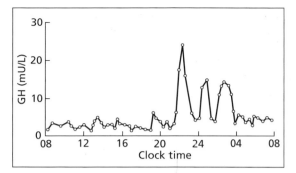

Figure 5.5 A 24-hour profile of serum GH in a normal 7-year-old child. Irregular pulses occur, which are greatest during sleep.

BOX 5.3 Assessing the GH–IGF1 axis

- GH release is pulsatile (Fig. 5.5)
  - random serum GH is a poor marker of GH activity
  - either dynamic testing or a profile is needed
- Circulating IGF1 levels are relatively constant
  - random serum IGF1 is a useful marker to assess GH 'status'

---

may be particularly important. Negative feedback has been proposed for IGF1, and for GH itself (Fig. 5.4). However, the axis lacks a single end organ that secretes a hormone with a clear negative feedback role (e.g. as for cortisol on ACTH). Instead, one positive influence (GHRH) coupled with a negative one (somatostatin) offers an alternative mechanism for regulation. GH pulses are virtually simultaneous with peaks of GHRH and low somatostatin levels; conversely, GH falls when somatostatin concentration rises. The pulsatile release of GH and its relatively short half-life of ~15 min means that basal serum levels are barely detectable (<1 mU/L). Although a circulating GH-binding protein slightly increases half-life, its physiological significance is unclear. Understanding the variable nature of circulating GH, in comparison to the more constant levels of serum IGF1, is important in assessing clinical GH status (Box 5.3).

Input from other axes
GH production from somatotrophs is dependent upon an adequate supply of thyroid hormone.

BOX 5.4 GH excess: a constellation of signs and symptoms due to bony and soft tissue overgrowth

- Gigantism: occurs prior to epiphyseal closure and causes increased stature
- Acromegaly: occurs after epiphyseal closure and causes progressive, cosmetic disfigurement

---

Hypothyroid children suffer from stunted growth. Glucocorticoids, as either endogenous cortisol or synthetic steroids given for inflammatory disorders (e.g. asthma), suppress GH secretion; while oestrogens sensitize the pituitary to the action of GHRH, so that basal and stimulated GH concentrations are slightly higher in women and rise earlier during female puberty.

Metabolic regulation
In addition to the regulation of GH by GHRH and somatostatin from higher centres, another important peptide regulator has been discovered. Ghrelin is secreted mainly by the stomach and acts as a potent GH secretagogue. It also stimulates hunger, in effect acting oppositely from leptin (see Chapter 15).

FFA and GH are involved in a classical feedback loop; GH induces lipolysis and a rise in FFA, which, in turn, inhibits GH secretion. Similarly, following a meal, the increase in FFA inhibits the secretion of GH at the same time that insulin secretion rises. The increased insulin suppresses lipolysis. With the fall in FFA concentrations as the individual moves back into the fasting state, GH secretion again increases. Longer periods of fasting and chronic malnutrition are associated with increased amplitude and frequency of GH secretion. In contrast, obesity is associated with reduced GH levels. The metabolic regulation of GH secretion is utilized in the clinical assessment of GH status (Fig. 5.6; Table 5.5).

Clinical disorders
Growth hormone excess—acromegaly and gigantism
Growth hormone excess is rare, affecting approximately 60 people per million (Box 5.4). It most commonly arises from tumourous expansion of the somatotroph cell type within the pituitary. In line with all pituitary tumours, these are virtually always benign adenomas rather than carcinomas.

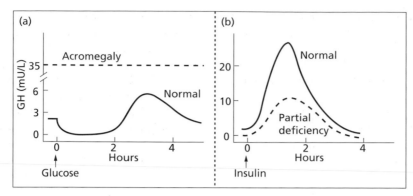

Figure 5.6 Dynamic tests of GH status. Oral glucose normally suppresses GH release, although it can rebound as blood glucose falls (as shown in (a)). In acromegaly, GH release is not suppressed (dotted line) and there may even be a paradoxical rise. Insulin injection reduces blood glucose, which stimulates GH release in normal subjects (as shown in (b)). This response is reduced in partial GH deficiency and lacking in patients with complete deficiency.

Table 5.5 Dynamic tests of GH status

Test	Results
75 g oral glucose load	Rapid suppression of GH secretion <2 mU/L if normal Remains high in acromegaly or gigantism
Insulin-induced hypoglycaemia (≤2.2 mmol/L)	Stimulation of GH secretion >20 mU/L if normal 9–20 mU/L partial deficiency <9 mU/L severe GH deficiency
Amino acid infusion (particularly arginine)	Stimulation of GH secretion (useful in patients where insulin-induced hypoglycaemia is undesirable)

Signs and symptoms. The appearance of bone growth differs depending on whether the patient presents prior to or after epiphyseal fusion. Before, the excess GH promotes increased linear velocity, which remains relatively proportional and results in extremely tall final stature—well over 2 m. Gigantism is relatively easy to recognize. After epiphyseal fusion, linear growth is no longer possible, leading to disproportionate growth and the features of acromegaly (Fig. 5.7). Of course, a patient with a GH-secreting adenoma that started before puberty and

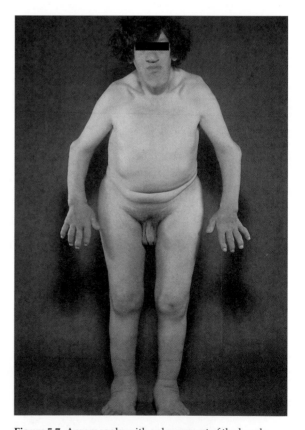

Figure 5.7 Acromegaly with enlargement of the hands, feet and jaw. The joints are abnormal and there is thickening of the soft tissues and fluid retention, which is manifested here by ankle oedema.

only presents after epiphyseal fusion will carry features of both syndromes. However, in isolation, acromegaly is more difficult to diagnose. The features are insidious, frequently causing a 10-year gap between the retrospective onset of symptoms and realizing the diagnosis (Box 5.5 and Case History 5.1). It is a cliché; however, the endocrinologist needs to think of the diagnosis before making it. The latter is important, as acromegaly increases mortality two- to three-fold, mainly due to cardiovascular complications.

Inspection of the patient discovers many of these features of bony and soft tissue overgrowth. However, examination should also include the cardiovascular system as blood pressure might be increased and there might be signs of congestive cardiac failure (e.g. ankle oedema, basal lung crepitations).

BOX 5.5 Signs and symptoms of GH excess

Musculoskeletal (acromegaly unless indicated)
- Increased stature (gigantism)
- Protruding mandible ('prognathia'), teeth separation on lower jaw
- Big tongue ('macroglossia')
- Enlarged forehead ('frontal bossing')
- Large hands and feet (carpal tunnel syndrome, tight rings, increasing shoe size)
- Osteoarthritis from abnormal joint loading

Cardiovascular
- Dilated cardiomyopathy → cardiomegaly → cardiac failure
- Hypertension

Metabolic
- Impaired glucose tolerance or potentially secondary diabetes (see Chapter 11)

Skin
- Irritating, thickened, greasy (increased sebum production)
- Excessive sweating

General
- Headaches
- Tiredness, often very disabling and lowers quality of life/ability to work

Local tumour effects
- See earlier anatomy section

Investigation and diagnosis. The hallmark of GH excess is loss of pulsatility due to autonomous production, such that a series of serum measurements detects continually high GH. IGF1 is also commonly elevated above the age- and sex-adjusted normal range. Using the 75 g oral glucose administration test, GH fails to suppress and remains >2 mU/L. These combined features diagnose GH excess. In all but exceptionally rare ectopic sources of GHRH, the cause is a GH-secreting pituitary adenoma. By MRI these tumours are usually greater than 1 cm diameter (i.e. a macroadenoma) and may have extended and eroded beyond the pituitary fossa at the time of diagnosis—see earlier section on local complications of pituitary tumours.

Treatment. Restoring normal GH status returns age-adjusted mortality to normal. The goal is a normal age-adjusted serum IGF1 and GH nadir on glucose loading of <2 mU/L. This is sometimes very difficult to achieve. There are several options (Table 5.6).

Normal somatotrophs respond to somatostatin via specific cell surface receptors by reducing GH secretion. Most GH-secreting adenomas retain this feature to some extent so that they can be treated by potent somatostatin analogue drugs delivered by monthly intramuscular injection. If these fail, dopamine agonists (see prolactinomas later) can sometimes be helpful, especially if the tumour also secretes prolactin. Pegvisomant antagonizes GH action at the GH receptor. Although it is a beautiful example of drug design (review Fig. 3.7), it has proved prohibitively expensive in the UK. A common management pathway sees a patient treated preoperatively with a somatostatin analogue if transsphenoidal surgery is not immediate. If surgery is not curative, drug treatment is continued and, to achieve better chances of final cure, radiotherapy is administered. Once radiotherapy has been effective, drug treatment can be stopped.

There is much debate over whether GH promotes bowel tumour formation and/or growth. Colonoscopy, at least once at diagnosis, can be considered to look for colonic polyps with malignant potential. Continued long-term surveillance is contentious, but may have a role, particular in patients who are not cured by the above modalities.

Table 5.6 Treatments of acromegaly

Advantages	Disadvantages
Transsphenoidal surgery — common first line	
Rapid effect	Invasive and requires general anaesthetic
Can restore vision in optic nerve compression	Noncurative for large, extrasellar tumours
Might be curative if complete resection	
Somatostatin analogue drugs lower GH — increasingly common first line	
Noninvasive	Monthly intramuscular injection
May shrink tumour	Expensive
Decreases GH in ~60% patients	Gastrointestinal side effects (commonly diarrhoea)
	Unlikely to be curative, i.e. continuous therapy needed
Radiotherapy — a good second line	
Noninvasive	Slow to act — may take up to 10 years
Likely to shrink tumour	Likely to cause hypopituitarism by destroying other pituitary cell types
Likely to reduce GH levels	May increase risks of cerebrovascular disease
Might be curative	

CASE HISTORY 5.1

A 45-year-old woman had attended her family doctor for a cervical smear. She was disappointed to be seen by a new doctor, whom she had not met before. She had known her previous doctor since she had been a little girl. The new doctor was concerned by the patient's coarse facial appearance and asked some questions. The lady was surprised to be asked about her shoe size but confirmed that most of her shoes were now a size larger than 10 years ago.

What is the diagnosis being considered?
What other questions should be asked?
What specific features of the examination should be sought?
What tests would confirm the doctor's suspicion?

Answers, see p. 77

Growth hormone deficiency

Like GH excess, insufficient GH presents differently at different times of life. Prior to final height, it comes to the attention of the paediatric endocrinologist as failure to grow ('falling off' height centile charts; Fig. 5.8). In adulthood, it presents insidiously, often in conjunction with other pituitary hormone deficiencies following surgery or radiotherapy to the anterior pituitary (Box 5.6).

Any pituitary space-occupying lesion can cause loss of the somatotrophs and growth hormone deficiency. In childhood, this may be a craniopharyn-gioma: in adults, most likely a nonfunctioning adenoma. Other childhood causes include congenital deficiency (review Box 3.6 and Fig. 3.9) or cranial irradiation for CNS tumours or haematological malignancy. In adults, loss of GH secretion is a physiological part of the ageing process and accelerated loss of GH secretion does not usually produce obvious clinical symptoms.

Lack of GH is diagnosed by stimulation testing and identifying a low serum IGF1 value (Fig. 5.6). It is treated by the daily subcutaneous injection of the recombinant hormone (oral peptides are degraded

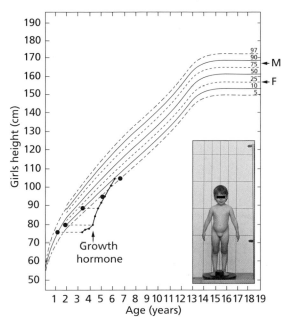

Figure 5.8 Short stature due to GH deficiency and the effect of growth hormone (GH) replacement. The height of this girl is shown compared to the reference growth charts, where the population is split into centiles (i.e. 50% of girls' heights lie below the 50th centile line, 5% below the 5th, etc.). Her height for her chronological age (·) is greatly reduced, but her skeletal maturity (or bone age) is also delayed. As a consequence, her height plotted for her bone age (●) falls within the centiles of normality. Bone age is determined by radiological examination of the epiphyses in the long bones in the hand. Comparison is made with standard radiographs to assess skeletal maturity. Serum GH was undetectable in a basal sample and no secretion could be elicited by dynamic testing. Secretion of other anterior pituitary hormones was normal. After GH replacement treatment was initiated, there was rapid catch-up of both height and skeletal maturity. M and F represents the mother's and father's height centile.

prior to absorption). In children with true GH deficiency, this results in a spectacular clinical effect, with a small child growing slowly into a normal adult. It is also used by paediatric endocrinologists to treat short stature of other causes (e.g. Turner syndrome/45,XO). Administration of GH in adequate dose will make any child grow more quickly in the short term.

Treatment in adulthood has been contentious due

> **BOX 5.6 Signs and symptoms of GH deficiency**
>
> • Decreased stature/cessation of growth (childhood)
> • Decreased exercise tolerance
> • Decreased muscle mass and strength
> • Increased body fat/decreased lean body mass
> • Centripetal fat distribution, increased waist : hip ratio
> • Hypertension and ischaemic heart disease
> • Decreased left ventricular mass
> • Dyslipidaemia (increased LDL cholesterol)
> • Osteoporosis
> • Poor quality of life

to historical underappreciation of GH physiology in adults. As the treatment is relatively expensive, it is important to demonstrate a clear benefit to the patient from its use. At present, in the UK this is achieved by a quality of life questionnaire to generate an Assessment of Growth Hormone Deficiency in Adults (AGHDA) score.

Prolactin

Human prolactin (PRL), synthesized in the lactotrophs, comprises 199 amino acids with three disulphide bonds. By weight, the normal human pituitary gland contains ~1% the amount of PRL as GH.

Effects and mechanism of action of prolactin

The most obvious action of PRL is to support the secretion of milk ('lactation') in the postpartum period (Fig. 5.9; also see the endocrinology of pregnancy in Chapter 7, Box 7.15). The mammary gland is rudimentary in young girls; during female adolescence, oestrogen, GH and adrenal steroids act together to stimulate the growth of the duct system. In parallel, alveolar growth is stimulated by oestrogen, progesterone, glucocorticoids and PRL with contributions from insulin and thyroid hormones. In boys, the process is largely inhibited by testosterone, however, some breast development may occur (see Table 7.3).

Following childbirth, with the decrease in both oestrogen and progesterone, PRL, in the presence of cortisol, initiates and maintains lactation. These roles

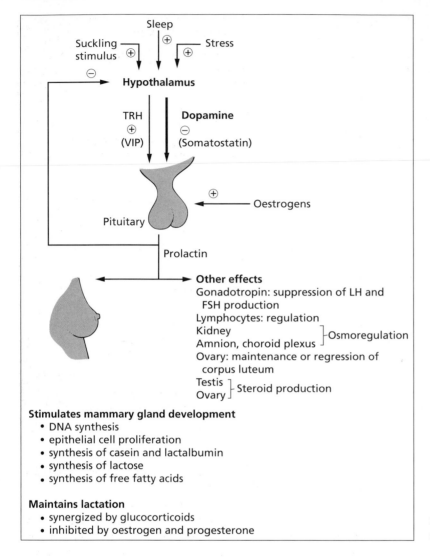

Figure 5.9 Summary of the regulation and effects of prolactin.

have been proven in experimental animals. Hypophysectomy leading to rapid loss of PRL results in the immediate cessation of milk secretion, whereas adrenalectomy leads to a gradual reduction. Other actions have been attributed to PRL in both male and female, although the physiological significance remains unclear (Fig. 5.9). Across species, PRL-like molecules are conserved: in birds, the hormone stimulates nest-building activity and crop-milk production; in reptiles, amphibians and some fish, it acts as an osmoregulator. Like GH, PRL signals through specific receptors that dimerize and recruit tyrosine kinase signalling pathways (review Chapter 3 and Fig. 3.8).

Regulation of prolactin production

The principles and features of PRL regulation are very similar to that of GH. PRL is under tonic inhibition by the negative factor, dopamine, with TRH able to stimulate prolactin release from lactotrophs (Fig. 5.9). Several inputs from higher centres (e.g. stress) feed onto these two regulatory hormones. Although the peaks are not as discrete as for GH, PRL is also released episodically with highest levels at night. The most profound changes in serum PRL occur during pregnancy and lactation. The concentration increases progressively, up to 10-fold, through pregnancy and remains elevated during lactation under the stimulus of suckling.

Pharmacological agents can also stimulate PRL release. For example, any drug that inhibits dopamine synthesis (e.g. L-methyldopa) or action (e.g. dopamine receptor antagonists used as antiemetics) can cause increased serum PRL and galactorrhoea (i.e. 'inappropriate' breast milk production). Conversely, dopamine agonists inhibit PRL release and are used to treat hyperprolactinaemia.

Clinical disorders

Hyperprolactinaemia

Signs and symptoms. Increased serum PRL is a common presentation to the endocrinologist (Case His-tory 5.2). It is most readily detected in women of reproductive age when it causes the very noticeable features of oligomenorrhoea or amenorrhoea, and, potentially, galactorrhoea. The raised PRL inhibits both the normal pulsatile secretion of luteinizing hormone (LH) and follicle-stimulating hormone (FSH) and the mid-cycle LH surge, resulting in anovulation. In contrast, men tend to present at a later age when the underlying pathology is more likely to be a larger macroadenoma. In this latter instance, presentation may reflect the consequences of a space-occupying lesion (see Box 5.1).

PRL rises with stress, such that poor venesection is sufficient to cause a rise above the normal range (normally <500 mU/L). To confirm true hyperprolactinaemia, several increased measurements are needed (perhaps over a few hours by the use of an indwelling cannula). Another issue is a laboratory one. On occasion, large forms of PRL circulate (called 'macroprolactin'—do not confuse with a macroprolactinoma). Although biologically insignificant, macroprolactins are detected by some assays and create the false impression of hyperprolactinaemia. Laboratory assays and methods exist to distinguish these different forms of PRL.

Having diagnosed hyperprolactinaemia, the major challenge is to tease apart the differential diagnosis (Box 5.7). The exclusion of pregnancy is one of

---

BOX 5.7 Hyperprolactinaemia

Commonly presents in women with amenorrhoea +/− galactorrhoea
Confirm hyperprolactinaemia on several stress-free blood tests
Differential diagnosis:
- Pregnancy
- Prolactin moderately raised (<2000 mU/L)
  - primary hypothyroidism ($\uparrow$ TRH drive to PRL secretion)
  - stress
  - drug treatment (e.g. dopamine receptor antagonists, neuroleptics, antidepressants and H2 antagonists)
  - chronic renal failure (reduced clearance)
  - idiopathic (PRL levels frequently return to normal)
  - stalk disconnection
  - acromegaly
- High prolactin (>3000 mU/L)
  - microprolactinoma
- Very high prolactin (>6000 mU/L)
  - macroprolactinoma
Treatment
- Dopamine agonist (e.g. cabergoline)
- Surgery and radiotherapy rarely needed

---

the first tests to perform in order to prevent any further unnecessary investigation.

The distinction between moderately raised and very high PRL is arbitrary, but some insight into the potential cause can be gained from the levels detected (Box 5.7). Very high levels are more likely to indicate a prolactinoma and can reach >100000 mU/L in large tumours. More modest elevations bring a host of other potential causes into consideration. For instance, primary hypothyroidism leads to inadequate feedback of thyroid hormone on TRH. In turn, raised TRH stimulates TSH but also modestly increases PRL (and FSH). Dopamine from hypothalamic neurones normally inhibits PRL. Therefore, anything that prevents these neurones reaching the lactotrophs will also cause a mild rise in PRL. This is called 'stalk disconnection' and can occur with pituitary tumours located in the stalk, previous surgery or trauma. Occasional pituitary tumours can cosecrete both GH and PRL, most likely reflecting the shared developmental origin of the somatotroph and lactotroph.

The past medical history and drug history are important (Box 5.7). Urea and electrolytes, pregnancy test and thyroid function test should be considered. Where pituitary pathology is suspected, other anterior pituitary axes need to be assessed for potential overactivity (e.g. acromegaly) and underactivity (due to the space-occupying effect of a tumour). For prolactinomas, MRI will delineate the size. Where there is extensive growth close to the optic chiasm, formal visual field assessment becomes very important.

Treatment. The major reasons for treating hyperprolactinaemia are to prevent inappropriate lactation, restore fertility and to prevent bone demineralization from inadequate oestrogen (or testosterone in men; see Chapter 7). It is treated by cause. If due to offending drugs, these can be withdrawn. Primary hypothyroidism is treated with thyroxine.

Although there has been 'escape' from the negative feedback of hypothalamic dopamine, prolactinoma cells remain exquisitely sensitive to potent dopamine agonists. Therefore, prolactinomas of all sizes should be treated with dopamine agonists in the first instance, even in the presence of optic chiasm compression. PRL falls, tumour cells shrink quickly and sight is commonly restored. Historically, bromocriptine has been used; however, it is frequently associated with nausea due to action on other dopamine receptor subtypes. Better alternatives now include cabergoline, taken orally, usually twice weekly. Surgery and/or radiotherapy are rarely required to control the tumours.

By using cabergoline for 5 years, the majority of microprolactinomas in young women are cured, that is PRL remains in the normal range after withdrawal of therapy. Conversely, extrasellar macroprolactinomas are unlikely to be cured and life-long treatment will be needed. The management of prolactinomas in pregnancy is potentially more difficult. Although there is little evidence of a teratogenic effect, dopamine agonists are usually stopped. However, the lactotroph population normally increases significantly during pregnancy and there is a risk of excessive tumour growth, especially from macroadenomas. One strategy is to conduct monthly visual field analyses. Headaches and visual disturbance are very important symptoms. If necessary, MRI scan and potential reinstitution of dopamine agonist therapy might be needed.

Hypoprolactinaemia
Although low serum prolactin might arise from loss of the lactotrophs, there is no known clinical consequence of hypoprolactinaemia, other than failure of lactation.

CASE HISTORY 5.2

A 16-year-old girl was referred to the gynaecologist with a history of primary amenorrhoea, tiredness and poor growth. She was receiving no medication. She was not sexually active. Apart from short stature, there were no other findings on examination. Investigations showed raised PRL (2000 mU/L) and MRI suggested a pituitary mass of 2 cm diameter. Her renal function was normal. A diagnosis of prolactinoma was made and she was treated with cabergoline. She started to have periods but did not grow. Repeat imaging of her pituitary showed no change. At this point she was referred to the endocrinologist who performed further investigations and realized that the initial diagnosis was wrong. Her treatment was altered and she started to grow. Her pubertal development continued and, furthermore, there was complete resolution of the abnormality on MRI.

What are the possible causes of hyperprolactinaemia?
What investigation clinched the diagnosis?
Why did the mass, visible on MRI, regress with treatment?

Answers, see p. 77

Adrenocorticotrophin

Adrenocorticotrophin (ACTH) is a short peptide of 39 amino acids. Residues 1 to 24 are highly conserved and confer full activity, such that synthetic ACTH(1–24) is used clinically to test adrenal function (see Chapter 6). ACTH comes from the *Pro-opiomelanocortin* gene (*POMC*), which initially encodes a much larger precursor protein (POMC; Fig. 5.10) that is cleaved enzymatically into many potential products. These include several species of melanocyte-stimulating hormone (MSH), which stimulate the synthesis of melanin in skin and can act as a hallmark of corticotroph overactivity (see below and the section on adrenocortical insufficiency in Chapter 6); and β-endorphin, which harbours morphine-like activities that may inhibit pain signals to the brain.

Effects and mechanism of action of ACTH

The actions of ACTH are largely confined to the adrenal cortex, where it stimulates several of the enzymatic reactions that convert cholesterol into either cortisol or adrenal sex steroid precursors (see Chapter 6). The hormone acts on the adrenocortical cell surface via a specific G-protein coupled receptor to increase intracellular levels of cAMP (review Chapter 3).

Regulation of ACTH production

ACTH is stimulated by CRH from the hypothalamus and inhibited by cortisol in a classical negative-feedback loop from the adrenal cortex. As biological significance lies with circulating levels of cortisol, details of axis regulation and its circadian rhythm are discussed in detail in Chapter 6 (Fig. 6.4). AVP also

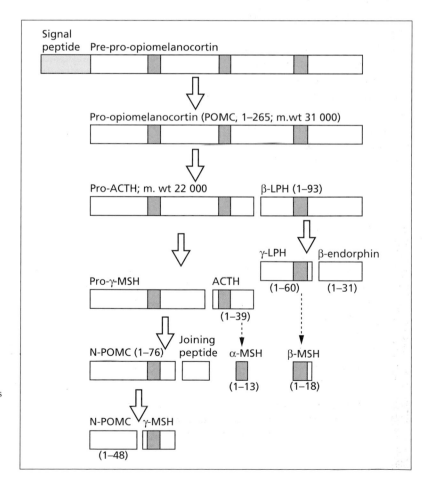

Figure 5.10 The cleavage of pro-opiomelanocortin (POMC). Shaded areas represent different species of MSH. The number of amino acids in each peptide unit is shown in parentheses. LPH, lipotrophic hormone; N-POMC, the amino-terminal sequence of POMC. M. wt refers to molecular weight in kilodaltons.

potentiates CRH action and may be particularly important during fetal life. Like PRL and GH, ACTH (and consequently cortisol) rises with stress following neural inputs from other brain centres. This includes hypoglycaemia, such that the administration of insulin has formed a clinical test of corticotroph function.

Clinical disorders

Excess ACTH and Cushing disease

An excess of cortisol is called Cushing syndrome (detailed in Chapter 6). When caused by excess ACTH from corticotroph adenomas, the disorder is specifically called Cushing *disease*, named after the endocrinologist who first described it. Too much ACTH overstimulates the adrenal glands, which become bilaterally enlarged, and cortisol increases to pathological levels. Clinically, the challenge is to recognize and diagnose glucocorticoid excess (i.e. Cushing syndrome); then to decipher whether the source is adrenal in origin (e.g. an adrenocortical adenoma; Fig. 4.7) or secondary. For the latter, excess ACTH comes either from the anterior pituitary (as in Cushing disease) or ectopically from rare tumours, such as small cell carcinoma of the lung or carcinoids. The tests, approach and treatment are described in Chapter 6.

Negative feedback is obviously inadequate in Cushing disease; however, it still exerts some effect. In particularly difficult operative cases and where pituitary radiotherapy has failed, a last resort is to remove the adrenal glands to solve the problem of excess cortisol. On occasion, this final removal of negative feedback causes uncontrolled growth of the pituitary adenoma and is called Nelson syndrome.

Interestingly, some 'nonfunctioning' adenomas, when removed, also display immunoreactivity for ACTH. It appears that these tumours pursue a slightly more aggressive course of recurrence and regrowth.

Excess ACTH due to adrenocortical insufficiency

Corticotroph overactivity can be physiological. In primary adrenocortical underactivity, negative feedback decreases and ACTH levels increase. Although this response is appropriate, in parallel, MSH is also generated from the increased *POMC* expression, so hyperpigmentation of the skin accompanies the raised circulating ACTH.

ACTH deficiency

In ACTH deficiency, cortisol and sex steroid precursor biosynthesis are lost, while aldosterone production by the zona glomerulosa is preserved (it is regulated by the renin–angiotensin system). Symptoms and signs are covered in Chapter 6. Historically, the diagnosis of hypoadrenalism due to pituitary dysfunction included use of the insulin stress test. Insulin was injected to produce hypoglycaemia, which, under normal circumstances, stimulates a prompt rise in ACTH and, thus, cortisol. The test is unpleasant and not without danger, requiring continuous medical supervision. It is contraindicated in patients with cardiovascular disease. More frequent today is the recognition that ACTH deficiency for longer than a few months leads to a withering of the adrenal cortex and an inadequate cortisol response to synthetic ACTH(1–24) (see Chapter 6). The important caveat remains that this latter test may miss recent corticotroph underactivity where the adrenal cortex can still respond to pharmacological stimulation.

Thyroid-stimulating hormone

TSH is a glycoprotein composed of two subunits (α and β). The α-subunit is shared for TSH, LH and FSH; hormone specificity is conferred by different, distinctive β-subunits. TSH is synthesized in the thyrotrophs, which constitute ~10% of all cells in the anterior pituitary.

Effects and mechanism of action of TSH

TSH is the major physiological regulator of the thyroid gland. It stimulates the biosynthesis and secretion of thyroid hormones (see Chapter 8). The hormone acts on the thyroid follicular cell surface via its specific G-protein coupled receptor to increase intracellular levels of cAMP (review Chapter 3).

Regulation of TSH production

TSH production is stimulated by TRH and acts to stimulate the biosynthesis and release of thyroid hormones—thyroxine (T_4) and triiodothyronine (T_3). Basal TSH secretion depends on tonic TRH release, such that rare hypothalamic lesions or transection of the pituitary stalk result in TSH deficiency and subsequent hypothyroidism. Conversely, the primary site for negative feedback by thyroid hormone is likely to be the anterior pituitary where it decreases the effectiveness of TRH, in part by reducing TRH receptor number. Somatostatin also inhibits TSH secretion from the anterior pituitary.

Clinical disorders
Excess TSH

Excess TSH is almost always a normal compensation to thyroid underactivity and is used as a screen for hypothyroidism in newborn babies (see Chapter 8). Interestingly, hypothyroidism also leads to increased TRH production when, in addition to TSH, it also stimulates FSH and PRL secretion, potentially causing increased testicular volume and galactorrhoea. Tumours that secrete TSH ('TSHomas') are very rare. They are most frequently macroadenomas and present with hyperthyroidism with inappropriately detectable TSH. The differential diagnosis is thyroid hormone resistance due to mutations in the thyroid hormone receptor. As one distinction, the latter condition is usually inherited and may be identified by a thorough family history; TSHomas are sporadic.

TSH deficiency

Any condition resulting in hypopituitarism (covered later) can cause TSH deficiency and clinical hypothyroidism (see Chapter 8).

Gonadotrophins — LH and FSH

Luteinizing hormone (LH) and follicle-stimulating hormone (FSH) are secreted from the gonadotrophs, which make up 10–15% of the cells in the anterior pituitary. As for TSH, the glycoproteins LH and FSH are composed of a common α-subunit and individualized β–subunit. Variation of the carbohydrate (i.e. the 'glyco-' part) leads to substantial microheterogeneity.

Effects and mechanism of action of LH and FSH

LH and FSH regulate gonadal function in males (testosterone biosynthesis and spermatogenesis in the testis) and females (the menstrual cycle and fertility in the ovary). All of these complex functions are described in detail in Chapter 7. Both hormones act through cell-surface G-protein coupled receptors linked to cAMP second messenger signalling.

Regulation of LH and FSH production

The production of gonadotrophins is stimulated by hypothalamic gonadotrophin-releasing hormone (GnRH), which binds to a cell-surface G-protein coupled receptor linked to cAMP second messenger signalling. Factors such as stress and prolactin act negatively. Like the hypothalamic–anterior pituitary axes regulating the adrenal cortex and thyroid, hormones secreted by the testis and ovary exert negative feedback actions on the production of both GnRH and gonadotrophins. These hormones are inhibin and the steroid sex hormones (see Chapter 7, Figs 7.8 and 7.12).

Clinical disorders
Excess gonadotrophins

Increased levels of gonadotrophins reflect loss of negative feedback from the testis or ovary. Usually, primary testicular or ovarian failure yields serum LH and FSH several times the upper limit of normal. The commonest cause of this gonadotrophin overactivity is physiological when ovarian depletion of ova ends cyclical hormone production at the female menopause. Excess gonadotrophin due to increased GnRH stimulation is rare. In contrast, inappropriately timed, rather than excessive production, causes central precocious puberty. These disorders are discussed in Chapter 7. A pituitary adenoma secreting functional LH or FSH is incredibly rare. Commonly however, nonfunctioning pituitary adenomas may stain by immunohistochemistry for the α-subunit, perhaps giving an indication of the developmental lineage, but little else.

Deficiency of the gonadotrophins

During childhood, it is normal for gonadotrophins to be low and relatively unresponsive to GnRH, although continued gonadotroph inactivity will ultimately cause delayed puberty. This can be tested by GnRH stimulation where serum LH and FSH are measured 30 min later. After puberty, loss of gonadotrophins causes secondary hypogonadism. In women, this is very common at some stage of the reproductive years as cyclical gonadotrophin secretion is exceptionally vulnerable to input from other

---

BOX 5.8 Hypogonadotrophic hypogonadism

Low or 'normal' gonadotrophins
+
Hypogonadal signs, symptoms and biochemistry
=
Hypogonadotrophic hypogonadism

BOX 5.9 AVP physiology, function and mechanism of action

Physiology
- Circulates largely unbound → rapidly removed from the circulation in the kidney → $t_{1/2}$ ~5 min

Function
- Regulates water excretion by the kidney—this is the main action at normal circulating AVP levels
  - Acts on the distal convoluted tubule → ↑ permeability to water → water resorption → ↑ urine concentration
- Potent vasoconstrictor

Cellular mechanism of action
- Distinct cell-surface G-protein coupled receptor (V) subtypes and second messengers
  - V_1 → phosphatidylinositol (PI) metabolism and ↑ intracellular Ca^{2+} → vascular smooth muscle contraction
  - V_2 → cAMP → renal water excretion

---

centres. Exercise, excessive dieting or, most commonly, stress of relatively minor proportions can be sufficient to temporarily silence the reproductive axis. As discussed earlier, a rise in prolactin levels is also sufficient to suppress LH and FSH production.

Clinically, it is important to realize that, in the face of significant hypogonadal symptoms and signs, or unequivocally low levels of sex hormones, gonadotrophins within the normal range are inappropriately low. In women, where significant fluctuation of gonadotrophins accompanies the normal menstrual cycle, this can be more difficult to identify. It tends to manifest as amenorrhoea with absent oestrogen. In both sexes the disorder is described as 'hypogonadotrophic hypogonadism' (Box 5.8).

Hormones of the posterior pituitary

The two hormones released from the posterior pituitary are oxytocin and AVP. Although structurally they are very similar, composed of nine amino acids, they have very different physiological roles (review Fig. 1.3). Damage to the posterior pituitary can occur quite commonly without AVP or oxytocin deficiency, so long as the hypothalamic neurones that transport them remain intact (see earlier anatomy section).

Arginine vasopressin

Clinically, this hormone is perhaps better known as antidiuretic hormone (ADH); scientifically it is more renowned as AVP. The basic science of AVP can be easily summarized (Box 5.9).

In the kidney, the presence of AVP and the high osmolality of the renal interstitium lead to water movement out of the final section of the distal convoluted tubule along the osmotic gradient. The effect can be truly remarkable. For example, a child weighing 30 kg needs to excrete a solute load of ~800 milliosmoles (mOsm) in 24 hours: at its most dilute (~50 mOsm/kg), this load requires 16 L of urine; under maximal AVP stimulation, it can be achieved in little over 700 ml (~1100 mOsm/kg).

The action of AVP on blood vessels has been utilized either directly or in analogue form to achieve haemostasis, for example in severe gastrointestinal bleeding or postpartum haemorrhage. It also acts on vascular 'tone' at normal physiological levels. As noted earlier, AVP can also act as an additional stimulus to ACTH release from corticotrophs.

Regulation of AVP production

The main physiological regulator of AVP release is osmolality of the blood, which is detected by osmoreceptors in the hypothalamus. Circulating volume is detected by baroreceptors in the carotid sinus and aortic arch, and by plasma volume receptors in the left atrium.

In addition to the factors listed in Box 5.10, hormones such as angiotensin II, epinephrine, cortisol and sex steroids (oestrogen and progesterone) can also modulate AVP release. The latter may explain the fluid retention that can occur in the latter part of the menstrual cycle. As with other hypothalamic hormones, the central nervous system plays an important part in the regulation of neurohypophyseal hormones. The pain and trauma associated with surgery cause a marked increase in the circulating concentration of AVP, as do nausea and vomiting. The activity of the neurohypophyseal system is also influenced by environmental temperature; a rise in temperature stimulates AVP release prior to any change in plasma osmolality.

Clinical disorders

Excess AVP/ADH: syndrome of inappropriate antidiuretic hormone

The syndrome of inappropriate antidiuretic hormone (SIADH) refers to the release of AVP when normal regulatory mechanisms should be restricting its secretion into the circulation (Case History 5.3).

Signs and symptoms. Symptoms are headache and apathy, progressing to nausea, vomiting, abnormal neurological signs and impaired consciousness. In very severe cases, there may be coma, convulsions and death. Generalized oedema is not a feature of excess AVP/SIADH because free water is evenly distributed across all body compartments.

Investigation, diagnosis and treatment. The cardinal features of SIADH are low serum osmolality, hyponatraemia and inappropriately high urine osmolality. Other common causes of hyponatraemia, especially in the elderly, are congestive cardiac failure and diuretic use. In SIADH, identifying

---

BOX 5.10 Regulation of AVP

Serum osmolality
- High (e.g. dehydration) $\rightarrow \uparrow$ AVP release $\rightarrow$ $\uparrow$ water retention $\rightarrow \downarrow$ osmolality
- Low (e.g. water intoxication) $\rightarrow \downarrow$ AVP release $\rightarrow$ $\downarrow$ water retention $\rightarrow \uparrow$ osmolality

Volume
- Fall in blood volume $\geq 8\%$ (e.g. haemorrhage) $\rightarrow$ $\uparrow$ AVP release $\rightarrow$ vasoconstriction

O_2 and CO_2 tension
- $\downarrow$ arterial O_2 partial pressure (P_aO_2) $\rightarrow \uparrow$ AVP release
- $\uparrow$ arterial CO_2 partial pressure (P_aCO_2) $\rightarrow \uparrow$ AVP release

---

BOX 5.11 SIADH = hyponatraemia + low serum osmolality (<270 mOsm/kg) with inappropriately high urine osmolality

Causes
- Tumours (e.g. small cell cancer of the lung)
- Any brain disorders (trauma, infection, tumour)
- Pneumonia
- Cytotoxic therapy (chemotherapy or radiotherapy)
- Narcotics and analgesics
- Hypothyroidism
- Hypoadrenalism

Treatment
- Identify and treat underlying cause where possible
- Restrict fluid intake (≤ 1 L) and replace sodium lost in the urine
- Demeclocycline may induce partial DI and be useful (see below)
- New V_2 receptor antagonists are being researched

CASE HISTORY 5.3

A 74-year-old man presented to the emergency medical service with a two-week history of a cough productive of bloody green sputum, fever, shortness of breath and pleuritic chest pain. He was a lifelong smoker. Serum sodium was 124 mmol/L; potassium, 3.6 mmol/L; urea, 2.7 mmol/L and creatinine 73 μmol/L. Serum osmolality was 258 mOsm/kg and urine osmolality was 560 mOsm/kg.

What is the most likely endocrine cause for the hyponatraemia and what acute condition underlies it?
What measures might be taken to rectify the situation?
What further investigations might you consider?

Answers, see p. 77

the underlying cause is important (Box 5.11). This is a difficult and dangerous clinical situation.

Deficiency of AVP: diabetes insipidus

The term 'diabetes insipidus' (DI) stems from when physicians used to taste urine and contrast it with the sweet urine of diabetes mellitus. Patients with DI pass extremely large volumes of low osmolality urine (potentially 20 L in 24 h). DI can occur due to deficient AVP production ('cranial') or deficient action at the V_2 receptor ('nephrogenic') (Table 5.7). In the former, the vast majority of AVP production needs to be lost (≥90%) before water balance is necessarily affected.

Signs and symptoms. Polyuria and nocturia are evidence that in DI the patient is unable to reduce the flow of urine. Clinically, problems arise when the patient is deprived of water as the plasma osmolality rises. These features form the basis of clinical investigation.

Investigation and diagnosis. Some centres have access to a vasopressin radioimmunoassay, when the diagnosis can be made by monitoring AVP concentrations after an infusion of hypertonic saline. Most endocrinologists still rely on the water deprivation test and the use of the AVP analogue, desmopressin (Table 5.7).

Treatment. Having diagnosed DI, it remains impor-

Table 5.7 Diabetes insipidus

Diabetes insipidus
  ↓ AVP secretion or action → large volume of low osmolality urine → clinical problems from high serum osmolality

Cranial DI	Nephrogenic DI
Causes	*Causes*
CNS tumours	Drugs (e.g. lithium, demeclocycline)
Head trauma	Familial X-linked recessive (i.e. males affected)
Infection (e.g. meningitis and encephalitis)	*V₂ receptor* gene loss-of-function mutation
Familial autosomal dominant	Autosomal recessive
Vasopressin gene mutation	*Aquaporin* 2 gene mutation
DIDMOAD syndrome (DI, diabetes mellitus, optic atrophy and	Chronic renal disease
deafness)	
'Idiopathic'	

Investigation
  Water deprivation test—conducted over 8 hours during the day
  Continued passage of dilute urine → rise in serum osmolality and fall in body weight
  Repeat osmolality measurements of serum and urine
  Terminate test if body weight falls ≥5% (dangerous) and allow the patient to drink

  DI diagnosed if:
  serum osmolality rises to ≥305 mOsm/kg (normal: 275–295 mOsm/kg) or urine remains ≤300 mOsm/kg

  Desmopressin (a synthetic AVP analogue) is given to distinguish between cranial and nephrogenic DI
  Cranial DI—urine now concentrates
  Nephrogenic DI—urine still fails to concentrate ≥800 mOsm/kg
  Hypokalaemia and hypercalcaemia can help to point to nephrogenic DI

  DI can be difficult to distinguish from psychogenic polydipsia (i.e. habitual excess water intake)

Treatment
  Ensure an intact thirst mechanism and free access to fluid
  Desmopressin can provide hormone replacement in cranial DI

tant to consider and investigate the underlying cause, which may be curable. Otherwise the management of DI relies on access to an adequate fluid intake and an intact thirst-sensing mechanism. For cranial DI, replacement of AVP is all that is required. Desmopressin, either by intranasal spray, tablet or injection, is a synthetic analogue that acts predominantly on the V_2 receptor and therefore causes minimal hypertensive effect. It is sometimes also used in normal children who suffer from nocturnal enuresis (bedwetting). Nephrogenic DI and psychogenic polydipsia can be harder to treat effectively. In the latter, the high urine flow rate tends to 'wash out' the solutes that create the counter-current exchange mechanism, that is the kidney loses its ability to concentrate urine.

Oxytocin

Oxytocin literally means 'quick birth' and is important for contraction of the uterine smooth muscles during labour and the myoepithelial cells that line the duct of the mammary gland (see Chapter 7). Oxytocin circulates in very low concentrations and is normally undetectable in the blood. It becomes elevated during lactation and parturition, when it peaks at delivery and facilitates expulsion of the placenta.

Effects and mechanism of action of oxytocin

Oxytocin has two sites of action: the uterus and the mammary gland. By increasing the contraction of the uterus, it aids in the expulsion of the fetus and the placenta. In addition to a possible role in regulating the release of oxytocin, ovarian steroid hormones may influence its action by altering uterine sensitivity. Progesterone appears to block and oestrogen appears to potentiate the response of the uterus to oxytocin. In the mammary gland, the myoepithelial cells surrounding the alveoli and ducts are sensitive to oxytocin and contract to expel milk from the breast. Like AVP, oxytocin circulates largely unbound and so is removed rapidly by the kidney ($t_{1/2}$ ~5 min). Oxytocin binds to G-protein coupled receptors on the cell surface and signals intracellularly via PI metabolism and calcium (review Fig. 3.16).

Regulation of oxytocin production

Vaginal stretch is an important factor controlling oxytocin release. A positive feedback mechanism operates when a fetus moves down the birth canal. Uterine muscular contraction, induced by oxytocin, distends the vagina, which further stimulates oxytocin secretion, until the baby is born. Other factors, such as the fall in progesterone and the presence of oestrogen, may play a part.

Stimulation of the nipple also causes release of oxytocin during suckling and leads to the ejection of milk. Even the sight and sound of an infant can stimulate milk ejection.

Clinical disorders

Syndromes of oxytocin excess and deficiency have not been described.

Hypopituitarism

The vast majority of pituitary hormone excess is restricted to one particular hormone. In contrast, deficiency in a patient more commonly includes several of the anterior pituitary hormones and, potentially, those of the posterior pituitary. This is termed 'hypopituitarism' and when all hormones are inadequate, 'panhypopituitarism'. In adult endocrinology, hypopituitarism is most commonly encountered due to compression from nonfunctioning pituitary adenomas or their treatment by surgery or radiotherapy. In paediatric practice, congenital absence or malformation of the pituitary gland becomes more prevalent. Other causes have already been mentioned throughout this chapter but are brought together in Box 5.12. Clinical investigation of the pituitary gland demands consideration of each hormone axis and its effects. History taking and examination needs to include all the features of hormone deficiency described in each of the preceding sections (e.g. hypogonadism, hypothyroidism and hypoadrenalism). For instance, diagnosing deficiency of LH and FSH, but missing concomitant ACTH deficiency might lead to a patient's death from hypoadrenalism (see Chapter 6 and Case History 5.4).

Mutations in several genes cause pituitary hypoplasia. Those responsible for earlier development tend to cause broader loss of anterior pituitary cell types and include malformation of other structures (e.g. absent corpus callosum and optic nerve underdevelopment in septo-optic dysplasia due to *HESX1* mutations). In contrast, isolated TSH deficiency is

BOX 5.12 Hypopituitarism—clinical suspicion requires investigation of all the hormone axes

Pituitary destruction
- Adenoma or other tumours (craniopharyngioma, meningioma, metastasis)
- Surgical treatment of pituitary tumour
- Radiotherapy of pituitary tumour
- Infarction

Congenital pituitary disorders
- Pituitary hypoplasia or aplasia
  - e.g. mutations in *POU1F1, PROP1, HESX1, LHX2*
  - *TPIT*—mutations tend to be restricted to the corticotroph lineage

Others
- Impaired secretion of hypothalamic hormones (e.g. loss of GnRH neurones in Kallman syndrome—see Chapter 7)
- Disconnection of the hypothalamopituitary axis (e.g. stalk tumour, trauma or infection)

rarely a problem. Because of relatively early divergence during development, corticotrophs also tend to be spared in some of the congenital causes of hypopituitarism.

In adult endocrinology, the hypothalamic–pituitary axes are particularly vulnerable to irradiation. Loss of pituitary hormones, especially GH, can become almost inevitable after cranial radiotherapy but may take up to 10 years to occur. In contrast, gonadotrophin secretion is particularly vulnerable to trauma such as surgery. Infarction of the pituitary is rare, although one well-described condition, Sheehan syndrome, is associated with the hypotension that follows major postpartum haemorrhage. The vascular insufficiency leads to sudden death of pituitary tissue.

CASE HISTORY 5.4

A patient has been diagnosed with acromegaly and referred to an endocrinologist. Visual field assessment reveals bitemporal hemianopia. MRI demonstrates a large pituitary mass extending to and compressing the optic chiasm. Serum PRL was 1200 mU/L, TSH was undetectable, fT_4 was 5.3 pmol/L and a short synacthen test gave a serum cortisol value at 30 min of 305 nmol/L.

What do these biochemistry results indicate?
What urgent treatments are needed?

Answers, see p. 77

KEY POINTS

- GH, PRL, ACTH, FSH, LH and TSH are the major hormones of the anterior pituitary
- Oxytocin and AVP are the major hormones of the posterior pituitary
- Pituitary tumours, especially nonfunctioning adenomas, are very common
- Hormone overactivity due to tumour can cause well-recognized endocrine syndromes
- Underactivity tends to affect multiple pituitary hormones, which require investigation
- Always consider local structural damage from pituitary tumours as well as hormonal consequences

Answers to case histories

Case history 5.1

The diagnosis under consideration is acromegaly. The insidious nature of this disorder means that those who know the patient well frequently miss it. Further questioning and the examination should include:

Identifying symptoms and signs relating to GH excess as listed in Box 5.5.

Does the patient or family recognize any differences in appearance from photographs during the previous 10 years?

Are there any symptoms or signs from loss of other pituitary hormones (e.g. hypoadrenalism or hypothyroidism) or a local mass effect? A sensitive question would interrogate potential loss of the menstrual cycle. Examination should look for potential visual field defects or diplopia.

Serum IGF1 should be measured. An oral 75 g glucose tolerance test (OGTT) should be considered or a serum GH day series conducted.

Case history 5.2

The differential diagnosis of hyperprolactinaemia is shown in Box 5.7. The presence of poor growth and tiredness suggests hypothyroidism.

A thyroid function test showed a markedly raised TSH with low T_4.

The lack of thyroid hormone feedback to the pituitary had led to an increase in TRH which, in turn, had promoted growth of lactotrophs. Once this stimulation was removed by treatment with thyroxine, the apparent mass regressed.

Case history 5.3

The man has SIADH. Although Addison disease might be considered in view of the hypona-traemia, the plasma osmolality is low. The SIADH is due to pneumonia, although an underlying lung malignancy cannot be excluded as a contributory factor at this stage.

After taking samples of sputum and blood for microbiology culture, antibiotics should be started and fluid intake restricted to ~1 L over the next 24 h with close attention paid to urine output and haemodynamic status (e.g. pulse and blood pressure). Tachycardia and hypotension would argue for high dependency medical and nursing care.

Other investigations directly related to his symptoms include arterial blood gas assessment (with oxygen given if the patient is hypoxic), chest X-ray and sputum analysis for tuberculosis and malignancy.

In this case, fever settled rapidly with antibiotics, the patient remained haemodynamically stable, serum sodium rose within 12 h to 132 mmol/L and, on continuing the same management, was 135 mmol/L (lower limit of normal) 36 h later. The man's other symptoms gradually improved. No evidence was obtained for lung malignancy and his electrolytes were normal at discharge.

Case history 5.4

The patient has secondary hypothyroidism and hypoadrenalism due to pituitary hormone loss. The PRL is minimally raised and is unlikely to represent tumour secretion of PRL with GH. It is more likely to indicate a small degree of stalk disconnection.

Because of the visual loss, the patient should be placed on hydrocortisone, then thyroid hormone, and immediately programmed for transsphenoidal surgery. The tumour should be 'debulked' to relieve pressure on the optic chiasm. Vision might be permanently lost if surgery is delayed. Surgery is highly unlikely to be curative and suitable secondary treatments include somatostatin analogues and/or radiotherapy.

6 The adrenal gland

LEARNING OBJECTIVES

- To appreciate the separate development of the adrenal cortex and medulla as two organs in one gland
- Adrenal cortex:
  — to understand the zone-specific biosynthesis and function of mineralocorticoids, glucocorticoids and sex steroid precursors
  — to understand the clinical consequences of underactivity, overactivity or disordered function of the adrenal cortex
- Adrenal medulla:
  — to understand the biosynthesis and function of adrenomedullary hormones
  — to understand the clinical consequences of tumourous overproduction of adrenomedullary hormones

This chapter integrates the basic biology of the adrenal gland with the clinical conditions that affect it

The adrenal cortex

Embryology, anatomy and vasculature

Understanding the development of the adrenal gland is needed to appreciate several features of adrenal disease (Box 6.1).

Epithelial cells that line the abdominal ('coelomic') cavity of the developing embryo form the adrenal cortex during the fifth week of development (Fig. 6.1). These cells proliferate to generate concentric functional layers called the outer definitive and the inner fetal zones of the adrenal cortex. This pattern is unique to higher primates and only begins its reorganization after birth into the more characteristic layers of the adult adrenal cortex (Fig. 6.2 and Box 6.2).

The adrenal gland lies immediately superior to the kidney (hence the anatomical name, 'suprarenal' gland). This arrangement is clinically significant for the investigation and operative approaches to the organ in hypersecretion or tumourous states. For instance, it can be necessary to sample from the veins that drain centripetally through the adrenal gland to measure hormone secretion. The adrenal gland and the kidney at least partially share their capsule. Removal of the kidney ('nephrectomy') almost always includes ipsilateral adrenalectomy. In contrast, either adrenal can be removed, increasingly by laparoscopic approaches, without disturbing the adjacent kidney. However, embryological variations can present challenges to the endocrine surgeon. Additional or unusual vascular supply, or embryological 'rests' of adrenocortical cells can lie outside the gland.

Biochemistry by zones

Although the determination and maintenance of these distinct regions remains unclear, understand-

BOX 6.1   Clinical consequences of embryology

- The adrenal cortex and medulla develop separately—clinical disorders almost always affect either cortex or medulla, but not both
- Forming the organ requires cell migration—adrenal disorders can occasionally cause trouble in unexpected places due to embryological 'rests' of cells
- The cells forming the adrenal cortex also form the steroidogenic cell lineages in the gonad—disorders of steroid production can affect both adrenal cortex and gonad at the same time

BOX 6.2   The zones of the adult adrenal cortex

- *Zona glomerulosa*, nests of closely packed small cells creating the thinnest, outermost layer
- *Zona fasciculata*, larger cells arranged in columns making up ~three-quarters of the cortex
- *Zona reticularis*, 'net-like' arrangements of innermost cells, formed at 6–8 years, heralding a poorly understood functional change called 'adrenarche'

ing the different adrenocortical zones is important because they define, and are defined by, very different biochemical activity (Box 6.3).

In addition to some cortisol, the zona reticularis makes weak androgens, dehydroepiandrosterone (DHEA) and androstenedione, that are converted into more potent sex hormones in peripheral target tissues. This compartmentalized function is all the more remarkable in light of the prevailing theory of adrenocortical aging whereby cells migrate from outer glomerulosa to innermost reticularis prior to undergoing apoptosis—steroid secretion being modified along the way.

The principles of steroidogenesis were introduced in Chapter 2. To recap, the steroid product depends on the complement of enzymes that catalyse the

BOX 6.3   Steroid hormone biosynthesis by zones

- Zona glomerulosa secretes: aldosterone
- Zona fasciculata secretes: cortisol (and sex steroid precursors)
- Zona reticularis secretes: sex steroid precursors (and cortisol)

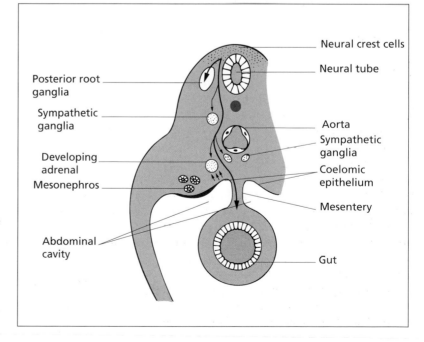

Figure 6.1 The development of the adrenal gland. The cortex is most likely derived from the epithelium lining the abdominal cavity. Neural crest cells migrate from the back of the embryo. Some give rise to posterior root and sympathetic ganglia, while others invade the adrenal cortex to form the medulla. The rim of coelomic epithelium shown in black also gives rise to the steroidogenic cells of the gonad.

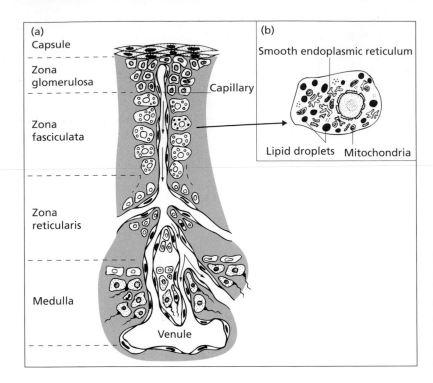

(a)
Capsule
Zona glomerulosa
Capillary
Zona fasciculata
Zona reticularis
Medulla
Venule

(b)
Smooth endoplasmic reticulum
Lipid droplets   Mitochondria

Figure 6.2 Section through the cortex of the adrenal gland. (a) The blood vessels run from outer capsule to medullary venule. (b) A zona fasciculata cell with large lipid droplets, extensive smooth endoplasmic reticulum and mitochondria.

sequential modification of cholesterol (Fig. 6.3 and Box 6.4). Many of these enzymes are members of the cytochrome P450 superfamily. Although the nomenclature for the corresponding genes has been unified, several other names remain in common usage (Table 6.1). Awareness of these names is important, as several of the genes are subject to mutation in congenital adrenal hyperplasia (CAH), one of the more common paediatric endocrine emergencies.

Function and regulation of the hormones

The adrenocortical hormones aldosterone and cortisol act in the cell nucleus by binding to steroid hormone receptors and functioning as transcription factors that influence target gene expression (review Chapter 3). The mechanism of action for DHEA remains unclear, other than serving as a precursor for extragonadal sex hormone biosynthesis.

Cortisol

Cortisol is the major glucocorticoid in humans. Like all steroid hormones, it is not stored but synthesized according to acute changes in demand. Its release

into the circulation influences cells in virtually every organ of the body. In the blood, cortisol is largely bound (>90%) to cortisol binding globulin (CBG). This is relevant, because, like thyroid hormones, it is only the free component that enters target cells. The free component is also able to pass into the urine—'urinary free cortisol' (UFC)—where its collection and assay over 24 h generates a biochemical assessment of glucocorticoid status (UFC is ~1% of cortisol production by the adrenal glands). Serum and saliva cortisol levels can also be useful measures of glucocorticoid status. However, both are variable, affected by stress and have a short half-life of ~1–2 h. Therefore, random measurement of a plasma or salivary cortisol is of limited clinical value. If measured during diagnostic testing, it should either be at 9 AM or late evening/near midnight (see Section on Cushing syndrome).

Regulation of cortisol biosynthesis and secretion—the hypothalamic–pituitary–adrenal axis
Regulation of the adrenal cortex comes largely from the anterior pituitary, via the production and circulation of adrenocorticotrophic hormone (ACTH), a

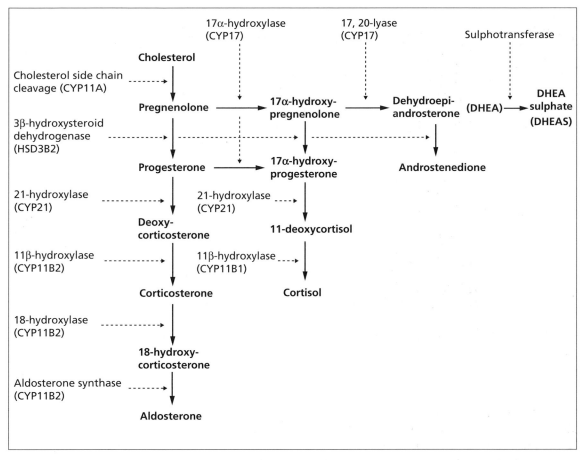

Figure 6.3 Biosynthesis of adrenocortical steroid hormones. The three steps from deoxycorticosterone to aldosterone are catalysed by the same enzyme, CYP11B2. These reactions were shown in more abbreviated form in Fig. 2.5.

BOX 6.4 Steroidogenesis can be summarized into a few key steps

- Transport of cholesterol into the mitochondrion by the steroid acute regulatory (StAR) protein
- Removal of the cholesterol side chain by CYP11A; the rate-limiting step of steroid hormone biosynthesis
- Shuttling intermediaries between mitochondrion and endoplasmic reticulum for further enzymatic modification
- Action of two key enzymes at branch points:
  — HSD3B2 steers steroid precursors away from the sex steroid precursors towards aldosterone or cortisol
  — CYP17 prevents the biosynthesis of aldosterone and commits a steroid to cortisol or sex steroid precursor

---

cleavage product of the *Pro-opiomelanocortin* (*POMC*) gene (review Chapter 5). In turn, ACTH is regulated by corticotrophin releasing hormone (CRH) from the hypothalamus (Fig. 6.4). By binding to cell surface receptors and activating cAMP second messenger pathways, ACTH increases flux through the pathway from cholesterol to cortisol, particularly at the rate-limiting step catalysed by CYP11A. This happens acutely such that a rise in ACTH increases cortisol levels within 5 min. Cortisol provides negative feedback to the anterior pituitary and hypothalamus to regulate CRH and ACTH production; thus, the hypothalamic–anterior pituitary–adrenal axis is established. Superimposed on this circuit is a circadian rhythm. Increased axis activity and cortisol levels coincide with awakening in the morning, remain moderate during the day, but decline so that by late evening/night time cortisol levels are low (Fig. 6.5).

Gene name	Alternative common enzyme names and abbreviations
CYP11A	Cholesterol side-chain cleavage enzyme (SCC) or desmolase
HSD3B2	Type 2 3β-hydroxysteroid dehydrogenase (Type 2 3β-HSD)
CYP21	21-hydroxylase
CYP11B1	11β-hydroxylase
CYP11B2	Aldosterone synthase
CYP17	17α-hydroxylase/17, 20-lyase

Table 6.1 Alternative names in common usage for steroidogenic enzymes

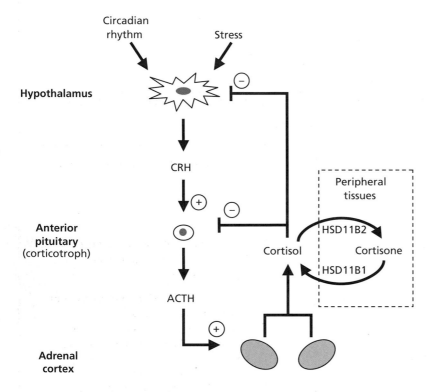

Figure 6.4 The hypothalamic–anterior pituitary–adrenal (HPA) axis. Higher brain function (e.g. circadian rhythm and stress) influences CRH synthesis and release, acting on the corticotroph of the anterior pituitary to make ACTH. Both CRH and ACTH are subject to negative feedback by cortisol, the levels of which are influenced in the periphery by the balance of activity of 11β-hydroxysteroid dehydrogenase (HSD11B) isoforms.

In contrast to these diurnal changes in steroid hormone biosynthesis, lengthier physiological events are more complex, but remain clinically relevant. Damage to the anterior pituitary can lead to a withering of the fasciculata and reticularis zones. In contrast, overactivity of the anterior pituitary induces a bilateral bulky increase in adrenocortical size. Unilateral growth occurs following adrenalectomy of the contralateral gland.

Cortisol is metabolized in peripheral tissues to inactive cortisone, which can, in turn, be converted back to active hormone; the two enzymatic reactions being catalyzed by type 2 and type 1 11β-hydroxysteroid dehydrogenase (HSD11B2 and HSD11B1) (Fig. 6.4 and Box 6.5).

Function of cortisol
Intermediary metabolism. The net metabolic effect of cortisol action is to raise circulating free fatty acids and glucose, the latter stimulating glycogen synthesis (Box 6.6). Excess cortisol also fosters an unfavourable serum lipid profile: raised total cholesterol and triglyceride with decreased HDL cholesterol. In addition, cortisol has a permissive

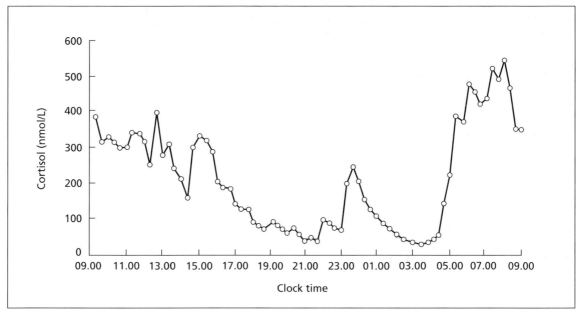

Figure 6.5 Typical diurnal variations in serum cortisol. Levels peak in the early morning and trough in the evening. In Cushing syndrome, diurnal variations are lost.

BOX 6.5 Important cortisol metabolism takes place in peripheral tissues-

- Cortisol and cortisone are interconverted by isoforms of 11β-hydroxysteroid dehydrogenase (HSD11B)
  - Type 2 (HSD11B2) inactivates cortisol to cortisone (the bulk of which occurs in the liver)
  - Type 1 (HSD11B1) reactivates cortisone to cortisol
- HSD11B1 is prevalent over HSD11B2 in visceral adipose tissue making fat a major steroidogenic organ
  - Excess glucocorticoid in centripetal obesity has been called 'Cushing disease of the omentum'

BOX 6.6 Cortisol, like glucagon, epinephrine and growth hormone, can be thought of as antagonistic to insulin

Cortisol tends to increase blood glucose levels by:
- Promoting gluconeogenesis
- Raising hepatic glucose output
- Inhibiting glucose uptake by muscle and fat
Other effects:
- Lipolysis from adipose tissue
- Protein catabolism to release amino acids

---

effect on epinephrine and glucagon, all of which creates a phenotype of 'insulin resistance', that is greater insulin secretion is needed to achieve the same metabolic effect. In the long-term, cortisol stimulates adipocyte differentiation, particularly in the viscera, predisposing to centripetal obesity.

Skin, muscle and bone. In skin, glucocorticoids inhibit keratinocyte division and collagen synthesis. In muscle, the catabolic effects reduce protein synthesis resulting in atrophy. Similar catabolic effects in bone shift the balance of activity from osteoblast (the bone forming cell type) to osteoclast (the bone resorbing cell type) predisposing to osteoporosis and the net flow of amino acids towards the liver (see Chapter 9).

Salt and water homeostasis and blood pressure. Glucocorticoids can potentially increase sodium resorption and potassium loss at the distal tubule through effects, not on the glucocorticoid receptor, but on the mineralocorticoid receptor (MR). More proximally, cortisol increases GFR and inhibits arginine vasopressin (AVP) to increase free water clearance. Cortisol increases blood pressure by several mechanisms including increased sensitivity of the vasculature to catecholamines.

Growth and development. Cortisol is an important hormone during growth and development of the fetus. It stimulates the differentiation of cell types to their mature phenotype. This is particularly evident in the lung, where it stimulates the production of surfactant, which reduces alveolar surface tension. This is one of the final steps in preparing the fluid-filled fetal airways for postnatal life. Too much glucocorticoid inhibits growth, evident to the paediatric endocrinologist as Cushing syndrome, and in keeping with its largely catabolic effects on the musculoskeletal system.

Central nervous system and psyche. The role of glucocorticoids in the brain is highly complex, matched by their potential to cause a range of emotional symptoms from euphoria to depression.

Anti-inflammatory effects. Glucocorticoid actions on inflammation and autoimmunity are among its most important, not so much physiologically, but from the use of potent synthetic steroids to treat a range of disorders. With glucocorticoid treatment, circulating T lymphocytes and eosinophils fall, however, neutrophils rise. This is a catch to remember for the patient with an acute exacerbation of asthma. It does not necessarily mean infection; it may simply reflect steroid treatment. In tissues, for instance the acutely inflamed joints of a patient with rheumatoid arthritis, glucocorticoids rapidly suppress inflammation by inhibiting cytokine production and antagonizing macrophage action.

Aldosterone and the renin–angiotensin system

Aldosterone circulates in ~1000-fold lower concentration and with a shorter half-life of ~20 to 30 min than cortisol. In part, this is due to diminished affinity for serum carrier proteins. It acts via binding to the nuclear MR to influence gene expression in target cells. Interestingly, the MR is not specific for aldosterone, binding cortisol with equal affinity. However, specificity is preserved by HSD11B2, which inactivates cortisol to cortisone, at the major sites of mineralocorticoid action, the distal tubule and collecting ducts of the kidney. Here, aldosterone acts on the Na-K-ATPase transporter to increase sodium resorption in exchange for potassium excretion (Box 6.7). The net effect is to increase osmotic potential within the circulation causing expansion of circulating volume. The direct effect of aldosterone to increase blood pressure comes from vasoconstriction.

The enzyme, renin, is synthesized predominantly in the kidney, in specialized cells of the juxtaglomerular apparatus. These cells surround the afferent arteriole before it enters the glomerulus (Figs 6.6 and 6.7) and form a sensing mechanism for intravascular volume—decreased volume stimulates renin biosynthesis. Renin acts upon its substrate, circulating angiotensinogen, to generate the decapeptide, angiotensin I, which is subsequently converted into angiotensin II (AII). It is this latter octopeptide that binds to the type 2 angiotensin II receptor in the zona glomerulosa cells to stimulate aldosterone biosynthesis and secretion. In addition, AII is a very potent 'pressor' agent, causing arteriolar vasoconstriction. Significant renin–angiotensin systems also exist within individual organs, for instance creating paracrine regulation of aldosterone secretion in the adrenal cortex. Furthermore, the volume of the zona glomerulosa layer influences its ability to generate mineralocorticoid. Thus, 'westernized' high salt

---

BOX 6.7 Aldosterone is the body's major mineralocorticoid

- It promotes sodium resorption from the urine and potassium excretion
- It increases blood pressure

In turn, aldosterone biosynthesis is regulated primarily by:

- The renin–angiotensin system (forming a negative feedback loop)
- Serum potassium concentration

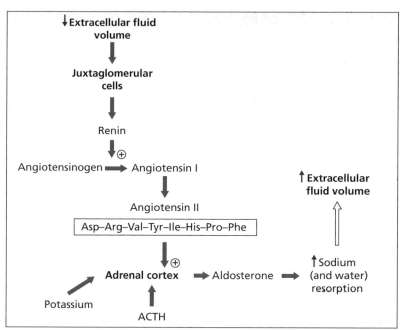

Figure 6.6 The renin–angiotensin–aldosterone axis. A fall in extracellular fluid volume produces increased activity in renal nerves, reduced sodium flux in the macula densa and a fall in transmural pressure. These activate the juxtaglomerular apparatus to increase renin production, which catalyses the beginning of the cascade that ends with angiotensin II-stimulated aldosterone secretion. High potassium, and to a lesser extent ACTH, also increase aldosterone production.

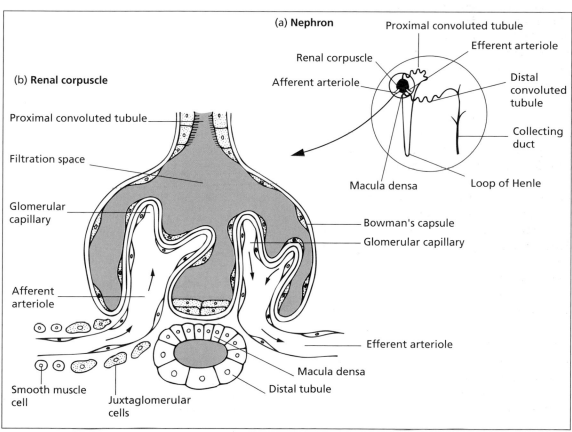

Figure 6.7 The structure of a nephron and the juxtaglomerular apparatus. (a) A nephron. The renal corpuscle, its blood supply and proximity to the distal tubule are shown in (b). (b) The structure of a renal corpuscle, its blood supply and the juxtaglomerular apparatus. Between the afferent and efferent arterioles lies the glomerular capillaries, which are surrounded by Bowman's capsule. The filtration space drains into the proximal tubule. The juxtaglomerular cells, containing renin granules, replace the smooth muscle cells of the afferent arteriole and are positioned next to the closely packed macula densa cells of the distal tubule.

diets, which expand the intravascular volume and raise blood pressure, suppress the renin–angiotensin system, leading to a shrivelled zona glomerulosa. High potassium also stimulates aldosterone biosynthesis (Fig. 6.6). Even ACTH plays a minor role, although its overproduction or underproduction carries no significant clinical impact on circulating aldosterone levels.

Sex steroid precursors from the innermost adrenal cortex

In the fasciculata and reticularis zones, the relative activity of CYP17 and HSD3B2 determines the production of cortisol versus DHEA. DHEA and its downstream derivative, androstenedione possess only weak androgenic activity; however, their peripheral conversion in other tissues can give rise to both androgen (e.g. testosterone) and oestrogen (e.g. oestradiol) (review Fig. 2.5). Therefore, they are much better termed 'sex steroid precursors'. Their biosynthesis, like cortisol, is primarily under the regulation of ACTH.

The function of these hormones is debated. During the second and third trimesters of fetal development, huge amounts of DHEA and its sulphated derivative, DHEAS, are generated. However, they are not essential. Postnatally, little androgen precursor is produced until adrenarche at 7–8 years, when the zona reticularis becomes functionally mature. Further metabolism of these hormones stimulates growth in middle childhood, sometimes accompanied with some pubic and axillary hair growth. Clinically, this is important, as it is physiological and needs to be distinguished from precocious puberty, the hallmarks of which include breast development in females and testicular enlargement in males (Table 7.5).

Clinical disorders

The major clinical disorders affecting the adrenal cortex arise from either too much or too little cortisol and aldosterone.

Hypoadrenalism

An underactive adrenal cortex leads to a shortage of cortisol (in all circumstances) and aldosterone (in primary causes). Primary hypoadrenalism arises from direct destruction of the adrenal gland, whereas secondary disease is a consequence of loss of the anterior pituitary corticotroph.

Primary hypoadrenalism—Addison disease
Worldwide, the commonest cause of adrenocortical deficiency comes from infection (either AIDS or tuberculosis) although in the western world this remains rare. In its place, autoimmune destruction of the cortex, first described by Thomas Addison in 1855, leads to deficiency of both aldosterone and cortisol. The disorder carries his eponymous title with the adjective 'Addisonian' used to refer to the clinical crisis that results from acute, severe cortisol (and aldosterone) deficiency. Other causes of underactivity are more unusual, although developmental abnormalities should not be discounted in a paediatric population (Case History 6.1).

Symptoms, signs and biochemical profile. Symptoms and signs relate to: diminished vascular volume and tone; renal sodium loss; bowel water and electrolyte loss; removal of negative feedback (causing pigmentation from MSH, see Chapter 5); and the loss of cortisol action on hepatic and peripheral metabolism (Box 6.8). The consequent classical laboratory findings are hyponatraemia (the vast majority) and hyperkalaemia (in most cases). Patients also carry an increased risk of other autoimmune endocrinopathies (see Box 8.7).

BOX 6.8 Signs and symptoms of hypoadrenalism

- Weight loss and anorexia
- Fatigue and weakness
- Nausea, vomiting, abdominal pain and diarrhoea
- Generalized wasting and muscle cramps
- Hypoglycaemia (especially in children)
- Dizziness and postural hypotension
- Loss of body hair
- Pigmentation of light-exposed areas, pressure points, scars and buccal mucosa (in primary disease)
- Vitiligo (associated with autoimmune adrenalitis)
- Circulatory shock (in acute circumstances)

Diagnosis. Plasma cortisol is highly variable, although a high enough level (>400 nmol/L) safely excludes Addisonian crisis. Similarly, ACTH tends to be high. The hallmark of diagnosis is dynamic testing, according to the principle *'if underactivity is suspected, try to stimulate it'*. Serum cortisol is measured 30 min after intramuscular or intravenous injection of synthetic ACTH. This contains the first 24 amino acids of biological ACTH. Tetracosactide is the generic name; however, it is better known by the tradenames, 'Synacthen' in the UK and 'Cortrosyn' in the USA, leading to the 'short Synacthen test (SST)' and 'Cortrosyn stimulation test'. Although lower-dose tests have been developed, the mainstay of adult endocrinology is to administer 250 μg. A serum cortisol level, 30 min later, greater than 525 nmol/L identifies the 5th percentile response (i.e. 95% of the population achieve higher values). In primary adrenocortical disease, plasma aldosterone may be low or normal; however, more tellingly, accompanying plasma renin activity and renin concentration will be elevated.

Treatment. 'If it is missing, replace it'. The mainstay of oral replacement therapy is hydrocortisone (the pharmacological term for cortisol—they are the same hormone) and the synthetic mineralocorticoid, fludrocortisone. Historically, endocrinologists have tended to over-replace cortisol, with detrimental side-effects similar to those for adrenocortical over-activity. The standard adult replacement dose is 20 mg hydrocortisone daily—10 mg on awakening and either 10 mg mid-afternoon or 5 mg at midday and a further 5 mg mid-to-late afternoon. This regime is relatively effective at replacing the normal circadian rhythm: high levels in the morning, low levels by bedtime. Disturbance to this profile can present as either difficulty or tiredness executing daily tasks (inadequate cortisol) and inability to sleep at night (too much cortisol). Fludrocortisone is much longer acting and therefore taken once daily (commonly 100 μg in adults).

Monitoring hydrocortisone treatment is contentious. Some endocrinologists advocate an intermittent series of serum measurements during the day (a 'cortisol day curve') although little evidence supports its value. In contrast, mineralocorticoid replacement is frequently overlooked. Normal renin concentration (or plasma renin activity) and normotension are valuable guides. Inadequate replacement causes raised renin levels whereas over-replacement tends to generate hypokalaemia and hypertension.

The major message for glucocorticoid replacement is that the patient is entirely dependent on tablets: the normal ability of the adrenal cortex to increase cortisol output during illness or stress is lost. Failure to advise the patient to double replacement dose when unwell risks an Addisonian crisis, a critical lack of glucocorticoid presenting as circulatory collapse, hyponatraemia, hyperkalaemia and hypoglycaemia. This medical emergency demands immediate treatment with intravenous hydrocortisone and well as large amounts of intravenous fluids. For these reasons, patients with adrenal insufficiency (either primary or secondary) should carry notification (Box 6.9).

Secondary hypoadrenalism

If the anterior pituitary corticotrophs are underactive, ACTH-dependent processes in the adrenal gland also suffer. This translates as cortisol deficiency and loss of adrenal sex steroid precursors, with retained aldosterone biosynthesis. The causes of this are covered in Chapter 5 on the anterior pituitary. However, the principles of glucocorticoid replacement therapy, and the consequences of its failure, are the same.

Hyperadrenalism

Adrenocortical overactivity most commonly relates to an excess of glucocorticoid or mineralocorticoid.

Glucocorticoid excess—'Cushing syndrome'

An excess of glucocorticoid is called Cushing syndrome, named after Harvey Cushing, who in 1912 described the first case characterized by obesity and hirsuitism. Twenty years later, its hormonal basis

---

BOX 6.9 Glucocorticoid replacement

- double the dose during illness
- carry a steroid alert card or bracelet

CASE HISTORY 6.1

A 35-year-old woman presented with tiredness and abdominal pain. She had fainted twice recently when unwell with vomiting and diarrhoea. Her sister takes thyroxine. On examination, she looked tanned with patches of skin depigmentation. BP was 90/60. Serum urea was slightly raised, however, creatinine was normal. Serum potassium was 5.5 mmol/L; serum sodium was low. Thyroid function tests were normal. The doctor also measured a full blood count. Haemoglobin was only 100 g/L with a mean cell volume (MCV) of 110 fl.

What is the diagnosis and what tests should be performed to confirm it?
What treatment should the patient be given?
What additional information should be provided?
What associated disorder should be considered to explain the haematological findings?

Answers, see p. 97

BOX 6.10 Signs and symptoms of Cushing syndrome

- Muscle wasting, relatively thin limbs
- Easily bruised, thin skin; poor wound healing
- Striae (purple or 'violaceous' rather than white)
- Thin (osteoporotic) bones that easily fracture
- Diabetes mellitus
- Central obesity, moon facies, buffalo hump
- Susceptibility to infection
- Predisposition to gastric ulcer
- Hypertension
- Disturbance of menstrual cycle; symptoms overlapping with polycystic ovarian syndrome (see Chapter 7)
- Mood disturbance (depression, psychosis)

was proposed. The commonest cause is from exogenous steroid drugs (e.g. as used in asthma). Discounting this, there are several endogenous causes of Cushing syndrome. However, despite greatly advanced knowledge, delays in detection remain problematic—the main hindrance being a failure of perception when presented with common, insidious symptoms. It most frequently occurs in women. (Case History 6.2).

Symptoms, signs and biochemical profile. The symptoms and signs of exaggerated cortisol action are shown in Box 6.10.

The first, most important step is to prove glucocorticoid excess. Three screening tests are commonly used. Autonomous production results in loss of diurnal variation with serum or salivary midnight cortisol values failing to drop. In moderate-to-severe Cushing syndrome, cortisol is also raised several-fold in the urine. The third test, the low-dose dexamethasone suppression test, is discussed below (Table 6.2). Random plasma cortisol estimations are not useful in diagnosing glucocorticoid excess. However, the sex steroid precursors, DHEA and androstenedione that can be converted to potent androgens causing hirsuitism and menstrual irregularities in women, may be elevated. Additional factors can increase serum cortisol and complicate the differential diagnosis of Cushing syndrome. This is called 'pseudo-Cushing syndrome' (Box 6.11).

Diagnosing the cause of glucocorticoid excess. Dynamic investigations offer confirmatory proof of glucocorticoid excess and then help to localize the site of the problem. They are based on the endocrine principle *'if overactivity is suspected, try to suppress it'*. Dexamethasone is a potent synthetic glucocorticoid, available orally, that inhibits normal ACTH production by the anterior pituitary and leads to decreased cortisol production in the adrenal. Two main tests, which should be used sequentially, interrogate this negative feedback loop (Table 6.2). There are two forms of the low-dose dexamethasone test. Using either, Cushing syndrome is excluded if cortisol is <50 nmol/L the following morning. Only if cortisol remains elevated, especially in conjunction with a raised UFC and absent diurnal variation, should the

Table 6.2 Dexamethasone suppression tests

Low-dose dexamethasone suppression test	High-dose dexamethasone suppression test
Defines glucocorticoid excess	Localizes glucocorticoid excess
0.5 mg × 8 doses 6-hourly ending at midnight or single 1 mg dose at midnight	2 mg × 8 doses 6-hourly ending at midnight
Positive diagnosis of Cushing syndrome: failure to suppress 9 AM serum cortisol the following morning to below 50 nmol/L	Anterior pituitary source: >50% suppression of 9 AM serum cortisol from pre- to post-test
	Extrapituitary 'ectopic' source of ACTH (or adrenal tumour): <50% suppression of 9 AM serum cortisol from pre- to post-test

---

BOX 6.11 Pseudo-Cushing syndrome

- Obesity
- Alcoholism
- Depression

Distinction from Cushing syndrome

- Diurnal variation is usually retained
- Cortisol falls on removal of alcohol abuse
- Cortisol tends to rise with insulin-induced hypoglycaemia

BOX 6.12 Cushing syndrome = glucocorticoid excess

- Cushing disease: anterior pituitary tumour, ACTH inappropriately normal or raised
- Ectopic ACTH: extrapituitary ACTH-secreting tumour; ACTH inappropriately normal or raised
- Adrenocortical tumour: ACTH suppressed (N.B. exogenous glucocorticoid drugs would also suppress ACTH)

---

next phase of investigation seek to locate the origin of the disease.

Primary adrenal Cushing syndrome most commonly arises as a benign adenoma of the zona fasciculata. The excess cortisol suppresses ACTH, usually to undetectable levels (Box 6.12). In contrast, ACTH-secreting tumours may not raise serum ACTH above the normal reference range, but the hormone is inappropriately present for the circulating levels of cortisol. The ACTH comes either from a corticotroph tumour of the anterior pituitary or from an ectopic source (e.g. small-cell carcinoma of the lung or a carcinoid tumour). The high-dose dexamethasone suppression test distinguishes between these options (Table 6.2). Baseline serum cortisol is assessed. ACTH-secreting pituitary adenomas usually retain significant negative feedback to high-dose dexamethasone, such that a fall of >50% from baseline points to a corticotroph adenoma, known correctly as 'Cushing disease'. A failure to suppress suggests either an ectopic source of ACTH or an adrenocorti-

cal tumour (when ACTH would be undetectable). Although less reliable, ACTH levels also tend to be higher when secreted by ectopic tumours rather than pituitary tumours.

Having defined the excess and gained clues to location, it is now appropriate to image either: the anterior pituitary by MRI; the adrenal glands by MRI or CT; or continue the search for the ectopic source of ACTH (potentially by CT of the chest or by uptake scans that might identify a carcinoid tumour). If further discrimination of an ACTH-secreting tumour is needed, the hormone can be measured in each inferior petrosal sinus following CRH stimulation ('inferior petrosal sinus sampling'). A clear gradient of ACTH from petrosal sinus to peripheral blood may point to the anterior pituitary and also help to lateralize the tumour within the pituitary fossa.

Treatment. Glucocorticoid excess causes premature mortality, predominantly from cardiovascular disease. The goal of treatment is to normalize

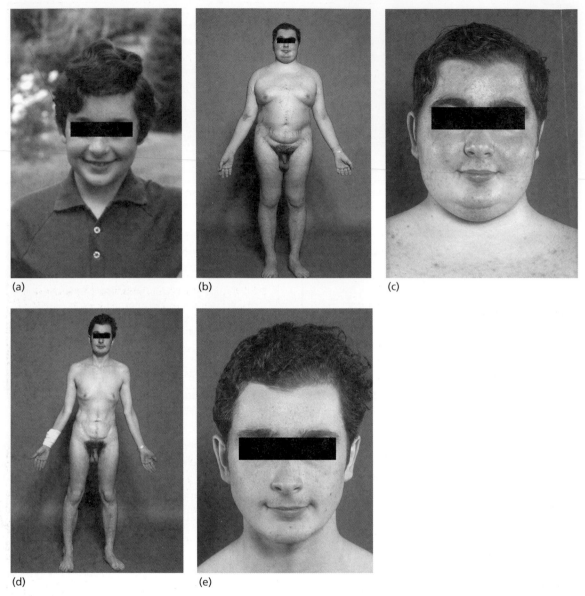

Figure 6.8 The effects of glucocorticoid excess in Cushing disease. (a) Normal appearance at 6 years. (b–c) Florid signs of excess cortisol by age 15: round face, greasy skin, severe acne, truncal obesity with stretch marks (striae) and bruising from a venepuncture site on the right arm. (d–e) Now aged 16, 1 year after transsphenoidal surgery and an operation to remove excess abdominal skin.

glucocorticoid production and diurnal rhythm. For adrenal adenomas, unilateral adrenalectomy is undertaken. For pituitary adenomas, transsphenoidal surgery is commonplace in major centres. The results of treating Cushing syndrome can be striking (Fig. 6.8 and Plate 6.1, facing p. 246).

Once the cause of excess glucocorticoid is removed, the hypothalamic–anterior pituitary–adrenal axis is so suppressed that endogenous cortisol cannot be detected in the immediate postoperative period—a marker of curative surgery. Furthermore, the body is so accustomed to high cortisol

---

CASE HISTORY 6.2

A 44-year-old woman had suffered symptoms, which she attributed to polycystic ovarian syndrome (PCOS), by virtue of reading articles on the internet. She went to see the doctor because of feeling generally unwell, having put on 10 kg in weight and due to a new feature of nocturia. She took no medication. The doctor suspected diabetes and, indeed, the patient's fasting blood glucose was 7.5 mmol/L. However, the doctor was more struck by the patient's appearance of a flushed round face, poor facial skin quality and purple stretch marks on the patient's abdomen. BP was 160/95. The doctor arranged several tests that confirmed the diagnosis. Serum ACTH was then measured and was undetectable.

What is the initial diagnosis and what tests were used to make it?

According to the undectable ACTH, where is the causative lesion and what imaging investigations might be considered?

Answers, see p. 98

---

levels, that the patient is commonly symptomatic of relative adrenal insufficiency, if not outright Addisonian crisis. Hydrocortisone therapy is needed for a sufficient period until the hypothalamic–anterior pituitary–adrenal axis functions normally. In those not fit for surgery, medical therapy, for instance with metyrapone, can directly inhibit glucocorticoid secretion. For inoperable pituitary adenomas or following failed surgery, either due to location or size, pituitary radiotherapy remains a valuable option.

Mineralocorticoid excess — Conn syndrome
Tumours of the zona glomerulosa result in excess aldosterone with relatively normal cortisol physiology.

Symptoms, signs and biochemical profile. Classically, too much aldosterone presents with hypokalaemic hypertension. The disturbance of salt balance may be unmasked or exacerbated by concomitant potassium-losing diuretic therapy, given for the hypertension (e.g. thiazides). Aldosterone excess also underlies a subset of normokalaemic hypertension, which, like all the more unusual causes of hypertension, demands a higher index of clinical suspicion (Box 6.13).

The symptoms tend to be vague. Hypertension may present with headaches and visual disturbances; hypokalaemia may cause muscle fatigue or tiredness. The incidence is higher in women in their third decade. If blood pressure is normal for age,

> **BOX 6.13 Remember to think of unusual causes of hypertension, especially in younger patients:**
>
> - Conn syndrome
> - Phaeochromocytoma
> - Renal artery stenosis
> - Coarctation of the aorta

> **BOX 6.14 Causes of hypokalaemia**
>
> - Vomiting (metabolic alkalosis)
> - Diarrhoea or other fluid loss from the lower bowel (e.g. ileostomy, villous adenoma of the rectum)
> - Insulin therapy
> - Diuretic use
> - Rare causes include renal tubular acidosis and Bartter syndrome

other causes of hypokalaemia merit consideration (Box 6.14).

Diagnosis. The diagnosis of aldosterone excess requires assessment of the renin–angiotensin–aldosterone axis in a salt-replete individual. The major confounding factor is the concomitant use of antihypertensives, many of which affect the hormone axis. Agents such as diuretics, beta-blockers and ACE inhibitors all require stopping for at least 2 weeks. Classically, testing has been performed supine (on wakening) and after 2h erect posture, although a single measurement in a semirecumbent position has also proved effective and easier. Potassium should be restored with oral supplementation in the days prior to testing.

A positive screening test detects a serum aldosterone that is greater than a threshold of ~200 pmol/L in the presence of a suppressed plasma renin concentration or activity. This combination generates a high aldosterone:renin (or aldosterone:plasma renin activity) ratio. A variety of options then offer supplementary evidence, such as challenge tests with fludrocortisone or detecting high urinary potassium excretion. Imaging with MRI or CT and, if needed, adrenal vein sampling helps to localize the potential source of mineralocorticoid excess.

Treatment. Aside from rare genetic causes, hyperaldosteronism usually occurs in two forms: a discrete adenoma and bilateral hyperplasia. The former is ideally treated by unilateral adrenalectomy, the latter by medical management. Spironolactone has been used for many years as an MR antagonist. Indeed, a clue to diagnosis can come with its use followed by a rapid fall in previously refractory high blood pressure. Unfortunately, the drug also antagonizes the androgen receptor (AR), necessitating contraceptive advice in fertile women to guard against feminizing a male fetus. Newer, more specific antagonists have just reached the market (eplerenone). This long-awaited development offers an additional approach to manage patients with Conn adenomas who are not fit for general anaesthesia, as well as bilateral adrenal hyperplasia.

Tumours involving the zona reticularis

In addition to cortisol, tumours from the fasciculata and reticularis zones can secrete sex steroid precursors. These steroids are converted in the periphery to androgens and, potentially, oestrogens that cause feminization in men (e.g. gynaecomastia). The tumours can be diagnosed by serum analysis of DHEA (or DHEAS), androstenedione, testosterone and assessment of glucocorticoid status, accompanied by imaging (CT, MRI). Where it is difficult to discriminate between an adrenal or gonadal source of the steroid excess, catheterization and sampling of the adrenal veins can be helpful. The tumours are treated surgically with removal of the offending adrenal gland.

Other tumours of the adrenal cortex

Adrenocortical carcinoma. The commonest malignant tumour of the adrenal cortex is metastatic. Primary adrenal carcinoma is rare. The vast majority are functional (80%), most of which secrete glucocorticoids or glucocorticoids plus sex steroid precursors. The clinical picture tends to be one of rapidly progressive Cushing syndrome and virilization accompanied by the more general effects of an aggressive tumour (e.g. weight loss, abdominal pain, anorexia and fever). Survival is poor, as most tumours have metastasized at the time of presentation so that adrenalectomy is no longer curative. Mitotane, an adrenolytic drug, palliates symptoms of hormone excess and can reduce tumour growth, but overall, no more than 20% of patients survive 5 years.

Incidentalomas. An increasing problem is the management of tumours identified on imaging for other reasons. Over 40 years of age, these 'incidentalomas' are common, potentially affecting 5% of individuals (Box 6.15).

Congenital adrenal hyperplasia

Congenital adrenal hyperplasia (CAH) is inherited as an autosomal recessive disorder. It is caused by

---

BOX 6.15 A pragmatic approach to adrenal incidentalomas?

- Exclude excess secretion of aldosterone, glucocorticoid, sex steroid precursor and catecholamines
- Assess likelihood that it is a metastasis, e.g. full history and examination; consider chest X-ray in smokers
- If >5 cm, risk of malignancy is increased, adrenalectomy more appropriate
- If <5 cm, hormone-negative and 'nonsuspicious' on imaging, annual follow-up and repeat investigation can be considered

mutations in the genes that encode enzymes in the pathway to cortisol (Fig. 6.3). This leads to cortisol deficiency, diminished negative feedback at the anterior pituitary and raised ACTH levels (Fig. 6.4). The high ACTH stimulates the remaining intact adrenocortical steroidogenic pathways. Mutations in *CYP21* account for 90% of CAH. The position of CYP21 in the biosynthetic pathway means that as well as decreased cortisol, the enzyme's substrate, 17-hydroxyprogesterone, is markedly increased. The high ACTH increases flux through the intact pathway to sex steroid precursors and results in elevated circulating androgens. The latter can cause: ambiguous genitalia in females at birth (Fig. 6.9); precocious puberty in males; and pronounced difficulties with hirsuitism, menstrual irregularities and fertility in women. Many patients also have inadequate aldosterone production ('salt wasting'); some do not ('simple virilizing').

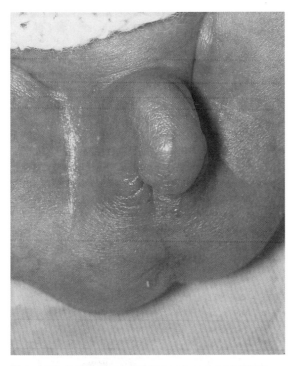

Figure 6.9 Ambiguous genitalia in a female with CAH. This 46, XX infant was virilized *in utero* and presented at birth with clitoral hypertrophy, fusion of the labia and a urogenital opening at the base of the phallus.

The diagnosis of CYP21 deficiency should be made in female neonates with virilized external genitalia, hypotension and hyperkalaemia. Basal ACTH is high. The diagnosis is confirmed on ACTH stimulation testing, when cortisol fails to rise significantly, but 17-hydroxyprogesterone increases a lot. Replacement is with glucocorticoid (+/− mineralocorticoid) to restore feedback and minimize androgen overproduction. This can be complex: one extreme of treatment is bilateral adrenalectomy and lifelong steroid replacement.

Therapeutic use of glucocorticoids

Glucocorticoid endocrinology lends potential therapeutic value throughout life. Dexamethasone is used in premature labour to stimulate fetal surfactant production. Postnatally, the immunosuppressive, anti-inflammatory effects of glucocorticoids lead to pharmacological doses of synthetic glucocorticoids being used in a range of autoimmune and inflammatory disorders. However, the lessons learned in this chapter on Cushing syndrome illustrate that these agents should only be used wherever possible on a short-term basis.

The adrenal medulla

Embryology

In contrast to the outer cortex, the adrenal medulla is derived from the neuroectoderm ('neural crest') cells that migrate in a forward direction from the vertebral column to the periaortic region (Fig. 6.1). These cells give rise to the sympathetic chain of ganglia that innervate much of the gut and blood vessels. However, some specialize by invading the adrenal cortex to form the chromaffin cells of the adrenal medulla; innervated by preganglionic sympathetic neurones that emanate from T7–L3.

Catecholamine biosynthesis

The adrenal medulla chromaffin cells are like postganglionic neurones. Rather than possess nerve terminals, they function in response to synaptic activation by releasing preformed catecholamine hormones into the circulation (Fig. 6.10). Norepinephrine (noradrenaline) comprises 20% of

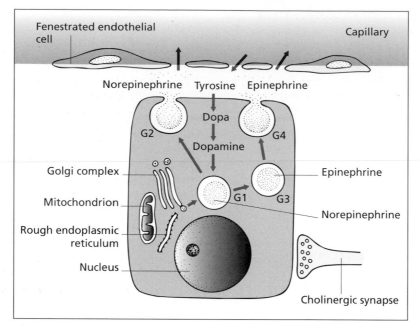

Figure 6.10 The synthesis, storage and release of catecholamines in the chromaffin cell of the adrenal medulla. The components of the storage granules (G), including the chromogranins, are synthesized on the rough endoplasmic reticulum and packaged in the Golgi complex. Dopamine enters a granule (G1) and is converted to norepinephrine, which can then be released exocytotically (G2). Alternatively, norepinephrine can be further converted to epinephrine (G3) and released by exocytosis (G4). Each cell has a cholinergic synapse where acetylcholine initiates the train of events leading to exocytosis. Individual chromaffin cells usually only secrete either norepinephrine or epinephrine.

circulating catecholamine, with an additional biochemical step generating the remaining 80% as epinephrine (adrenaline). Much of the chromaffin cell is made up of secretory granules, which contain the stored catecholamines and proteins called chromogranins. The latter can serve as a clinical marker of endocrine tumours, such as phaeochromocytoma, carcinoid tumour or a gut endocrine tumour (see Chapter 10).

The biosynthesis of catecholamines occurs in four steps (Fig. 6.11). The hydroxylation of tyrosine is rate-limiting and subject to negative feedback by the downstream hormone products, norepinephrine and dopamine. The two biosynthetic steps to dopamine are the same as occur in the substantia nigra cells of the brain stem—the cells that are lost in Parkinson disease. The last step, converting norepinephrine to epinephrine reflects the unusual embryological development of the adrenal medulla.

Robust expression of phenylethanolamine N-methyl transferase, the enzyme required for epinephrine production, depends upon high concentrations of glucocorticoid that are only present in the adrenal medulla because of the centripetal drainage of venous blood from the outer adrenal cortex.

Stimulation of the chromaffin cell by preganglionic neurones is mediated by acetylcholine, and to a lesser extent, by serotonin and histamine. This releases the catecholamine hormones, which then diffuse the short distance into the adjacent blood vessels (Fig. 6.10).

Terminating catecholamine action
Ending the effect of catecholamines relies on several different mechanisms (Fig. 6.11). The most efficient method sees norepinephrine taken up by postganglionic sympathetic nerve terminals, where it can be metabolized by monoamine oxidase (MAO). Similar

mechanisms take up mainly epinephrine into platelets. Circulating catecholamines are also metabolized in either neuronal or nonneuronal tissues (e.g. the liver) and the metabolites excreted in urine. The collection and assay of urine over 24 h closely reflects adrenal medulla activity and serves as a valuable clinical test (see below).

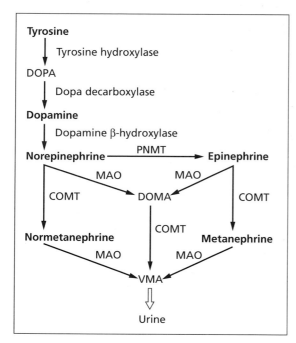

Figure 6.11 The synthesis and degradation of the catecholamines. DOPA, 3,4-dihydroxyphenylalanine; dopamine, 3,4-dihydroxyphenylethylamine; PNMT, phenylethanolamine *N*-methyl transferase; MAO, monoamine oxidase; COMT, catechol-*O*-methyl-transferase; DOMA, 3,4-dihydroxymandelic acid; VMA, vanillylmandelic acid (3-methoxy-4-hydroxymandelic acid).

Physiology

Epinephrine and norepinephrine are major stress hormones responsible for the body's 'fright, fight and flight' responses following provocation (Table 6.3). The subtle differences reflect affinities for the different adrenoreceptors, predominantly α and β subtypes 1 and 2. Norepinephrine stimulates α and $\beta1$ receptors, thus does not cause bronchodilation, a $\beta2$ response. In contrast, the distribution of α and $\beta2$ receptors in skeletal muscle beds can actually cause vasodilation (i.e. increased muscle blood flow) compared to vasoconstriction in the gut. Thus, the combined effects of both catecholamines raise blood pressure, divert nutrients away from nonessential organs and promote delivery to the muscles that are active in the 'fight or flight' responses to danger. The hormones also play important metabolic roles. Both hormones raise blood glucose by stimulating glycogenolysis in liver and muscle, and hepatic gluconeogenesis. Fatty acid release is increased. All of these actions increase energy substrate available to the body in a way that counteracts the effects of insulin (see counter-regulatory mechanisms in Chapter 12).

Clinical disorders

Catecholamines from the adrenal medulla are dispensable. In bilateral adrenalectomy, glucocorticoid replacement is mandatory, but catecholamine replacement is not required.

Phaeochromocytoma
The most important clinical disease of the adrenal medulla is overactivity due to a tumour of the chromaffin cells called 'phaeochromocytoma'. (Case History 6.3).

Table 6.3 The effects of catecholamines

Epinephrine	Norepinephrine
Systolic blood pressure and heart rate rise	Systolic and diastolic blood pressure rise (increasing mean arterial pressure)
Gut motility decreases	Heart rate decreases
Circulation diverted to limb muscle beds and away from the gut	
Bronchodilation; mucus secretions reduce	
Piloerection	
Mydriasis (pupil dilation)	

Symptoms, signs and features. These rare tumours can occur sporadically or as part of familial syndromes (see 'multiple endocrine neoplasia' in Chapter 10). As a teaching aid, a '10% rule' has been described: 10% are malignant and 10% are extra-adrenal. These points serve as useful reminders that the vast majority of phaeochromocytomas are benign and may occur outside the adrenal along the sympathetic chain. It used to be said that 10% were inherited, although, with the wider availability of molecular genetic testing and greater knowledge of causative mutations, this appears an underestimation (see below). Excessive unregulated catecholamine release occurs at inappropriate times resulting in unusual and distinctive symptoms (Box 6.16). Hypertension is the most common finding (90–100% of cases), which may be constant (in ~50%, frequently children) or episodic.

The frequency of symptomatic events can vary from daily to monthly, which can make diagnosis difficult. If suspicion is high, investigation should be repeated at intervals. Less commonly, tremor, angina or nausea can be apparent. In the experience of the authors, the most bizarre symptom heralding the onset of catecholamine release was sneezing 'fits'.

Diagnosis. Secretion is episodic. The best screening test to detect excess catecholamines is measurement in the urine over 24 h. This can be done randomly or, with infrequent symptoms, immediately after an attack. Most laboratories will measure a range of metabolites: metanephrine and normetanephrine, vanillylmandelic acid and possibly the parent hormones epinephrine, norepinephrine with their precursor, dopamine. This combined approach is important. It is exceptionally rare for patients to present with a phaeochromocytoma that over-secretes only one of these hormones or metabolites in the absence of the others. Occasionally, very large or extra-adrenal phaeochromocytomas escape the normal influence of cortisol on PNMT and secrete an increased proportion of norepinephrine. Once a biochemical diagnosis has been made, imaging, ideally by MRI, aids localization for surgical intervention. In very specialized centres, uptake scans with meta-iodobenzylguanidine (mIBG) may be possible (see Plate 4.1, facing p. 246).

Treatment. Managing phaeochromocytoma focuses on two aspects: blocking the effects of catecholamine excess using α and β adrenoreceptor blockers, and then surgical removal of the offending adrenal gland. It is important to provide α blockade first to avoid a potential hypertensive crisis from unopposed α adrenoreceptor stimulation. Successful surgery requires this good preparation as manipulation of the tumour at operation can result in catastrophic release of stored catecholamines.

Familial syndromes including phaeochromocytoma
Like all tumours, phaeochromocytomas arise due to genetic abnormalities in the affected cell-type. In ~25% of phaeochromocytomas, these mutations are inherited via the germline when every cell in the body is affected. Two syndromes of 'multiple endocrine neoplasia (MEN)' have been described in particular detail (see Chapter 10). Phaeochromocytoma most commonly associates with Type 2 MEN. The syndrome is rare, but bilateral or extramedullary tumours, or phaeochromocytomas at a young age, should raise suspicion and instigate a thorough family history, additional examination, and biochemical testing. Phaeochromocytoma is also a part of Von Hippel Lindau syndrome and Von Recklinghausen neurofibromatosis syndrome.

Therapeutic uses of catecholamines
Based on their physiology, catecholamines, particularly epinephrine, are useful in clinical scenarios that range from the trivial to the profoundly serious. In intensive care medicine, catecholamine infusions can maintain blood pressure in septic shock. In every day life, similar vasoconstriction makes catecholamines useful nasal decongestants.

BOX 6.16 The triad of classical symptoms in phaeochromocytoma

- Hypertension
- Throbbing bilateral headaches
- Palpitations

CASE HISTORY 6.3

A 44-year-old man attended his doctor because of headaches. His partner attended the consultation and also commented on several occasions during the last few months when he had gone extremely pale and appeared ill at ease. Closer questioning elicited the presence of palpitations during these events, which lasted ~15 min. Examination was unremarkable except for a blood pressure of 180/110. The man was not overweight, took plenty of exercise and had no significant past medical history.

What diagnosis should be considered?
What investigations are appropriate?

Answers, see p. 98

KEY POINTS

- The adrenal cortex and adrenal medulla develop as separate organs
- The major adrenocortical hormones are aldosterone, cortisol and the sex steroid precursors
- Overactivity and underactivty of adrenocortical hormone biosynthesis causes important endocrine syndromes
- The major hormones from the adrenal medulla are the catecholamines, epinephrine and norepinephrine
- Phaeochromocytomas are tumours that oversecrete adrenomedullary hormones

---

Answers to case histories

Case history 6.1

The patient has Addison disease due to autoimmune destruction of the adrenal cortex. Decreased circulating volume has caused hypotension associated with dehydration and raised serum urea. The pigmentation is due to inadequate negative feedback from cortisol leading to corticotroph overactivity and increased POMC production, which gives rise to ACTH and, as a by-product, MSH. The pale areas are vitiligo, another autoimmune condition.

Addison disease is diagnosed by an ACTH stimulation test (known in the UK as a 'short Synacthen test') with a serum cortisol measured at 30 minutes. A normal response is >550 nmol/L; lower values increasingly raise suspicion of Addison disease. Serum ACTH may be measured at time zero and would be expected to be elevated. Plasma renin concentrations or activity levels may also be increased due to aldosterone deficiency.

Once diagnosed, the patient should be commenced on hydrocortisone and, potentially, fludrocortisone. If there is concern over Addisonian crisis, treatment should be started before diagnostic testing. The patient should be given a steroid alert card and informed about steroid alert bracelets. Advice should be given to double hydrocortisone doses during illness. If unable to take tablets (e.g. if vomiting due to gastroenteritis), the patient needs intravenous treatment.

This patient has an increased risk of autoimmune disease affecting other endocrine organs and cell-types. This is exemplified by the vitiligo and family history of thyroid disease. The haematology results are suspicious of pernicious anaemia. Autoimmune destruction of the cells in the stomach that make intrinsic factor prevents vitamin B_{12} absorption. This causes defective red blood cell biosynthesis with the presence of large red cells in the circulation ('macrocytosis'). Hypothyroidism is another cause of macrocytosis, however this was excluded. Serum vitamin B_{12} levels should be measured.

Case history 6.2

The patient has signs and symptoms of glucocorticoid excess—Cushing syndrome—that has precipitated diabetes mellitus, centripetal weight gain and the cardinal feature of purple abdominal 'striae'. On closer examination, thin bruised skin and proximal myopathy might be evident.

Initial investigations aim to demonstrate glucocorticoid excess; 24-h urine collections on three occasions, midnight cortisol estimation and low dose dexamethasone suppression tests can all be used to confirm glucocorticoid excess and diagnose Cushing syndrome.

In the absence of steroid medications, the undetectable ACTH means that the Cushing syndrome is of adrenal origin. CT or MRI imaging should be considered (review Fig. 4.7). CT scans can even suggest whether the lesion is lipid-rich, consistent with a functional adrenocortical adenoma.

Case history 6.3

The history and the finding of hypertension are suggestive of phaeochromocytoma; 24-h urine collection for excreted catecholamines should be undertaken on several occasions. In addition, an ECG and echocardiogram might be considered. The latter may show left ventricular hypertrophy. Only if catecholamine excretion is increased, should the adrenal glands be imaged by CT or MRI. Although more restricted in availability, mIBG scans demonstrate the uptake of labelled marker by phaeochromocytoma tissue.

Reproductive endocrinology

LEARNING OBJECTIVES

- The male reproductive system:
  — to understand normal male development
    and the regulation and function of the testis
  — to understand the clinical consequences
    of an underactive male reproductive
    axis
- The female reproductive system:
  — to understand normal female development and
    the regulation and function of the ovary

- to understand the hormonal consequences of
    pregnancy
- to understand the clinical consequences of a
    dysregulated female reproductive axis
- To appreciate reproductive endocrinology and its
  clinical disorders during different phases of life
- To develop an understanding of how to approach,
  counsel and treat the subfertile couple

This chapter integrates the basic biology of the reproductive system in males and females with the clinical conditions that affects it

Embryology of male and female development

Reproductive development *in utero* can be broken down into two processes: sex determination and sexual differentiation.

Sex determination

Chromosomal sex depends on whether the fertilizing spermatozoon bears an X or a Y-chromosome.

However, the translation of chromosomal sex into either the male testis or female ovary depends on events during the first two months of gestation (Box 7.1). Initially, there is no morphological difference between XX and XY gonads (Fig. 7.1a). However, at ~7 weeks of development, the cells of the male gonad start to express critical genes. The first is *SRY* (*Sex-determining Region of the Y* chromosome), followed by a cascade of others that eventually leads to the creation of a testis. During this period, called 'sex determination', the cells of 46,XX embryos undergo little change. This relative absence of activity defines development of an ovary.

The future function of the gonad also relies on the presence of germ cells that give rise to either spermatozoa or ova. Prior to, and during sex determination, primordial germ cells migrate from the wall of the yolk sac through the gut mesentery into the gonad. In males, the formation of testicular cords sends the germ cells into mitotic arrest. In the female, they continue proliferation for a few more weeks combined with atresia and entrance into the first stage of meiosis. The summation of these processes determines the total germ cell number for female postnatal life.

Sexual differentiation

Sexual differentiation occurs from two pairs of ducts, which form the internal genitalia, and the urogenital sinus, which forms the external genitalia (plus the terminal urethra and prostate in the male). In the male, events progress rapidly so that the major events are largely complete by the end of the first trimester. In the female, the future is determined by an absence of male development and pursuit of the default pathway.

The internal genitalia originate as the Müllerian (also called mesonephric) duct system that drains the primitive kidney (the mesonephros) and the Wolffian duct system that forms along the length of the urogenital ridge (Fig. 7.1b). In each sex, the duct that is

not required regresses and the other matures into recognizable parts of the adult anatomy (Box 7.2). In the male, anti-Müllerian hormone (AMH), also known as Müllerian inhibiting substance (MIS), from the Sertoli cells of the testicular cords causes regression of the Müllerian duct (Fig. 7.1c). In its place, testosterone, secreted by the interstitial Leydig cells, virilizes the Wolffian duct system into the structures that transport and mature spermatozoa from their origin in the testicular cords to the seminal vesicles and prostate (Fig. 7.2). In the female, absence of AMH and testosterone allows the growth of the Müllerian ducts and Wolffian regression (Fig. 7.1c).

The urogenital sinus also differentiates down a female path if male hormones are absent. 5α-dihydrotestosterone (DHT), formed in target tissues by the action of type 2 5α-reductase on testosterone, virilizes the external genitalia and stimulates prostate formation. Under this influence, the urethral folds fuse in the midline and the primitive genital tubercle expands and elongates to form the male phallus. The labioscrotal swellings also fuse to form the scrotum into which the testes eventually descend (Fig. 7.3). In the female, the absence of androgen lessens growth of the genital tubercle as the clitoris and retains the patency of the urethral and labioscrotal folds as the labia minora and majora, respectively (Fig. 7.3). The events are largely complete by 12 weeks of development, after which the phallus continues to enlarge and the testes descend, under the dual influence of insulin-like 3 and androgen.

Disturbances at any point in these pathways carry major clinical consequences. Mutation or altered dosage of the genes that form the gonad, a failure of hormone biosynthesis or loss of action at its target receptor all potentially result in 'intersex' or 'sex reversal' phenotypes. Such ambiguity of the genitalia at birth causes major parental distress and creates a diagnostic challenge to the paediatric endocrinologist.

Disorders of sex determination and sexual differentiation

The more severe the disruption or complete the sex reversal, the earlier *in utero* the problem occurred, with the extreme being a total failure of gonad formation. Clinical nomenclature is also based on the very rare disorder of hermaphroditism—the presence of

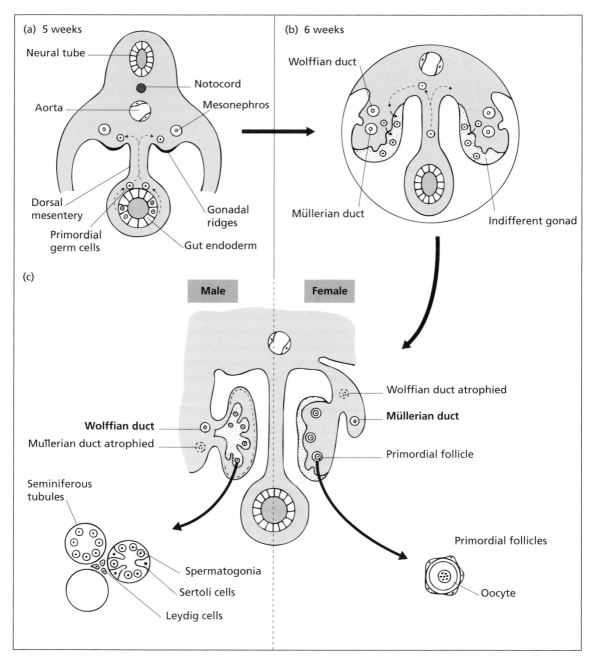

Figure 7.1 Sex determination and sexual differentiation. (a) Cross-section of a human embryo showing the primordial germ cells migrating via the dorsal mesentery to invade the developing gonads. (b) The appearance of the Wolffian and Müllerian ducts at ~6 weeks. (c) In the male, seminiferous tubules differentiate containing spermatogonia and Sertoli cells with Leydig cells interspersed between the tubules. The Müllerian duct regresses. In the female, primordial follicles develop and the Wolffian duct regresses.

both functional testicular and ovarian tissue. These true intersex cases possess both male and female sexual development. Derived from this term, 'pseudohermaphroditism' describes either abnormal male or female sexual development (Box 7.3).

Clinical features
The approach to an infant with ambiguous genitalia is a general one (Box 7.4).

Male pseudohermaphroditism. Deficiencies of any of the enzymes in the biosynthetic pathway to testosterone, its conversion to DHT or mutations of the androgen receptor can cause inadequate androgen action. Human society ascribes sexual phenotype

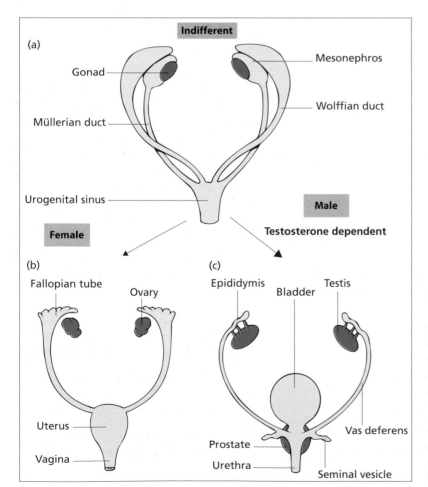

Figure 7.2 Sexual differentiation of the internal genitalia. (a) The indifferent stage when both the Müllerian and Wolffian ducts are present. (b) Female differentiation, which in males is antagonized by AMH. (c) Male differentiation. Testosterone virilizes the Wolffian ducts to form the rete testis, epididymis, vas deferens and seminal vesicle.

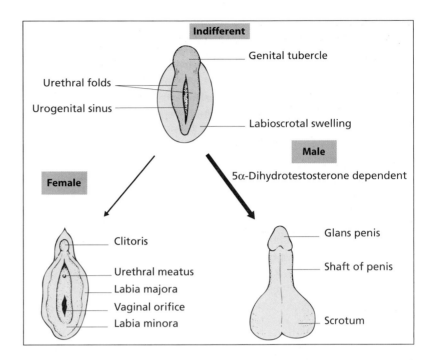

Figure 7.3 Fetal development of the external genitalia.

BOX 7.3 Disorders of sex determination and sexual differentiation

- Failure of gonadal differentiation
  - Turner syndrome (45,XO)
  - Klinefelter syndrome (47,XXY)
- Male pseudohermaphroditism: female phenotype in 46,XY individual
  - failure of testicular determination (e.g. mutation in *SRY*)
  - failure of steroidogenesis (mutation of enzyme in biosynthetic pathway to testosterone)
  - failure of dihydrotestosterone biosynthesis (5α-reductase mutation)
  - androgen insensitivity (androgen receptor mutation)
  - maternal consumption of antiandrogen drugs (e.g. spironolactone)
- Female pseudohermaphroditism: male phenotype in 46,XX individual
  - congenital adrenal hyperplasia (usually 21-hydroxylase deficiency—see Fig. 6.9)
  - maternal androgen excess (e.g. androgen-secreting tumour or anabolic steroid abuse)

BOX 7.4 Defining the diagnosis in genital ambiguity

- What is the extent of the sex reversal?
  - Complete—an early fetal influence
  - Incomplete
    Female, e.g. clitoral enlargement
    Male, e.g. hypospadias
- Are there associated clinical emergencies (salt-wasting hypoadrenalism in congenital adrenal hyperplasia (CAH))?
- Are there other congenital abnormalities?
- Is there a family history of other affected relatives, e.g. CAH?

Two questions are important:
- What is the karyotype?
  - Is it male or female pseudohermaphroditism? (Also needed to confirm clinical suspicion of Turner syndrome)
- In male pseudohermaphroditism, is there a uterus?
  - Yes—deficient action of both androgen and AMH
  - No—defect restricted to androgen pathway, i.e. AMH acted appropriately

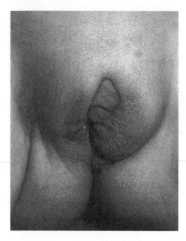

Figure 7.4 Genitalia of a 2-year-old male with 5α-reductase deficiency. Note the genital ambiguity and swelling in the left 'labium' due to a testis.

BOX 7.5 Contentious issues in the management of disorders of sexual differentiation

- To what extent is the developing human brain virilized in 46,XX fetuses with androgen excess and with what consequences? Indeed, our knowledge of this is limited during normal 46,XY male development.
- To what extent should surgery reconstruct the external genitalia, at what age and under whose consent?
  - reduction of clitoral size in CAH may create a visually more 'normal' female external genitalia, but it can nullify future sexual sensation

---

discretely—male or female—with grades of intersex considered abnormal. The example in Fig. 7.4 illustrates how distressing these disorders can be to parents and, later, to the patient. There are highly contentious issues in both male and female pseudo-hermaphroditism (Box. 7.5).

Female pseudohermaphroditism. Exposure to androgens before week 12 of pregnancy causes virilization by fusing the labia of a female fetus. The conse-

quences of later exposure of the external genitalia are limited to growth of the phallus, causing postnatal clitoromegaly. These features occur most commonly in CAH (see Chapter 6). As there is no abnormality in the ovary or internal genitalia, reproductive function may be possible after appropriate treatment.

The male reproductive system

Testicular morphology and function

The testis can be thought of as two compartments: sperm-producing testicular cords ('seminiferous tubules')—the structures, which largely determine testicular volume—interspersed within lipid-laden, interstitial steroidogenic Leydig cells (Fig. 7.5 and Box 7.6). The seminiferous tubules contain two types of cell: the germ cells and the Sertoli cells (Fig. 7.6). Tight junctions between adjacent Sertoli cells produce two compartments: a basal compartment with the spermatogonia, and an adluminal compartment for the spermatocytes, spermatids and spermatozoa. The tubules of each testis lead via the rete testis to the epididymis, where maturation of the spermatozoa occurs, and on to the vas deferens.

Androgen biosynthesis, secretion and metabolism

The principles of steroidogenesis were introduced in Chapter 2. Leydig cell steroidogenesis mirrors the process by which cholesterol is converted to the weak androgen, androstenedione, in the inner adrenal cortex (review Fig. 6.3). In the testis, the additional presence of type 3 17β-hydroxysteroid dehydrogenase (HSD17B3) generates the potent androgen, testosterone (Fig. 7.7). The testis is the major site of androgen synthesis, with only a small contribution (<5%) from the adrenal. Testosterone acts in its own right as a hormone, virilizing the inter-

---

BOX 7.6 The male gonad has two important functions:

- The synthesis of the male sex hormones—androgens
- The production of gametes—spermatogenesis

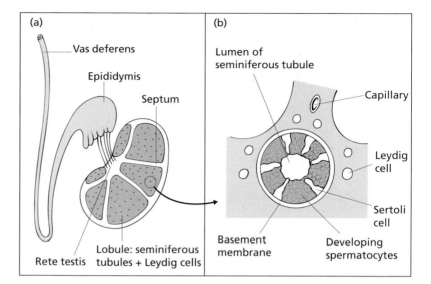

Figure 7.5 A testis in cross-section. (a) The testis is organized into lobules, in which lie the seminiferous tubules and the Leydig cells. Efferent ducts lead from the rete testis into the epididymis. (b) The organization of the seminiferous tubules and the interstitial Leydig cells.

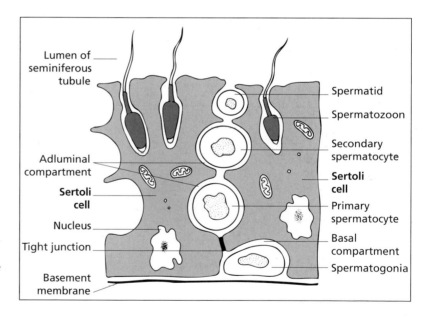

Figure 7.6 The structure of the wall of a seminiferous tubule. Sertoli cells (light shading) span the thickness of the tubule from the outside basement membrane to the central lumen. Tight junctions between adjacent Sertoli cells separate the spermatogonia in the basal compartment from the later stages of spermatogenesis in the adluminal compartment.

nal genitalia and acting anabolically on muscle cells. However, in other target tissues the action of the microsomal enzyme 5α-reductase forms the more potent DHT (Fig. 7.7). DHT binds with greater affinity than testosterone to the androgen receptor (AR). The DHT–AR complex then mediates androgen action by regulating the transcription of downstream target genes (review Figs 3.18 and 3.20).

Many clinical laboratories measure total serum testosterone. However, in the circulation, testosterone is largely protein-bound to albumin and sex hormone binding globulin (SHBG) with only a tiny fraction circulating free. In practice, these dynamics mean that ~50% of circulating testosterone is able to enter target cells. Testosterone secretion also carries a minor but significant diurnal variation with lower

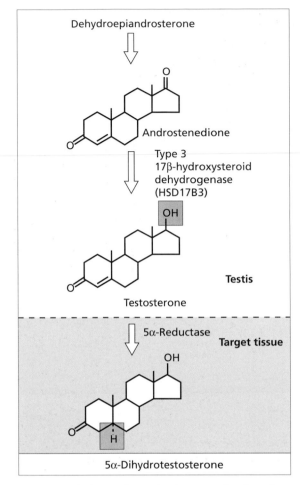

Dehydroepiandrosterone

Androstenedione

Type 3
17β-hydroxysteroid
dehydrogenase
(HSD17B3)

OH

Testis

Testosterone

5α-Reductase   **Target tissue**

OH

H

5α-Dihydrotestosterone

Figure 7.7 The biosynthesis of androgens in Leydig cells.

BOX 7.7 Major functions of the gonadotrophins

• FSH: spermatogenesis
• LH: androgen biosynthesis

spermatocytes then undergo the first meiotic division to form haploid secondary spermatocytes (review Fig. 2.1). The second meiotic division produces spermatids, which gradually mature into spermatozoa. An intimate association with the Sertoli ('nurse') cells is essential for this process. The spermatozoa are extruded into the lumen of the tubule and pass to the epididymis, following which they become mixed with the secretions of the seminal vesicle and prostate at the time of ejaculation.

Regulation of testicular function — the hypothalamic–anterior pituitary–testicular axis

The testis is regulated by the two pituitary gonadotrophins, follicle-stimulating hormone (FSH) and luteinizing hormone (LH), both of which act via cell surface G-protein coupled receptors linked to adenylate cyclase second messenger systems (review Chapter 3). Testosterone biosynthesis is stimulated by pulsatile LH, particularly at the rate-limiting step of cholesterol side-chain cleavage. This LH-induced testosterone, diffusing from the Leydig cells, acts along with FSH on the Sertoli cells to stimulate spermatogenesis (Box 7.7).

The secretion of LH and FSH is regulated by gonadotrophin-releasing hormone (GnRH; also known as LHRH), a decapeptide released by the hypothalamus in pulses every 90 min (Fig. 7.8). Without this pulsatility, gonadotrophin release fails; so much so that continuous GnRH can be used clinically to 'shut down' the reproductive endocrine axis in both men and women. Serum testosterone feeds back negatively to inhibit the release of LH (more than FSH), with a minor contribution from oestradiol and DHT.

The secretion of FSH from the gonadotrophs is selectively inhibited by the Sertoli cell protein, inhibin. Inhibin is comprised of α- and β-peptide chains, linked by disulphide bonds. Different types of β-chain generate two forms of the whole protein

values later in the day. Clinical measurements should be performed at 9 AM. As well as forming DHT, testosterone may also be aromatized to oestradiol in target cells; or, alternatively, metabolized to degradation products that are excreted in the urine.

Spermatogenesis

The primordial germ cells that invade the embryonic gonad enter mitotic arrest as spermatogonia until puberty, after which they continuously augment their numbers by mitotic division (Fig. 7.6). The basal stem cell population renews itself, whereas a second cohort moves into the adluminal compartment and divides to form primary spermatocytes. Primary

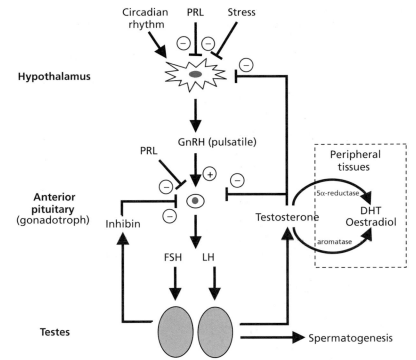

Figure 7.8 The hypothalamic–anterior pituitary–testicular axis. Negative feedback at the gonadotroph and hypothalamus is complex and involves: DHT and testosterone on LH; and inhibin, testosterone and oestrogen on FSH. Prolactin (PRL) exerts a negative influence on gonadotrophin release, probably via altering GnRH pulsatility and action.

called inhibin A and inhibin B. Inhibin B is of major physiological relevance, produced under stimulation by FSH to create a true negative feedback loop.

Phases of testicular function and reproductive development after birth

Only by understanding normal development can the endocrinologist correctly diagnose abnormality.

Neonatal life and childhood

During the first year of life gonadotrophin levels rise providing a surge in testosterone and inhibin secretion of uncertain significance. During childhood, gonadotrophin secretion is low due to very sensitive negative feedback from the testis. At adrenarche, minor signs of androgen action, such as some axillary and pubic hair growth, are normal (review Chapter 6). Occasional nocturnal pulses of LH and FSH occur in young children, the frequency and amplitude of which gradually increase with the advancing years. By 9–11 years, children normally experience regular nocturnal pulses of gonadotro-

phins due to increased GnRH secretion and gonadotroph sensitivity. Ultimately, sufficient sex steroid is present to initiate secondary sexual development and entrance into puberty.

Puberty

The onset of puberty can be detected by an increase in penis size and testicular volume, the latter due to maturation of the seminiferous tubules and the onset of spermatogenesis (Fig. 7.9). The Leydig cells also increase in number and size, and are stimulated to synthesize testosterone (Box 7.8).

Adulthood and old age

The effects of puberty are largely permanent—a broken voice does not regress if a patient becomes hypogonadal. Others, such as maintenance of muscle mass and sexual drive, require an ongoing supply of androgen. Beard growth is only likely to slow rather than stop if androgen is lost later in life. In old age testosterone usually remains in the normal range. However, levels do fall slightly and the circadian rhythm is diminished.

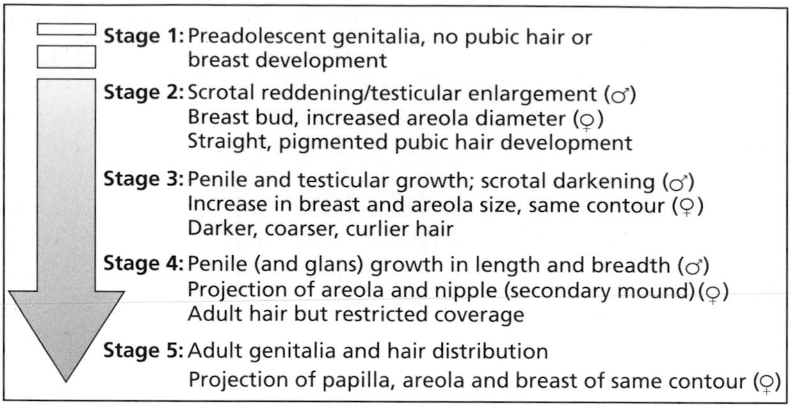

Stage 1: Preadolescent genitalia, no pubic hair or
breast development

Stage 2: Scrotal reddening/testicular enlargement (♂)
Breast bud, increased areola diameter (♀)
Straight, pigmented pubic hair development

Stage 3: Penile and testicular growth; scrotal darkening (♂)
Increase in breast and areola size, same contour (♀)
Darker, coarser, curlier hair

Stage 4: Penile (and glans) growth in length and breadth (♂)
Projection of areola and nipple (secondary mound) (♀)
Adult hair but restricted coverage

Stage 5: Adult genitalia and hair distribution
Projection of papilla, areola and breast of same contour (♀)

Figure 7.9 Tanner stages of pubertal development in males and females.

Box 7.8 The consequence of rising androgens

- Skeletal muscle growth
- Development of the larynx/deepening of the voice
- Pubic hair and beard growth
- Sebaceous gland activity, odorous sweat
- Thickened and pigmented skin over external genitalia
- Prostate, seminal vesicles and epididymis increase in size
- Epiphyseal fusion and termination of linear growth

BOX 7.9 Clinical features of male hypogonadism

- Postpuberty
  - loss of libido
  - subfertility/decreased sperm count
  - decreased muscle mass and exercise tolerance
  - decreased shaving frequency
  - smooth skin, loss of pubic hair
  - small, soft testes
  - gynaecomastia
  - osteoporosis
- At (or dating back to) puberty
  - failure of voice to 'break'
  - failure of testicular enlargement and penile growth
  - lack of scrotal pigmentation
  - eunuchoidism (arm span > height)
  - delayed bone age

Clinical disorders of the male reproductive system

The major clinical disorder of the testis is underactivity — 'hypogonadism'. Its presentation in adults may be due to primary (i.e. testicular), secondary (i.e. pituitary) or tertiary (i.e. hypothalamic) causes. In practice, the latter two sites can be considered together (Case History 7.1).

Primary hypogonadism

History and examination. From the normal physiology of androgen action and testicular function, it is possible to predict the consequences of hypogonadism (Box 7.9). The history should take care in documenting earlier development, including whether virilization was complete at birth. For instance, hypospadias might indicate androgen deficiency *in utero* (a useful question asks whether the patient

had to sit down to pass urine as a child). Similarly, it is important to ascertain whether testicular descent was complete or whether surgical intervention was necessary. Did the patient enter and progress through puberty at the same time as his peers? Examination should assess virilization and determine the existence and size of both testes correctly positioned in the scrotum.

Investigation and diagnosis. Assessment of the hypothalamic–anterior pituitary–testicular axis and the principles of negative feedback determine whether hypogonadism is primary or secondary/tertiary

(Box 7.10). Serum testosterone should be measured at 9 AM along with SHBG. An unusually low SHBG (e.g. in obesity or hypothyroidism) lowers total testosterone and can cause diagnostic confusion. Semen analysis would most probably show a diminished count in true hypogonadism (either azoospermia or oligospermia). After confirming primary hypogonadism, a precise diagnosis is needed (Box 7.11). Obtaining the karyotype may define chromosomal disorders. In addition, bone densitometry (a 'DEXA' scan) will assess the consequence of androgen deficiency on bone mineralization (see Chapter 9).

BOX 7.10 Distinguishing primary from secondary/ tertiary male hypogonadism

Low testosterone/ high LH and FSH = testicular problem (primary)
Low testosterone/ normal or low LH and FSH = pituitary/hypothalamic problem (secondary/tertiary)

BOX 7.11 The causes of male primary hypogonadism/ testicular failure

- Maldescended or undescended testes
  — common cause
  — 10% risk of malignancy
- Inflammation
  — mumps orchitis
  — trauma
- Postchemotherapy or postradiotherapy—semen storage advisable pretreatment
- Drugs—very rare, however, can occur with commonly used HMGCoA reductase inhibitors ('statins')
- Alcohol
- Chronic illness
- Autoimmune disorder
- Chromosomal disorders
  — Klinefelter syndrome (47,XXY; 1 : 500 males), possible intellectual impairment
  — Others rare (47,XYY; 46,XX with *SRY* translocation)
- Idiopathic/ unknown

Treatment. If it is missing, replace it: give testosterone. Due to first pass metabolism through the liver, oral preparations are relatively ineffective at delivering testosterone into the systemic circulation. The mainstay has been depot intramuscular injection, which lasts between 2 and 4 weeks. Newer preparations are designed to last longer. Other routes are transdermal (most effective as new gel preparations) or even absorption via the buccal mucosa. Monitoring replacement therapy should aim for a serum testosterone in the normal range and, most importantly, normalization of LH.

Supraphysiological androgen replacement is not without risk. Polycythaemia (a raised red blood cell count) increases the risk of thrombosis (monitor the full blood count and haematocrit); and stimulation of the prostate may promote prostatic hypertrophy or accelerate androgen-dependent prostatic cancer (prostate specific antigen has been used as a marker).

Secondary/tertiary hypogonadism

If the anterior pituitary gonadotrophs are underactive for any reason, failing FSH- and LH-dependent processes in the testis will cause androgen deficiency and oligospermia or azospermia. Commonly, this occurs as part of a wider syndrome of hypopituitarism (review Chapter 5); however, some conditions are specific to the hypothalamic–anterior pituitary–testicular axis. Kallman syndrome is due to mutation in a range of genes that results in aberrant migration of the GnRH-producing neurones and a failure of smell (anosmia). Specific causes of secondary hypogonadism include the use of anabolic steroids (when androgen deficiency would be spared), haemochromatosis or Prader–Willi syndrome.

In diagnosing secondary/tertiary hypogonadism, even normal gonadotrophin levels are inappropriate when accompanied by a low serum testosterone (i.e. the physiological response should be raised LH and FSH). All the other anterior pituitary hormone axes should be investigated. Although rarely performed, a GnRH test, where GnRH is injected and LH and FSH measured at baseline and after 30 min, distinguishes hypothalamic/tertiary (LH and FSH respond) from pituitary/secondary (no LH or FSH response) causes of hypogonadism.

CASE HISTORY 7.1

A 35-year-old man was referred to the endocrinologist after his partner made an appointment with the doctor. His partner had commented that the patient had no interest in sex, had lost interest in social life and was commonly asleep in the evenings. Total serum testosterone was 3 nmol/L with an SHBG at the upper end of normal. Both gonadotrophins were three times the upper limit of normal. On further questioning, the man, who was tall, had never really felt much sexual drive. His beard growth was patchy and he only needed to shave once a week. On examination, bilateral gynaecomastia was noted and both testes were small and soft.

> To where does the disorder localize?
> What further investigations are needed?
> What might the diagnosis be?
> What treatment and advice are needed?
> What would a DEXA scan indicate?

Answers, see p. 125

BOX 7.12 Testicular tumours of germ cell origin

- Embryonal carcinoma or teratocarcinoma, tends to affect children
- Seminoma, tends to affect in early adulthood or old age

Testicular tumours

Testicular tumours occur at all ages and may present to the endocrinologist. The type of tumour is age-dependent and incidence is raised in undescended testes (~5-fold) or ones that are dysfunctional (e.g. gonadal dysgenesis) (also see Chapter 10). Testicular germ cell tumours are associated with extra copies of the short arm of chromosome 12, where several genes important for germ cell proliferation are located (Box 7.12). Tumours of somatic cell types are less common (e.g. Sertoli or Leydig cell tumours).

Tumours usually present as painless enlargement of the testis but metastasize early. Failure to present to a physician is common and education to self-examine is as important for men as breast-care is for women. For functional Leydig cell tumours, abnormal sex steroid production is usually obvious as virilization (e.g. precocious puberty) or feminization (e.g. gynaecomastia). For nonseminomatous germ cell tumours, serum human chorionic gonadotrophin (hCG) and α-fetoprotein (AFP) are very useful as they fall with successful treatment and can be used as clinical markers.

Orchidectomy is important, if only for debulking, and may need to be bilateral. Chemotherapy is very successful and combinations of vinblastine, bleomycin, etopiside and cisplatin cure most tumours. If possible, cryopreservation of sperm allows future *in vitro* fertilization if surgery and chemotherapy render the patient infertile.

Gynaecomastia

Gynaecomastia, the development of breast tissue greater than 2 cm in males, can be physiological or represent an abnormal balance of sex steroid production or metabolism (Table 7.1). An enlargement of breast tissue at birth due to oestrogens of either placental or maternal origin is short-lived. A similar increase commonly follows puberty. It can be unilateral and painful, although it usually involutes by the end of the teenage years. Gynaecomastia can also occur in old age due to a variety of factors: a rise in SHBG; reduced androgen availability; or increased aromatization to oestrogen (review Fig. 2.5). During the latter two phases, the diagnosis of normal physiological variation should be one of exclusion, especially if onset is rapid and persistent. History (especially drug history), examination and investigation are important. Treatment is most commonly one of reassurance, withdrawal of offending medications or cosmetic surgery.

Table 7.1 Gynaecomastia

Causes of gynaecomastia	Investigations to consider
Physiological	General investigations:
Neonatal	serum testosterone, LH, FSH,
Pubertal	prolactin, thyroid function test,
Old age	urea and creatinine
Any cause of hypogonadism, e.g. Klinefelter	Karyogram
syndrome (47, XXY)	
Adrenal or testicular tumours secrete	Serum hCG, DHEA(S),
oestrogen or androgen (with peripheral	androstenedione, oestrogen
aromatase activity)	imaging
Liver disease	Liver function tests
Inadequate clearance and altered metabolism	
of steroid hormones	
Alcohol	
Drugs	
Oestrogens, antiandrogens (spironolactone),	
cimetidine, ACE inhibitors	

The female reproductive system

Puberty in females heralds the beginning of the female menstrual cycle when one mature germ cell usually reaches full maturity at intervals of ~28 days. This cycle has limited lifespan as only ~400 germ cells reach full maturity and ovulation. The cycle is associated with concordant changes in ovarian steroidogenesis that, in turn, influence the reproductive tract.

Ovarian morphology and function

Oogenesis begins in the fetal ovary, when, late in the first trimester, the germ cells enter the first stage of meiosis and arrest in prophase (review Fig. 2.1). Termed primary oocytes at this stage, they are surrounded by a layer of steroid-producing granulosa cells and together constitute 'primordial follicles' (Fig. 7.10). There are ~6 to 7 million primordial follicles at 20 weeks of gestation, following which their number declines inexorably. At birth, there are ~2 million, and by puberty only 300 000. Menopause marks the depletion of germ cells within the ovaries.

Formation of the Graafian follicle

At the beginning of a menstrual cycle, the granulosa cells in 10 to 20 early follicles proliferate to form pri-

mary and then secondary follicles (Fig. 7.10). In any one menstrual cycle, usually only one of the follicles matures fully. Stromal cells become arranged around the outside to form the well-vascularized 'theca'. At midcycle, the Graafian follicle ruptures ('ovulation') and the oocyte is liberated and enters the fimbriated opening of the Fallopian tube. If the ovum meets a spermatozoan and is fertilized, embryonic development starts. Arrival into the uterine cavity is aided by the ciliated wafting of the inside of the Fallopian tube. By this time, the embryo has usually reached the blastocyst stage, at which point it implants into the uterine endometrium. If the ovum is not fertilized, it dies.

Formation of the corpus luteum

The remaining structures of the ruptured Graafian follicle play a critical role for the second half of the menstrual cycle. The cells proliferate, enlarge and fill the collapsed antrum of the follicle. This new structure becomes a solid, round mass of steroidogenic cells called the corpus luteum; initially red, but which matures to a yellowish colour (Fig. 7.10). If fertilization and blastocyst implantation do not occur, the corpus luteum, having been active for ~2 weeks, dies. The luteal cells cease synthesizing steroids and undergo programmed cell death ('apoptosis'), and the whole structure is replaced with scar tissue (the

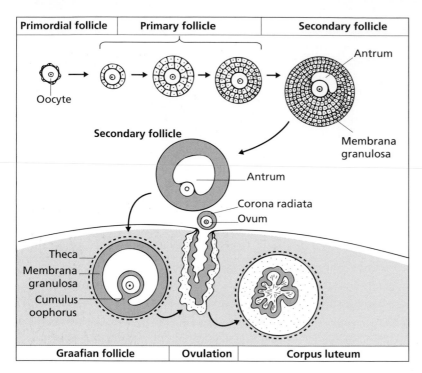

Primordial follicle	Primary follicle	Secondary follicle

Oocyte

Secondary follicle

Antrum

Membrana granulosa

Antrum

Corona radiata

Ovum

Theca

Membrana granulosa

Cumulus oophorus

Graafian follicle	Ovulation	Corpus luteum

Figure 7.10 Follicle growth, maturation and ovulation. The entire process takes place close to the ovarian surface. The outer steroid-producing granulosa cells divide and grow to form a multilayered membrana granulosa. The appearance of a liquid-filled antrum defines the transition from primary to secondary follicle. The antrum enlarges creating a stalk of cells (the 'cumulus oophorus'), by which the oocyte remains attached to the membrana granulosa. Stromal cells form the outer steroidogenic theca cell layer. The entire structure is now termed a Graafian follicle, which ruptures at ovulation, expelling the ovum surrounded by a layer of cells, the corona radiata. The collapsed follicle becomes the corpus luteum.

corpus albicans). However, if implantation occurs, the corpus luteum increases in size and remains active during the early weeks of pregnancy until the placenta assumes steroidogenic function. As such, the corpus luteum maintains the uterine endometrium in early pregnancy.

Ovarian steroidogenesis, the hypothalamic–anterior pituitary–ovarian axis and the menstrual cycle

During reproductive years, ovarian hormone production accompanies egg development on an approximate 4-week cycle (Box 7.13). In the absence of fertilization, the cycle is terminated by the restricted lifespan of the corpus luteum.

The most potent oestrogen in humans is oestradiol. Its biosynthesis relies on two somatic cell types, the theca cell and the granulosa cell, packaging steroidogenesis within the developing follicle (Fig. 7.11). Oestradiol can also be generated from oestrone by HSD17B1 activity. Progesterone biosynthesis is relatively straightforward. Removal of the cholesterol side chain generates pregnenolone in theca

> **BOX 7.13 Ovarian hormone action during the menstrual cycle: 'a cycle of two halves'**
>
> - Oestrogen: prepares the egg for release during the 1st half—the follicular phase
> - Progesterone: maintains pregnancy ('progestational') in the 2nd half—the luteal phase
>
> Therefore, the timing of clinical assessment is important:
>
> Day 1: first day of vaginal bleeding from preceding cycle
> Day 2–5: the time to measure FSH, LH and oestradiol
> Day 21: the time to measure progesterone

cells, which is converted to progesterone by HSD3B activity (review Fig. 2.5).

The follicular phase: the control of follicle development. The menstrual cycle is regulated by the hypothalamic–anterior pituitary–ovarian axis and intraovarian mechanisms (Fig. 7.12). At the beginning of each

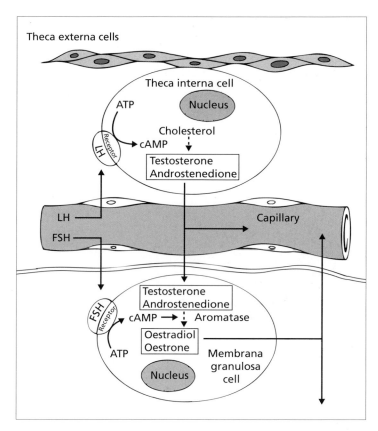

Figure 7.11 The two-cell biosynthesis of oestrogens. LH stimulates receptors on the theca interna cells via cAMP to synthesize testosterone and androstenedione. These either pass into the local capillaries or cross the basement membrane into the adjacent granulosa cells. The granulosa cells are stimulated by FSH to aromatize testosterone and androstenedione to oestradiol and oestrone, respectively. These female hormones enter the circulation or pass into the antrum of the follicle and act on the oocyte. The formal name for aromatase is CYP19 (review Fig. 2.5).

cycle, under FSH stimulation, a cohort of ~20 primary follicles begin to develop into secondary follicles, which produce oestradiol. In turn, oestradiol increases FSH receptor expression on the surface of the proliferating granulosa cells. Now is the time for clinical investigation of serum LH, FSH and oestradiol levels (Box 7.13). The oestradiol and inhibin secretion begin to suppress FSH production from the anterior pituitary. As the concentration of FSH falls (Fig. 7.13), only the ripening follicles with the highest concentration of FSH receptors are able to sustain development, while the rest undergo atrophy and regress. Thus, progressively, one dominant follicle is selected, around which theca cells develop under the influence of LH.

Ovulation. Midcycle is associated with a surge of LH and, to a lesser extent, FSH from the pituitary (Fig. 7.13). The LH surge lasts ~36h, allowing for the final

maturation of the oocyte and the stimulation of factors that aid follicle rupture. The principal cause for the gonadotrophin surge is an alteration in oestradiol feedback at the pituitary. In general, pulsatile GnRH stimulates gonadotrophin release, while inhibin (both types A and B) and oestradiol are restrictive. However, this alters temporarily at midcycle. As the dominant follicle ripens, oestrogen output increases and at ~day 12, a threshold of oestradiol is exceeded. If maintained for a further 36h, feedback temporarily switches at the gonadotroph from negative to positive. Now, high levels of oestradiol drive further gonadotrophin secretion, creating the surge that culminates in ovulation.

The luteal phase. After ovulation, the corpus luteum contains theca interna cells trapped between granulosa cells. This structure produces progesterone under the stimulus of low level LH. Indeed, a serum

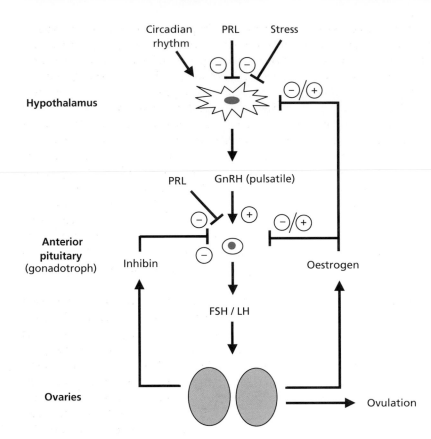

Figure 7.12 The hypothalamic–anterior pituitary–ovarian axis and its variable feedback.

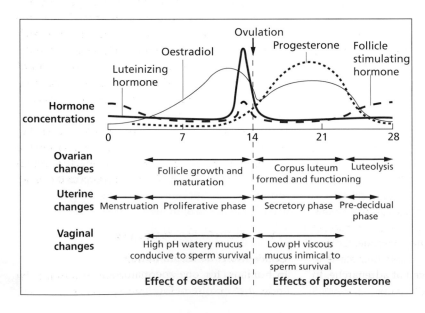

Figure 7.13 Changes in the 28-day menstrual cycle. The start of menstruation is day 1 of a new cycle.

progesterone measurement at day 21 that exceeds 30 nmol/L is a valuable marker of preceding ovulation (Box 7.13). However, the corpus luteum also secretes oestradiol, which resumes negative feedback on LH and FSH output (Fig. 7.12). By ~day 25, the falling LH is no longer able to maintain adequate steroidogenesis. The fall in progesterone leads to loss of the endometrium and menstruation follows. This drop in oestradiol and progesterone also removes negative feedback from the pituitary, which, under the ongoing stimulus of GnRH pulses, resumes secretion of FSH and LH. So begins the next cycle.

If implantation of a blastocyst occurs at ~day 20, the resulting trophoblast begins to secrete hCG, a glycoprotein hormone that acts like LH at the LH receptor. hCG maintains the corpus luteum and, in the face of continuing oestradiol and progesterone, menstruation is postponed.

Cyclical effects on the uterus and vagina. The changing ovarian steroid output causes cyclical alterations in the uterine endometrium and the rest of the female genital tract (Figs 7.13 and 7.14). The increased secretion of oestradiol at the start of a cycle stimulates the repair and proliferation of the endometrium and the expression of receptors for progesterone and oestradiol. After ovulation, the rise in progesterone prepares the endometrium for potential implantation. It doubles in thickness, and the simple tubular glands become tortuous and saccular. However, with corpus luteum failure ('luteolysis'), the endometrium breaks down, sloughs off and causes menstrual bleeding. The cyclical hormones also alter the consistency and pH of the cervical mucus.

Phases of ovarian function and reproductive development after birth

Puberty. Puberty sees the transition from immature to fully developed, fertile female endocrinology (Table 7.2). Although the start of the growth spurt comes first, the most obvious sign is breast development (classified by the endocrinologist Tanner; Fig. 7.9). Stages 1 to 4 are dependent on oestrogen; the last phase, Stage 5, also requires progesterone. Coincident with breast development, pubic hair starts to grow. This may have commenced at adrenarche. In fact, pubic hair growth is actually largely under the influence of androgen from both adrenal precursors and the ovary, however, it usually progresses in parallel with oestrogen-stimulated breast development. There are also oestrogen-dependent changes in vaginal size, mucosal appearance and pH. The labia thicken and 'rugate', a similar process to that which occurs in male scrotal skin. Menarche, the onset of periods, usually occurs during Tanner Stage 4.

Puberty in females also marks a transition from nocturnal pulsatile secretion of gonadotrophins to the 24-h pulsatility that is necessary for reproductive capacity. The first few cycles after menarche are potentially anovulatory and slightly irregular, but a regular pattern should emerge relatively quickly. Its absence is a strong indicator to support the diagnosis of polycystic ovarian syndrome (see later).

Menopause. Fertility tends to decline progressively once a woman has entered her thirties. Thus, the menopause may be preceded for a number of years by less regular ovarian function. Some cycles release multiple ova interspersed with spells of anovulation. During this premenopausal stage, gonadotrophin levels can become somewhat increased, providing a clinical indicator of 'ovarian reserve' and a marker for the likely success of IVF therapy. All of which is normal, or a variation thereof, and culminates in the menopause, defined as the last menstrual period, usually near 50 years of age. At this juncture, the ovaries cease to function cyclically due to an exhaustion of primordial follicles. The decline in oestrogen and inhibin relieves negative feedback and concentrations of LH and FSH rise several-fold.

The fall in oestradiol production causes atrophy of the vaginal mucosa and breasts and, for reasons that are not entirely clear, bone mass begins to decline more rapidly. When acute, the loss of oestrogen causes characteristic flushing attacks. After the menopause, the only source of oestrogen is from the adrenal substrate androstenedione, which is aromatized by CYP19 in peripheral locations to the weak oestrone.

The endocrinology of pregnancy

Conception and implantation

In humans, for one spermatozoon to fertilize the ovum, ~25 to 30 million are ejaculated as a few

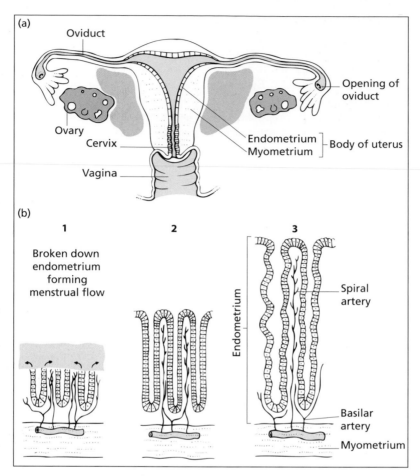

Figure 7.14 Changes in the uterine endometrium during the menstrual cycle. (a) The female reproductive organs. The body of the uterus consists of an inner endometrial layer and a surrounding smooth muscle myometrium. (b) Changes in the uterine gland during the menstrual cycle. (1) Breakdown of the endometrium (days 1–3) when the outer two-thirds is shed to form the menstrual flow. The basal third of the endometrium persists and its cells divide and grow over the exposed tissue (arrows) to repair the endometrium. (2) During the oestrogenic proliferative phase (days 3–14), the uterine glands grow in length as the endometrioum thickens. (3) During the progestational secretory phase (days 14–28), the uterine glands double in length and become tortuous and sacculated. Stromal oedema increases to a maximum by day 21, the approximate time of blastocyst implantation. During the last 2–3 days of this phase, the spiral blood vessels vasoconstrict and rupture. Lakes of blood form in the stromal tissue. Endometrial breakdown follows.

millilitres of semen into the vagina. From here, they traverse the cervix and body of the uterus en masse (referred to as the 'sperm train' in some species) to reach the fallopian tube and encounter the ovum. Hydrolytic enzymes from the acrosomes of many spermatozoa loosen the corona radiata (Fig. 7.10). However, as soon as one sperm has entered the ovum, a series of reactions block multiple penetra-

tions ('polyspermy'). The fertilized ovum is transported along the fallopian tube by peristaltic contractions and the action of ciliated epithelial cells, during which time local environmental factors are likely to be important (Box 7.14) and, if all goes well, mitosis has created a morula of ~16 cells. The window period for fertilization is relatively short, probably 72 hours or so, based on: favourable cervical mucus for sperm

Table 7.2 Different phases of ovarian function and its effects

Phase	Oestrogen	Progesterone
Puberty	Stimulates the growth of the uterus and breast; determines the female figure via fat deposition Contributes to closure of the epiphyses Exerts important effects on personality and sexual responsiveness	Aids transition from Tanner Stage 4 to 5
Menstrual cycle	Follicular phase: Causes endometrial proliferation and secretion of clear, high pH cervical mucus; conducive to sperm survival Matures the vaginal epithelium Causes positive- and negative-feedback on the hypothalamus and anterior pituitary	Luteal phase: Causes a rise in body temperature; the production of a secretory endometrium; and secretion of thick, low pH cervical mucus — not conducive to sperm survival Negative-feedback on the hypothalamus and pituitary
Pregnancy	Causes growth of the breast duct system and myometrial hypertrophy together with fluid retention and increased uterine blood flow	Causes a reduction of contractions and reduced smooth muscle tone Causes a rise in body temperature and growth of the alveoli of the breasts
General cellular effects	Enhances receptors for progesterone (i.e. oestrogen is needed for progesterone to exert its intracellular actions)	Stimulates HSD17B isoforms, which leads to inactivation of oestradiol to weak oestrone

---

BOX 7.14 Local environmental factors for early embryo growth and implantation

- A good fallopian and intrauterine nutritional/metabolic milieu (e.g. euglycaemia)
- A 'receptive' endometrium for implantation

Failure of these attributes is likely to contribute to subfertility

---

penetration; the lifespan of the spermatozoan in the female genital tract; and the presence of the ovum in the fallopian tube.

The fetoplacental unit

Successful implantation leads to development of the trophoblast, which begins to secrete the 'LH-like' hCG into the maternal bloodstream (Fig. 7.15). hCG

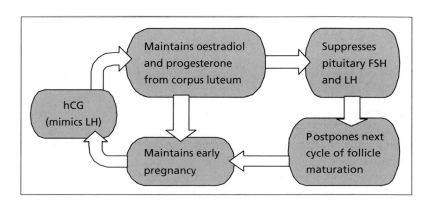

Figure 7.15 The role of hCG in postponing menstruation.

is excreted into the maternal urine, where it forms the basis of most pregnancy tests. Levels are sufficient to be detected by urine strip assays soon after a period is 'missed' (i.e. equivalent to ~3 weeks of embryo development). The date of pregnancy ('gestation') is from the last menstrual period (LMP). Thus for ~4-week menstrual cycle:

LMP age = true fetal age + 2 weeks

Towards the end of the first trimester, a variety of steroidogenic activities takes place in the fetus. This 'fetoplacental unit' synthesizes pregnenolone in both the placenta and the fetal adrenal cortex (Fig. 7.16). From pregnenolone, the fetal adrenal synthesizes DHEA and its sulphated derivative, DHEAS. DHEA serves as substrate for a variety of enzymatic reactions that give rise to the different oestrogens: oestradiol, oestrone and oestriol. The latter can be detected from week 12 in maternal urine (Fig. 7.16). With the onset of steroid production by the placenta, the corpus luteum gradually regresses. Levels of progesterone and oestriol continue to rise throughout pregnancy.

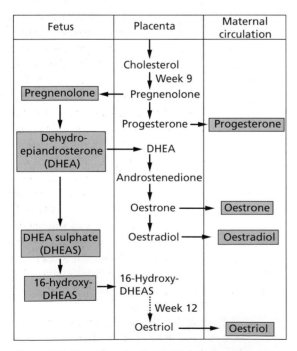

Figure 7.16 Steroid production in the fetoplacental unit.

Endocrine changes during pregnancy, parturition and lactation

Whereas the need for placental function is irrefutable, the function of the fetal adrenal is intriguing. Fetuses with congenital absence of the adrenal cortex develop normally *in utero*, implying that it is dispensable. Nevertheless, it is incredibly active, synthesizing large quantities of sex steroid precursors and, approaching term, cortisol (Box 7.15). Cortisol stimulates the synthesis of surfactant proteins, which decrease surface tension in the lungs. This allows the fluid-filled alveoli to expand with air at birth and permit efficient gas exchange. The mechanism is so important that dexamethasone, a synthetic gluco-

---

> **BOX 7.15 Endocrine alterations during pregnancy, parturition and lactation**
>
> Pregnancy
> - Maternal:
>   - increased heart rate / cardiac output rises by ~30–50% due to the hormonal milieu and placental circulation
>   - hypertrophy / hyperplasia of lactotrophs synthesizing prolactin
>   - thyroid volume increases, possibly due to hCG (partially mimics TSH)
>   - increased pancreatic islet size / increased beta cells
>   - increased adrenal cortisol output
> - Fetal:
>   - development and growth due to the thyroid, insulin and GH–IGF axes
>   - 'maturation' of the fetal lung by cortisol near term
>
> Parturition
> - Oxytocin from the posterior pituitary increases by positive feedback as the fetus descends the birth canal and distends the vagina
> - Local prostaglandins stimulate the early uterine contractions
>
> Lactation
> - High oestrogen and progesterone during pregnancy inhibit lactation
> - Postpartum, lactation relies on continued prolactin (and cortisol)
> - Oxytocin, released in response to the suckling reflex, stimulates milk ejection

corticoid that crosses the placenta, is administered to the mother in premature labour to decrease the incidence of respiratory distress syndrome.

Breast development, called 'thelarche', had started ~2 years before menarche, under the influence of ovarian oestrogens, which stimulate the proliferation of the duct system and the accumulation of fat in the breast. In early pregnancy, oestrogens stimulate further growth of the ducts and breast tissue. Later on, glucocorticoids from the adrenal, prolactin from the anterior pituitary and placental lactogen (a prolactin-like hormone from the placenta) are required for the induction of enzymes needed for milk production (Box 7.15). So long as breast-feeding is continued, the elevated prolactin inhibits pituitary gonadotrophin release, thus reducing fertility. Even though it is unreliable for an individual, globally it is an important contraceptive.

The signal for parturition after ~ 9 months is still not entirely clear. However, as progesterone levels fall, two factors, oxytocin and prostaglandins, are important for expulsion of the fetus (Box 7.15).

Clinical disorders of the female reproductive system

Endocrine disorders that affect the ovary tend to manifest with loss of ovulatory cycles and absence of the periods (amenorrhoea) (Box 7.16 and Case History 7.2). Although somewhat arbitrary as the same pathology can cause both, amenorrhoea can be classified as either primary or secondary.

BOX 7.16 Amenorrhoea

In the UK:
- ~95% of girls have undergone menarche by 15 years
- ~50% have done so by 12½ years

The absence of periods is called amenorrhoea:
- Primary amenorrhoea if menstruation has not started by the age of 16
- Secondary amenorrhoea if, after starting, menstruation has been absent for >6 months

The first question to address: is oestrogen present or absent?

The commonest cause is temporary hypothalamic secondary amenorrhoea when oestrogen is absent

---

Amenorrhoea with absent oestrogen

History, examination and investigation. The commonest cause of amenorrhoea is hypothalamic, and is usually secondary and transient. The human female body has evolved to suboptimal or challenging conditions, as subtle as athletics training or 'stress' (for instance, exams or bullying), by altering GnRH pulsatility and silencing the reproductive cycle. Remove the cause of the problem and the menstrual cycle returns. Questioning such matters requires time and sensitivity from the endocrinologist. Broader questioning of endocrine pathology addresses the other pituitary axes, including potential galactorrhoea from excess prolactin (Table 7.3). Assessment is needed of whether the ovaries ever functioned. Are there menopausal symptoms, most clearly demonstrated by hot flushing, due to the acute withdrawal of oestrogen? Is there any breast development? Are there features of Turner syndrome (shield chest/widely spaced nipples, webbed neck, and increased carrying angle)?

Oestradiol may be very low or undetectable:

- *If the aetiology is ovarian,* lack of negative feedback causes a pronounced rise in gonadotrophins into the post-menopausal range (several-fold the upper limit of normal; Table 7.3). Ultrasound can determine the presence and structure of the ovaries. A karyogram excludes gross chromosomal abnormality (e.g. Turner syndrome) and screening is increasingly available for other causes of premature ovarian failure (menopause before 40 years of age), such as fragile X syndrome.

- *If the pathology is in the hypothalamus or anterior pituitary,* gonadotrophin values are low or inappropriately normal (Table 7.3; review Chapter 5). Whether they rise adequately after GnRH administration might distinguish pathology in the hypothalamus (they do) from the anterior pituitary (they do not). In younger patients, congenital deficiency needs to be excluded, as does craniopharyngioma, a histologically benign but erosive tumour of the cells thought to have lined Rathke's pouch. The anterior pituitary is best delineated by magnetic resonance imaging (MRI; see Fig. 4.8).

Treatment. If it is missing, replace it. Lack of oestrogen for prolonged spells leads to bone demineralization and risk of future osteoporosis. If persistent for 6

Table 7.3 Approaching amenorrhoea with absent oestrogen

History and examination
Compassion and time are needed to elicit features of anorexia or bulimia nervosa, or bullying. Is there excessive physical exercise? Is there undiagnosed systemic illness, e.g. coeliac disease? Have the ovaries ever functioned? Question for a history of menopause-like flushing and look for evidence of breast development.

Differential diagnosis

Categories	Examples
Hypothalamic or anterior pituitary deficiency— indicated by low or normal LH and FSH	Simple constitutional delay (i.e. not pathological)
	Transient, hypothalamic inhibition from 'higher' centres (e.g. excessive exercise, anorexia nervosa or stress)
	Head trauma
	Cranial irradiation
	Kallman syndrome (associated anosmia)
	Congenital hypopituitarism
	Tumour of the pituitary gland region (e.g. craniopharyngioma, non-functioning adenoma, or hormone-secreting tumour)
	Hyperprolactinaemia (e.g. dopamine antagonist drugs, prolactinoma or stalk compression)
Ovarian (i.e. lack of follicles)—indicated by high LH and FSH, consider investigating the karyotype	Absent or rudimentary ovaries, e.g. Turner syndrome (45,XO) or disorders of sex determination
	Damage, e.g. chemotherapy, radiotherapy or autoimmune destruction
	Premature exhaustion of follicles, e.g. fragile X syndrome

CASE HISTORY 7.2

A 25-year-old woman is referred because of galactorrhoea that occurs spontaneously and has become socially embarrassing. Her periods have stopped and she is sexually inactive. Serum prolactin is found to be 4500–6000 U/L on repeat 'stress-free' investigations.

What other questions need to be asked?
What is the most likely diagnosis?
Would serum oestradiol be high or low?
What other investigations need to be considered?
What drug treatment will lower the prolactin and most likely stop the galactorrhoea?

Answers, see p. 125

---

months or more, the reproductive hormones should be replaced, most commonly by using female sex hormones as hormone replacement therapy (HRT). Unopposed oestrogen increases the risk of endometrial carcinoma: if the uterus is present, HRT must include a progestogen. Specific details for treating anterior pituitary pathology are covered in Chapter 5.

The endocrinologist needs to be mindful of the emotionally charged reaction that loss of fertility can precipitate. If amenorrhoea is ovarian and permanent (i.e. no ova left) before the age of 40 years, it is called 'premature ovarian failure (POF)'. However, the uterus may still be capable of carrying a pregnancy following egg donation. Alternatively, if the problem is in the anterior pituitary or hypothalamus, the ovaries may still release ova upon stimulation. Both scenarios require referral to fertility specialists.

Amenorrhoea with oestrogen present

Polycystic ovarian syndrome and other causes

The commonest cause of decreased or irregular menstrual frequency with detectable oestrogen is polycystic ovarian syndrome (PCOS). Although its defining criteria remain controversial, it is encapsulated by amenorrhoea with relative clinical or biochemical androgen excess in the absence of other causes (Table 7.4).

The syndrome is linked to insulin action. The incidence of impaired glucose tolerance (IGT), gestational (GDM) and type 2 diabetes (T2DM) is increased in individuals with PCOS, although care is needed not to miss the overlap with Cushing syndrome. The pathology of PCOS is incompletely understood; however, it includes ovarian 'insulin resistance', detected more broadly by an increased circulating insulin and C-peptide level. Although PCOS associates with increased weight, simple obesity alone raises insulin resistance and is associated with decreased menstrual frequency and relative subfertility. This leads to difficulty distinguishing a common scenario of simple weight gain in the woman's twenties from a true genetic predisposition to PCOS. A key question to address this is whether, prior to weight gain, periods were regular. A persistent tendency to irregular periods is found in PCOS.

Investigations should exclude other curable endocrinopathies. No test is diagnostic of PCOS; however, the ratio of LH to FSH tends to be increased. Low SHBG associates with hyperinsulinism, but is also prevalent in simple obesity. The androgen excess of PCOS is both ovarian and adrenal in origin. However, a particularly high DHEA or DHEAS may suggest an adrenal tumour. A serum testosterone >4 nmol/L significantly increases the risk of tumour, especially if supported by true virilization, which is very uncommon in PCOS (Table 7.4). Ultrasound can help to exclude ovarian tumours (the best views of the pelvic anatomy are transvaginal). Observing multiple, small cysts, as 'PCOS' suggests, is not discriminatory. Similarly, absence of cysts does not exclude the diagnosis of PCOS.

Treatment is largely tailored according to the patient's needs (Table 7.4); however, the need for regular shedding of the endometrial lining is particularly important. Progesterone is lacking due to anovulation. Chronic 'unopposed' oestrogen increases the risk of endometrial carcinoma ~sixfold. 'Withdrawal bleeds' can be induced by a weeklong course of progesterone every 3 to 4 months. At the end of each course, the fall in serum progesterone simulates the normal end to the menstrual cycle and provokes endometrial breakdown. Fertility treatment can begin with metformin, although if this is insufficient, specialist referral is warranted (see later).

Other female reproductive endocrinology referrals

Hirsuitism

Excess hair growth in women ('hirsuitism') is a common referral to the endocrinologist. The first distinction is between androgen-dependent and independent growth. In the latter instance, hypothyroidism and causative drugs (e.g. phenytoin) should be excluded, after which effective treatment can be difficult.

As with PCOS, it is critical to exclude curable endocrinopathies, such as androgen-secreting tumours, by thorough history and examination that searches for signs of virilization. Some forms of the combined oral contraceptive pill possess androgenic activity. Serum 9 AM testosterone helps to distinguish between androgen-secreting tumours (usually >4 nmol/L) and increased sensitivity to normal circulating testosterone (<2.5 nmol/L).

Individuals vary in their sensitivity to androgens. Total serum testosterone is a blunt measure of androgen action in target cells. Not only is type 2 5α-reductase required for conversion to the more active DHT (Fig. 7.7), but the AR also varies between individuals due to variability ('polymorphism') in its first exon. Blocking DHT production (e.g. by 5α-reductase inhibitors, such as finasteride) or AR occupancy (e.g. by antagonists, such as spironolactone) can be effective. Waxing, plucking, laser therapy and the application of new creams that inhibit hair follicle cell division are also valid strategies that are free from systemic side-effects.

Galactorrhoea

Inappropriate milk production outside of breastfeeding is common in young women and results

Table 7.4 Polycystic ovarian syndrome

The key principle

Exclude other curable endocrinopathies with overlapping phenotype

This requires a full history, examination and investigations. Never miss pregnancy as a cause of amenorrhoea in the presence of circulating oestrogen.

Making the diagnosis and treatment

Were periods ever regular?	
No	Supports the diagnosis of PCOS
Yes	Suspicion raised of:
	An androgen-secreting ovarian or adrenal tumour, especially if the patient is virilized, e.g. deepened voice and clitoromegaly
	Cushing syndrome (see Chapter 6), especially if physical stigmata, hypertension or glucose intolerance are present
	Hyperprolactinaemia
	Thyroid dysfunction
Other features to detect:	
Amenorrhoea/oligomenorrhoea and reproduction	Loss of ovulatory cycles decreases fertility
	Suboptimal metabolic milieu increases spontaneous abortion even if pregnancy is achieved
Relative androgen excess	Acne
	Hirsuitism—commonly on face, chest and above the 'bikini line' to umbilicus
	Frontal hair loss
Insulin resistance	Obesity or significant difficulty keeping an ideal body mass index
	Positive family history for type 2 or gestational diabetes
	Acanthosis nigricans
Investigations:	
To exclude other causes	A pregnancy test
	Low-dose dexamethasone suppression test or 24-hour urinary free cortisol (Cushing syndrome)
	Serum 17α-hydroxyprogesterone (late onset congenital adrenal hyperplasia)
	Thyroid function test (hypo or hyperthyroidism)
	Serum prolactin (hyperprolactinaemia)
	Ovarian ultrasound (helps exlude an androgen-secreting tumour of the ovary)
To characterize biochemical hyperandrogenism	Serum testosterone, SHBG, androstenedione, DHEA(S)
To characterize any wider metabolic disturbance	Fasting glucose or oral glucose tolerance test (IGT or T2DM)
	Liver function tests—hepatitic markers (e.g. ALT)
	Liver ultrasound may show fatty infiltration
	Fasting lipid analysis—mixed dyslipidaemia common
Treatment options and advice:	
According to patient's wishes. . . .	
Regular menstruation and contraception	Combined oral contraceptive pill
To restore the normal cycle or improve fertility	Insulin sensitizers, e.g. metformin (may also help weight loss)
Hirsutism	See later section
Simple reassurance	Exclude other curable endocrinopathies
Promoted by the endocrinologist. . . .	
Uterine 'health'	Regular shedding of the endometrium every 3–4 months
Health education/information for the future	The decline in fertility with age is exacerbated in PCOS, plan pregnancy earlier rather than later
	Maximal 'cardiovascular fitness' and weight control will improve symptoms and minimize risk of future IGT, GDM and T2DM

from excess prolactin or increased sensitivity to its action. Hyperprolactinaemia requires assessment of the anterior pituitary (see Chapter 5) and the exclusion of pregnancy. Galactorrhoea with normal serum prolactin is due to increased breast sensitivity and responds well to dopamine agonists, such as cabergoline.

Hormone-dependent gynaecological disorders
Covered in greater depth in *Essential Reproduction*, endometriosis and uterine fibroids (leiomyomata) are hormone-dependent and prevalent in women during the reproductive lifespan.

Endometriosis is the presence of endometrial tissue outside of the uterine cavity and may affect the ovaries, broad ligament, or other peritoneal surfaces. The tissue contains oestrogen receptors that mediate proliferation and hypertrophy. This can cause chronic pelvic pain or, if affecting the fallopian tube, subfertility. In addition to surgery, decreased oestrogen production (e.g. by continuous GnRH agonist or the progesterone-only contraceptive pill) can help.

Fibroids are benign tumours of the myometrium (the muscle layer of the uterus) and respond to oestrogen and, potentially, progesterone. Hormone modulation is most likely of short-term benefit, whereas surgery offers more definitive treatment. Total hysterectomy ends fertility. However, local laparoscopic resection can preserve the uterus, albeit with increased risk of rupture in future pregnancy.

Menopausal issues and hormone replacement therapy
HRT in the menopausal period can overcome the acute symptoms of oestrogen withdrawal, typified by hot flushes. The duration and relative benefit of HRT therapy is contentious (Box 7.17). Recent studies suggest that it is best limited to no more than 5 years; otherwise, the increased risk of cardiovascular disease and breast cancer may outweigh potential benefits. In the presence of a uterus, oestrogen needs to be combined with progesterone, which reduces ER

BOX 7.17 HRT is not protective against future osteoporosis and fracture risk

- Bone mineral density is preserved during HRT, but rapidly lost upon cessation

---

number in target cells and increases inactivation of oestradiol to oestrone. Given intermittently, this combined therapy can produce withdrawal bleeding.

Pubertal disorders

Children with endocrine abnormalities causing pubertal precocity or delay must be distinguished from those who simply represent the extremes of the normal range. Even where observation may be appropriate in the latter group, there are major psychosocial consequences of puberty occurring out of keeping with the patient's peer group. Early puberty, subject to ethnic differences, also induces the growth spurt, which ultimately causes early epiphyseal fusion and short adult height.

Precocious puberty

Precocity can be due to either the normal process, driven by GnRH pulses, occurring abnormally early ('central' or 'true') or aetiology extrinsic to the hypothalamic–anterior pituitary–gonadal axis that results in sex steroid biosynthesis (Table 7.5). Precocity may even be due to oestrogen in boys and androgen in girls, leading to inappropriate feminization or virilization respectively ('contrasexual precocity'). The goal is to treat underlying causes and avoid significant disruption of psychosocial development or the attainment of predicted final height. It needs to focus on the individual cause. For true precocity, continuous GnRH can be used to suppress the pituitary gonadotrophins. For isolated premature breast development ('thelarche'), reassurance is appropriate.

Delayed puberty

As well as entry into puberty being slow, delay may also occur within pubertal stages (Box 7.18). The commonest cause is constitutional or chronic illness when puberty may be late, but bone age is also appropriately delayed. Delayed puberty may also be a reflection of gonadal failure when serum gonadotrophins are raised and sex steroids are low. Ovarian ultrasound may show streak gonads and a karyogram might indicate Turner syndrome (45,XO). Secretion of pituitary gonadotrophins can be assessed in response to GnRH. In boys, a rise in testosterone after hCG injection indicates normal testicular function. If necessary, treatment is with sex steroids to induce pubertal changes with close monitoring of pubertal progression and growth. In females, progesterone is added once uterine bleeding starts (Case History 7.3).

BOX 7.18 Delayed puberty defined as >2 standard deviations above the mean age

Boys = >16 years of age
Girls = >14 years

Table 7.5 Precocious puberty

Definition	>2 standard deviations below the mean age
	    Boys = <9 years of age
	    Girls = <7 years

Types	'True' or 'central'
	    Idiopathic
	    Disruption to the central nervous system (e.g. tumour/infection/trauma)
	Gonadotrophin-independent isosexual
	    hCG-secreting tumour
	    Androgen excess in males, e.g. CAH or tumour of the adrenal cortex or testis
	    Genetic, e.g. McCune–Albright syndrome
	Gonadotrophin-independent contrasexual
	    Male, e.g. a tumour with aromatase activity that generates oestrogens
	    Female, e.g. androgen excess due to CAH or a tumour of the adrenal cortex or ovary

History	Age and order of onset, e.g. breast growth/body odour/genital enlargement/menstruation Are there other medical conditions? Is it familial? Has there been a recent growth spurt or weight gain?
Examination	Are there signs of secondary sexual development, e.g. breast or pubic hair growth? Are the changes out of keeping with the child's sex? Full neurological examination 'Café-au-lait' spots (patches of brown skin pigment) may indicate McCune–Albright syndrome (review Fig. 3.14)
Investigation	Serum testosterone, oestradiol, androstenedione and DHEA or DHEAS 17α-hydroxyprogesterone (to exclude CAH due to 21-hydroxylase deficiency) GnRH test—LH and FSH at 0 mins and 30 mins after GnRH Tumour markers, e.g. AFP and hCG X-ray to estimate bone age

CASE HISTORY 7.3

A 15-year-old girl was referred because of a failure to commence periods. At consultation, her mother frequently interrupted her daughter and strongly wished for 'something to be done'. The patient declined examination but was noted to be generally well looking if rather short for predicted family height. She agreed to some blood tests, which revealed LH and FSH below the normal range and undetectable oestradiol. Thyroid function, karyotype and serum prolactin were normal.

Does anything need to be done instantly?
What other questioning might be insightful?

Answers, see p. 125

Subfertility

Subfertility is defined as the failure of the female partner to become pregnant despite a year of unprotected regular intercourse with her male partner. Always assess both partners (Table 7.6).

Male factor treatment

Treatment depends on cause. In secondary hypogonadism, testicular function can be restored with injections of hCG and, if needed, human menopausal gonadotrophin (hMG) to mimic endogenous LH and FSH. In the event of unlikely spontaneous fertilization *in vivo* or *in vitro*, the spermatozoa can be assessed for intracytoplasmic sperm injection (ICSI).

Female factor treatment

Gaining a regular ovulatory cycle of ~28 days is im-
portant. In overweight individuals or those with PCOS, increased cardiovascular exercise and weight reduction may be sufficient to generate regular ovulatory cycles. An insulin sensitizer, such as metformin, can be useful. The importance of fitness and weight control prior to pregnancy cannot be overemphasized: patients with PCOS are already at higher risk of first trimester miscarriage; and obesity links with GDM and difficulties in labour.

Other methods of ovulation induction increase the risk of multiple pregnancies, which, in turn, increases maternal and fetal morbidity. Blocking oestrogen feedback at the gonadotroph (most commonly with clomiphene) is the simplest. Ovulation induction using hCG and hMG is used to recover ova for *in vitro* fertilization (IVF) or ICSI. Other aspects of fertility management are described in *Essential Reproduction*.

Table 7.6 An approach to subfertility

Female factor subfertility	Male factor subfertility
Was there normal development at birth? Was childhood normal? Did the individual enter puberty at the appropriate time?	
Consider PCOS, pituitary, thyroid or adrenal disease	All the potential causes of primary or secondary hypogonadism need consideration
Pelvic inflammatory disease (PID) can block the fallopian tubes—symptoms include discharge and pain	Examination: Is testicular size normal (20–25 ml)?
What is the cycle length and regularity? A regular 28-day cycle is likely to be ovulatory	Is there a varicocoele? Are the external genitalia structurally normal?
Biochemical profile and investigation	
Day 2–5: serum LH, FSH, oestradiol, prolactin and thyroid function tests	LH, FSH, testosterone, SHBG, prolactin and thyroid function tests
Consider investigations related to PCOS (Table 7.4)	Consider testing for other anterior pituitary disorders
Day 21: progesterone to assess ovulation	Consider karyogram to exclude Klinefelter syndrome (46,XXY)
BMI—fertility declines with obesity	Semen analysis—volume, concentration, motility and morphology
Swab for pelvic inflammatory disease, e.g. Chlamydia	
Consider a hysterosalpingogram or laparoscopy to assess tubal patency	

Answers to case histories

Case history 7.1

Serum testosterone is very low. LH and FSH are high. The diagnosis is primary hypogonadism with the problem located in the testes. A karyogram is needed because of the suspicion of Klinefelter syndrome (47,XXY).

The patient should be commenced on testosterone, initially at low dose. This can be given effectively by intramuscular injection or gel preparation. If diagnosed by karyogram, he should be offered information about the Klinefelter support group. The correct maintenance dose of testosterone is the one that normalizes LH. The patient can anticipate increased beard growth, improved energy levels and sexual drive. The gynaecomastia might persist, at least in part, at which point cosmetic correction should be offered. A DEXA scan would demonstrate bone demineralization and quite possibly osteoporosis due to the hypogonadism (see Chapter 9). Performing this investigation at diagnosis offers a 'benchmark', against which replacement therapy might be monitored.

Case history 7.2

A drug history should be obtained. Chronic medical illnesses should be excluded. Pregnancy is ruled out if the patient is sexually inactive. Thyroid function tests should be performed although the prolactin level is rather high for primary hypothyroidism. At this level, a microprolactinoma is by far the most likely diagnosis. Oestradiol would be low and may well be undetectable. An MRI scan of the pituitary gland is indicated, which may appear normal as some lactotroph tumours are tiny and below the resolution of an MRI scan.

Once a microprolactinoma has been diagnosed, the patient should be reassured that these tumours are benign and offered treatment with cabergoline, a dopamine agonist. She should be warned that periods and fertility are likely to return with treatment. The galactorrhoea is likely to stop within a matter of weeks. After 5 years, ~60% of patients with microprolactinomas can stop treatment and retain a normal serum prolactin level. Further details relevant to this case are provided in Chapter 5.

Case history 7.3

In the absence of major signs of pituitary disease (e.g. no visual disturbance, normal prolactin), nothing needs to be done instantly. Although a reluctant patient has compromised the history, examination and investigation, all features are consistent with simple constitutional delay. It would be helpful to know whether menarche had tended to occur slightly later than the norm in other family members.

In this particular case, the follow-up appointment was attended with grandparents when the patient was more communicative and willing to be examined with a chaperone and relatives present. Breast development was noted to be Tanner stage 3. She had grown since the last appointment. Six months later, periods had commenced and were regular. The patient was discharged.

LEARNING OBJECTIVES

- To appreciate the development of the thyroid gland and its clinical consequences
- To understand the regulation, biosynthesis and metabolism of thyroid hormones
- To understand the function of thyroid hormones
- To understand the clinical consequences of underproduction and overproduction of thyroid hormone

This chapter integrates the basic biology of the thyroid gland with the clinical conditions that affect it

The thyroid gland sits in the neck and is responsible for the concentration of iodine and the biosynthesis of thyroid hormones from tyrosine. Thyroid hormones play major roles in regulating the body's metabolism and affect many different cell types. Understanding the basic science and associated clinical conditions of the thyroid gland, therefore, is of major importance.

Embryology

Understanding the development of the thyroid gland and its anatomical associations allow the correct surgical approach to the gland in the treatment of thyroid overactivity or enlargement. In the fourth week of development, the thyroid begins as a midline thickening at the back of the tongue. This endodermal out-pouching of the oral cavity stretches downward and soon forms a solid mass of cells weighing 1 to 2 mg (Fig. 8.1). This thyroid primordium migrates past the front of the larynx and by 7 weeks is bilobed. It remains attached to its origin by the thyroglossal duct. The descent of the thyroid brings it into close proximity with the developing parathyroid glands (Fig. 8.1; see Chapter 9). In adulthood, these small, pea-sized structures are situated on the back of the thyroid as pairs of upper and lower glands and are responsible for calcium homeostasis. The lower parathyroids start out higher in the neck than the upper glands and only achieve their final position by also migrating downwards. The thyroid gland comes into contact with other cells during its migration. From the lower part of the developing pharynx, the future C-cells that secrete calcitonin mix with the descending thyroid and eventually comprise ~10% of the gland (see Chapter 9).

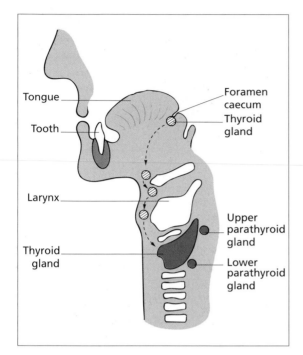

Figure 8.1 The thyroid gland and its downward migration. The point of origin in the tongue persists as the foramen caecum. Common sites of thyroglossal cysts (⌀) and the final position of the paired parathyroid glands are indicated (Modified from K. L. Moore, *The Developing Human*, W.B. Saunders, Philadelphia).

Towards the end of the second month, the thyroglossal duct and the thyroid gland lose contact. The duct atrophies in all but ~15% of the population, in whom its lowest portion differentiates into the pyramidal lobe as an upward, finger-like extension of thyroid tissue. Laterally, two distinct lobes form on either side of the trachea. These are connected in the midline by the narrow isthmus in front of the trachea, just below the larynx—a convenient landmark for locating the 'bowtie-shaped' thyroid gland during clinical examination (see Box 8.12). The cells are grouped into clusters, which by ~11 weeks have organized themselves into a single layer of epithelial cells surrounding a central lumen. This signals the first ability of the gland to trap iodine (as iodide) and synthesize thyroid hormone, although it only responds to thyroid-stimulating hormone (TSH) from the anterior pituitary towards the end of the second trimester.

> **BOX 8.1 Embryological abnormality and clinical consequences**
>
> Failure of the gland to develop → congenital hypothyroidism
> *Under* or *over*migration of the thyroid → lingual or retrosternal thyroid
> Failure of thyroglossal duct to atrophy → thyroglossal cyst

On occasion, embryology does not take place normally with several clinical consequences (Box 8.1). Thyroglossal cysts are located in the midline and can be distinguished clinically by upward movement on tongue protrusion. Congenital absence of the thyroid due to mutation in genes, such as *PAX8*, requires immediate detection and treatment with thyroid hormone in order to minimize the severe and largely irreversible neurological damage that could occur in the infant.

Anatomy and vasculature

The adult thyroid gland weighs 10 to 20 g. Commonly, the right lobe is larger than the left and the entire gland is bigger in women and in areas of the world with iodine deficiency. It enlarges during puberty, in pregnancy and during lactation.

The outer part of the capsule is not well-defined, but attaches the thyroid to the trachea. The parathyroid glands are situated between this and the inner capsule, from which trabeculae of collagen pervade the gland and carry nerves and a rich vascular supply to the cells (Fig. 8.2). The thyroid receives ~1% of cardiac output from superior and inferior thyroid arteries, which branch off the external carotid and subclavian arteries respectively. Per gram of tissue, this disproportionately large supply is almost twice that of the kidney. Supply is increased further during some conditions of overactivity and may be evidenced by a bruit on auscultation (Box 8.2 and Box 8.12).

Histologically, the functional unit of the thyroid is the follicle (Fig. 8.2). This consists of cuboidal epithelial ('follicular') cells arranged as spheres, the central lumen of which contains colloid. Colloid is com-

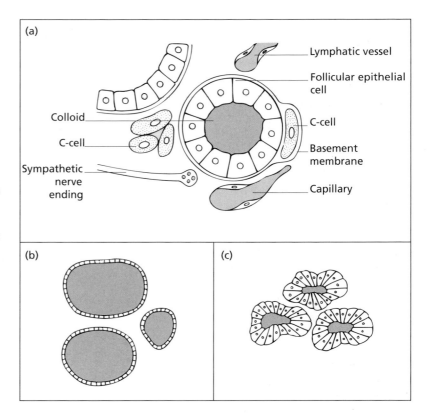

Figure 8.2 Histology of the human thyroid gland. (a) Euthyroid follicles are shown, consisting of 'hollow' spheres of cuboidal epithelium, the lumens of which are filled with gelatinous colloid that contains stored thyroid hormones (complexed in thyroglobulin). Surrounding each follicle is a basement membrane enclosing parafollicular C-cells within a stroma containing fenestrated capillaries, lymphatic vessels and sympathetic nerve endings. (b) Underactive follicles with flattened thyroid epithelial cells and increased colloid. (c) Overactive follicles with tall, columnar epithelial cells and reduced colloid.

BOX 8.2 The adult thyroid gland

- Enlargement = a 'goitre'
- The gland is encapsulated
  - breaching the capsule is a measure of invasion in thyroid cancer
- The thyroid receives a large arterial blood supply
  - may cause a bruit in Graves disease

---

posed almost entirely of the iodinated glycoprotein, thyroglobulin, which turns an intense pink on periodic acid-Schiff (PAS) staining. The normal human follicle varies in diameter from 20 to 900 μm. Many thousands are present in the gland interspersed with blood vessels, an extensive network of lymphatic vessels, connective tissue and the parafollicular calcitonin-secreting C-cells. The blood flow through the fenestrated capillaries is controlled by postganglion-ic sympathetic nerve fibres from the middle and superior cervical ganglia.

When the gland is quiescent, as occurs in an iodine-deficient hypothyroid state, the follicles are distended with colloid and the epithelial cells are flattened with little cytoplasm. In an overactive gland, the follicular cells are columnar and contain colloid by light microscopy—a sign of intense activity (Fig. 8.2).

Thyroid hormone biosynthesis

There are two active thyroid hormones: thyroxine (3,3′,5,5′-tetraiodothyronine), frequently abbreviated to T_4, and triiodothyronine (T_3)—the subscript 4 and 3 representing the number of iodine atoms attached to each thyronine residue (Fig. 8.3). These thyroid hormones are generated from the sequential iodination and coupling of the amino acid tyrosine. They are inactivated by deiodination and modification to 'reverse T_3' (rT_3; 3,3′,5′-triiodothyronine) and

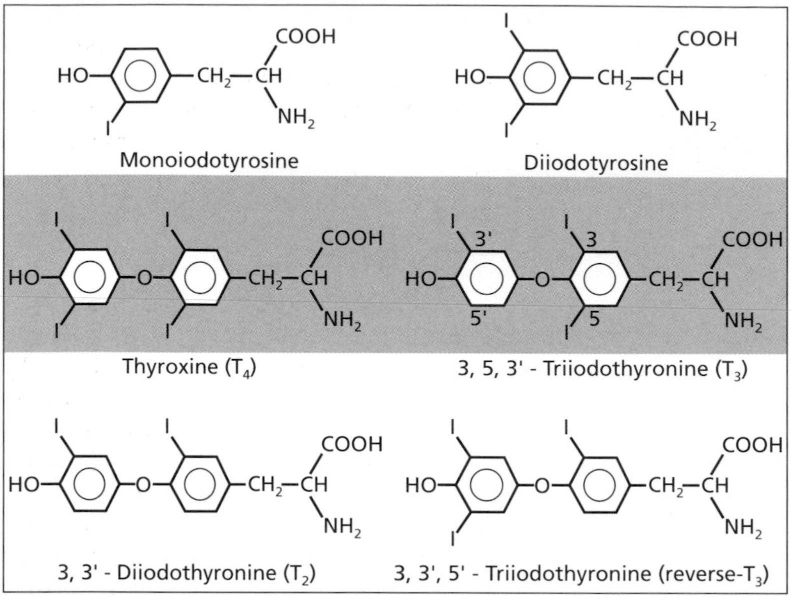

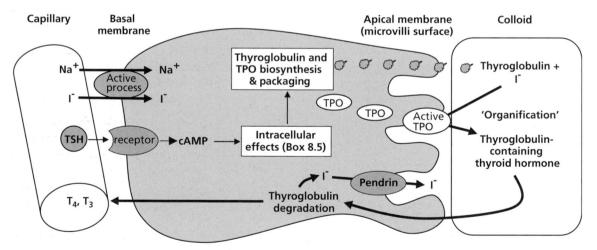

Figure 8.3 The structures of active and inactive thyroid hormones and their precursors. Monoiodotyrosines and diiodotyrosines are precursors. Thyroxine (T_4) and triiodothyronine (T_3) are the two thyroid hormones, of which T_3 is the biologically more active. Reverse T_3 and T_2 are inactive metabolites formed by deiodination of T_4 and T_3 respectively. The numbering of critical positions for iodination is shown on the structure of T_3.

Figure 8.4 Thyroid hormone biosynthesis within the follicular cell. Active iodide import is linked to a Na^+/K^+ ATPase pump. Thyroglobulin is synthesized on the rough endoplasmic reticulum, packaged in the Golgi complex and released from small, Golgi-derived vesicles into the follicular lumen. Its iodination is also known as 'organification'. Cytoplasmic microfilaments and microtubules organize the return of thyroglobulin as endocytotic vesicles into the cell. The thyroglobulin now contains thyroid hormone, which is released upon degradation. Modified from Williams Textbook of Endocrinology, 10th edition, Saunders, 2003. Chapter 10, page 332.

diidothyronine (T_2). The balance in the formation of these different molecules determines overall thyroid hormone activity. The synthesis of thyroid hormones can be broken down into several key steps described over the next few pages and depicted in Fig. 8.4.

Uptake of iodide from the blood

The synthesis of thyroid hormone relies on a constant supply of dietary iodine (as iodide). When the element is scarce the thyroid enlarges to form a goitre (see Box 8.3). Iodide enters the follicular cell by active transport from the circulation through the basal cell membrane. The sodium/iodide (Na^+/I^-) pump is linked to the activity of an ATP-driven sodium/potassium (Na^+/K^+) pump. This process concentrates iodide within the thyroid gland ~20 to 100 times that of the remainder of the body. This selectivity allows the organ-specific use of radioiodine both diagnostically and therapeutically (covered in later sections). Several structurally related anions can competitively inhibit the iodide pump. For example, large doses of perchlorate (ClO_4^-) can be employed clinically as a short-term measure to block iodide uptake by the gland (e.g. in accidental ingestion of radioiodine). The pertechnetate ion incorporating a γ-emitting radioisotope of technetium is also taken up by the iodide pump and allows the thyroid gland to be imaged diagnostically.

The synthesis of thyroglobulin

Thyroglobulin is synthesized within the follicular cell from many tyrosine residues. It is ~1% iodine by weight and serves as the substrate for the synthesis of T_4 and T_3. Thyroglobulin is a glycoprotein and contains ~10% carbohydrate, some of which includes the sialic acid that is responsible for the intense pink PAS staining of colloid. Thyroglobulin is transcribed, translated, post-translationally modified in the Golgi apparatus and then packaged into vesicles within the follicular cell (Fig. 8.4 and review Chapter 2). These vesicles move to the apical membrane, with which they fuse, and then release their contents into the follicular lumen.

Iodination of thyroglobulin

Thyroid peroxidase (TPO) catalyses the iodination of thyroglobulin. Like thyroglobulin, the enzyme is synthesized and packaged into vesicles at the Golgi complex. At the apical cell membrane, TPO becomes activated. Active TPO binds the iodide and thyroglobulin at different sites. The enzyme oxidizes iodide, which is then transferred to an exposed tyrosine residue of thyroglobulin. The enzyme is particularly efficient at iodinating fresh thyroglobulin; as the reaction proceeds, the efficiency of adding further iodide decreases. Drugs inhibiting TPO and iodination are used to treat hyperthyroidism (Box 8.4).

BOX 8.3 Iodine deficiency

Some areas of the developing world remain iodine-deficient, which can cause hypothyroidism and particularly large goitres (Plate 8.1, facing p. 246). Thyroglobulin in the normal human thyroid stores ~2 months supply of thyroid hormone. When dietary iodide is limited (<50 µg per day), less is incorporated into thyroglobulin, which consequently releases a higher proportion of the more active T_3 to T_4. However, eventually thyroid hormone biosynthesis can no longer keep up. Diminished negative feedback increases TSH secretion, which induces thyroid enlargement, a compensatory mechanism to increase the capacity for iodide uptake. This may permit sufficient thyroid hormone biosynthesis under normal circumstances; however, during pregnancy, the supply of iodine and thyroid hormones will not be sufficient for a developing fetus. The fetus is at risk from severe neurological damage and may develop a goitre. Postnatally, the syndrome of intellectual impairment, deafness and diplegia (bilateral paralysis) has been termed 'cretinism' and affects many millions of infants worldwide. Decreased iodine intake with a marginal but chronic elevation of TSH may also result in an increased incidence of thyroid cancer, especially if irradiation is involved, as with the Chernobyl accident.

Prophylaxis with iodine supplements has reduced the incidence of cretinism, although tends not to shrink adult goitres very much. Supplementation of common dietary constituents such as salt or bread has been undertaken in many countries but is not always practicable. In extremely isolated communities, depot injections of iodized oils can provide the thyroid with supplies for years.

BOX 8.4 Antithyroid drugs—effective at suppressing the synthesis and secretion of thyroid hormones

- Carbimazole
- Methimazole (active metabolite of carbimazole; used in USA)
- Propylthiouracil (PTU)

Some naturally occurring substances, such as chemicals from well water, the milk of cows fed on certain green fodder and the brassicae vegetables (cabbages, sprouts), can inhibit the iodination of thyroglobulin and hence the synthesis of thyroid hormones. Negative feedback is diminished at the anterior pituitary and TSH secretion increases (Fig. 8.5). Prolonged stimulation results in thyroid hyperplasia and a goitre, hence the chemicals are known as 'goitrogens'.

The production of thyroid hormones

The process of iodination is also important for initiating the formation of thyroid hormones (Figs 8.3 and 8.4). Within the thyroglobulin structure, diiodotyrosine couples to either a monoiodotyrosine (to gener-

ate T_3) or to another diiodotyrosine (to generate T_4). This coupling occurs during the TPO-mediated iodination reaction so no additional enzyme is necessary. The iodinated thyroglobulin protein now contains thyroid hormone stored as colloid in the lumen of the thyroid follicle.

The secretion of thyroid hormones

The thyroglobulin-containing thyroid hormone returns into the follicular cell (Fig. 8.4). Microvilli on the apical cell membrane envelop the thyroglobulin ('endocytosis') to form colloid droplets within the cell. The cytoskeleton steers these vesicles away from the apical membrane and facilitates fusion with lysosomes. The enzymes from the lysosomes break down the thyroglobulin, releasing thyroid hormones and degradation products. The latter, including iodide, are recycled within the gland. The transporter, Pendrin, moves iodide back into the follicular lumen. Mutations in the *Pendrin* gene cause a congenital form of hypothyroidism (Pendred syndrome). The thyroid hormones move across the basal cell membrane and enter the circulation, ~80% as T_4 and 20% as T_3.

Regulation of thyroid hormone biosynthesis

The activity of the thyroid gland is controlled by TSH from the anterior pituitary, which in turn is regulated by thyrotrophin-releasing hormone (TRH) from the hypothalamus (review Chapter 5). Thyroid hormones, predominantly via the more active T_3, complete the negative feedback loop by suppressing the production of TRH and TSH (Fig. 8.5). TSH binds to its specific G-protein coupled receptor on the surface of the thyroid follicular cell and activates both adenylate cyclase and phospholipase C (review Chapter 3). The former appears to be the dominant effect and the second messenger cAMP mediates most of the actions of TSH (Box 8.5). The net effect increases fresh thyroid hormone stores and, within ~1 h, increases the release of thyroid hormones. The most recently synthesized thyroglobulin is the first to be resorbed as it is nearest to the microvilli. This thyroglobulin has also had less time to be iodinated than the mature, centrally positioned store, such that it releases

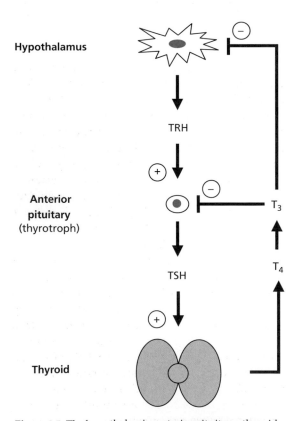

Figure 8.5 The hypothalamic–anterior pituitary–thyroid axis. The more active hormone, T_3, provides the majority of negative feedback.

BOX 8.5 Consequences of TSH stimulation on the follicular cell

- $\uparrow$ intracellular cAMP concentration
- $\uparrow$ iodination of thyroglobulin
- $\uparrow$ microvilli number and length at luminal cell surface
- $\uparrow$ in intracellular volume and endocytosis of colloid droplets
- $\uparrow$ thyroid hormone release
- $\uparrow$ iodide influx into the cell (relatively late effect as activation of the iodide pump requires protein synthesis)
- $\uparrow$ cellular metabolism
- $\uparrow$ protein synthesis (including thyroglobulin)
- $\uparrow$ DNA synthesis (in fact, mitosis and cell division are rather limited in the adult thyroid)

BOX 8.6 Circulating thyroid hormones

- Thyroid hormones are almost entirely bound to the following serum proteins (in order of decreasing affinity):
  - thyroxine-binding globulin (TBG)
  - thyroxine-binding prealbumin (TBPA)
  - albumin
- The unbound fraction is tiny, yet critical—*only free thyroid hormone enters cells:*
  - free T_4 (fT_4) ~0.015% of total T_4
  - free T_3 (fT_3) ~0.33% of total T_3
  - circulating half-life T_3, ~1–3 days—needs to given several times a day if used clinically
  - circulating half-life T_4, ~5–7 days—can be given as single daily dose
  - Both fT_4 and fT_3 are measured by immunoassay (see thyroid function tests later)
- T_3 is more potent than T_4 (~2 to 10-fold depending on response monitored)

thyroid hormones with a relatively higher T_3 to T_4 ratio and, consequently, greater activity.

Circulating thyroid hormones

Once the serum concentrations of thyroid hormones have settled to constant values ~3 days after birth, little change occurs in normal individuals throughout the remainder of life. Thyroid hormones are strongly bound to serum proteins (Box 8.6). Only the tiny amount of free hormone can enter cells and function. T_3 is bound slightly less strongly than T_4 to each of the three principal serum binding proteins, of which albumin is a relatively nonspecific binder of circulating thyroid hormone. Some drugs, such as salicylates, phenytoin or diclofenac, which structurally resemble the iodothyronine molecule, can compete with thyroid hormone for protein binding. Starvation or liver disease alters the concentration of binding proteins. In either scenario, readjustment of total circulating hormone levels ensures that the free concentrations remain unaltered.

Metabolism of thyroid hormone: the conversion of T_4 to T_3 and rT_3

As already alluded to, T_3 is the more active hormone. However, only 20% of the thyroid's output is T_3. To

generate more requires the removal of one iodine atom from the outer ring of T_4, a process called deiodination (Fig. 8.3 and Fig. 8.6). This step is catalysed by selenodeiodinase enzymes, which contain selenium that accepts the iodine from the thyroid hormone. Selenium deficiency in parts of western China or Zaire can be a rare contributory factor to hypothyroidism. The type 1 selenodeiodinase (D1) predominates in the liver, kidney and muscle and is responsible for most of the body's circulating T_3. It is inhibited by the antithyroid drug propylthiouracil (PTU) (Fig. 8.6). The type 2 enzyme (D2) is predominantly localized in the brain and the pituitary, key sites for regulating T_3 production for negative feedback at the hypothalamus and thyrotroph. There is a third selenodeiodinase, type 3 (D3), which deiodinates the inner ring and catalyses the conversion of T_4 to reverse T_3 (rT_3; Fig. 8.3 and Fig. 8.6). rT_3 is biologically inactive and cleared very rapidly from the circulation (half-life ~5 hours). The same degradative action on T_3 is one method by which the similarly inactive T_2 is generated. These combined steps are important. It is suggested that, when a given cell has sufficient T_3 for its metabolic requirements, it switches to produce rT_3, which is then rapidly cleared. At least in part, T_4 can

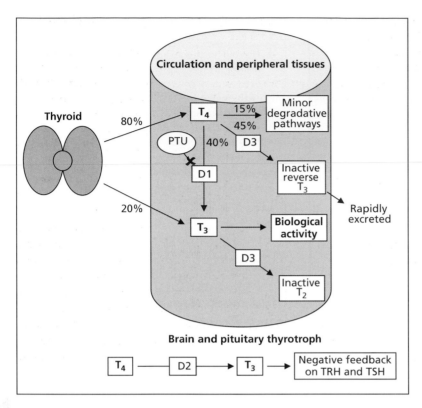

Figure 8.6 Metabolism of thyroid hormone in the circulation. Four times more T_4 is produced by the thyroid gland than T_3. Under normal 'euthyroid' physiology, ~40% of circulating T_4 is converted to active T_3 by type 1 selenodeiodinase (D1) and ~45% of T_4 is converted to rT_3 by the type 3 selenodeiodinase (D3). The remaining 15% of T_4 is degraded by minor pathways, such as deamination. The conversion of T_3 to T_2 by D3 is shown, although other pathways also exist for this reaction. The type 2 selenodeiodinase (D2) is predominantly located in the brain and pituitary gland where it catalyses the production of T_3 for negative feedback within the hypothalamic–anterior pituitary–thyroid axis.

thus be thought of as a 'prohormone', its presence required only to maintain a constant supply of T_3.

Function of thyroid hormone

Thyroid hormones affect a vast array of tissue and cellular processes, most obviously increasing the body's metabolic rate. In other species, effects can be more diverse, such as regulating metamorphosis in *Amphibia*.

T_3 acts in the nucleus of the target cell where it binds to the thyroid hormone receptor (TR) with 15-fold greater affinity than T_4. This predominantly explains why T_3 is more potent than T_4. The consequence is altered gene expression (review Fig. 3.20). In this way, within the anterior pituitary, thyroid hormone can activate growth hormone (GH) production by the somatotroph and repress TSH production by the thyrotroph (part of the negative feedback loop of thyroid regulation). This predominantly genomic action explains why most actions of thyroid

hormone are relatively slow, days rather than minutes-to-hours.

The TR is not identical in all target tissues. There are two predominant isoforms, TRα and TRβ, each encoded by different genes and each subject to alternative promoter use and/or mRNA splicing (review Fig. 2.2). This creates a number of additional subtypes, all of which perform the basic activities of binding thyroid hormone, binding DNA and influencing target genes. However, they achieve these actions with subtly different efficacy. This layer of complexity helps to explain why different tissues respond differently to the same circulating thyroid hormone. Clinically, this can be evidenced in the very rare condition of thyroid hormone resistance due to mutations mostly located in the TRβ gene. A striking combination of thyroid overactivity can be observed in some tissues (e.g. tachycardia), while the thyrotroph in the pituitary responds as if thyroid hormone activity is inadequate (i.e. TSH secretion is maintained).

Thyroid hormones influence the actions of other hormones, but these effects can be difficult to discriminate from the generalized increase in cell metabolism. One of the most important effects clinically is the ability of T_3 to synergize with catecholamines to increase heart rate, causing palpitations in thyrotoxicosis.

Thyroid function tests

Clinical investigation of the thyroid gland hinges upon immunoassay of circulating thyroid hormones and TSH, combined as the 'thyroid function test'. Together, they inform the endocrinologist as to whether the patient's thyroid gland is overactive ('hyperthyroid'), underactive ('hypothyroid') or normal ('euthyroid') (Table 8.1). Now that robust assays are available, thyroid hormones are measured unbound to protein as fT_4 and fT_3. fT_3 concentrations are ~30% those of fT_4. Serum TSH is the critical parameter as, in the absence of pituitary disease, it illustrates the body's response to its own thyroid hormone levels. Ideally all three, fT_4, fT_3 and TSH, should be measured.

Biochemical assessment can be invaluable as thyroid disease can be insidious, especially primary hypothyroidism in the elderly. Commonly, it is difficult to act on borderline test results, such as subclinical hypothyroidism and hyperthyroidism. These are discussed in the following sections.

Pituitary underactivity can reduce TSH levels and cause hypothyroidism when it is very important to consider the other hormone axes, which might also be underactive. Similar thyroid function test results may be seen in patients suffering from physical (or in some instances psychiatric) illnesses that do not directly involve the thyroid gland. Severe illness in a patient is usually obvious, when total and free T_3 and T_4 may fall below normal without a compensatory increase in TSH. The body's type 1 selenodeiodinase activity is low. This condition is referred to as the 'sick euthyroid' syndrome. Although contentious, treatment is not normally undertaken. If recovery occurs, T_3 and T_4 return to normal of their own accord. In

Table 8.1 Interpretation of thyroid function tests

Test results			Interpretation
TSH	fT_4	fT_3	
Normal	Normal	Normal	Euthyroidism
Low	High	High	Primary hyperthyroidism
Low	(High) normal	(High) normal	Subclinical primary hyperthyroidism or pregnancy
Low	Normal	High	T_3-toxicosis
High/normal	High	High	Pituitary (secondary) hyperthyroidism or TR mutation; both exceptionally rare
High	Low	Low	Primary hypothyroidism
High	(Low) normal	(Low) normal	Subclinical primary hypothyroidism
Low	Low	Low	Consider secondary hypothyroidism (assess other pituitary hormone axes)
Normal/low	Low	Low	'Sick euthyroid' syndrome

For simplicity, higher axis disorders have been listed as secondary, i.e. pituitary, although tertiary hypothalamic disease is possible.
In effect, serum TSH = a bioassay of thyroid hormone action in the body.

pregnancy, TSH might decline, particularly in the first trimester, as human chorionic gonadotrophin (hCG) from the placenta is capable of mimicking TSH action.

Clinical disorders

The major clinical disorders affecting the thyroid gland arise from either too much or too little thyroid hormone, benign goitrous overgrowth causing local symptoms or malignant tumourigenesis.

Hypothyroidism

Lack of thyroid hormone occurs most commonly due to disease of the thyroid itself (primary hypothyroidism) and, less frequently, from lack of TSH from the pituitary (secondary hypothyroidism) (Box 8.8 and Case History 8.1). Tertiary hypothyroidism, due to hypothalamic dysfunction, is rare.

Primary hypothyroidism

The commonest presentation of thyroid underactivity in the western world is from autoimmune destruction of the gland. It is sixfold more common in women and incidence increases with age (up to 2% of adult women). Attempts have been made to classify the disorder according to goitre with its presence signifying 'Hashimoto thyroiditis', its absence 'primary myxoedema' or 'atrophic thyroiditis'. As we understand more about the pathogenesis, this clinical distinction becomes blurred; indeed, the disease process even overlaps with that of hyperthyroidism due to Graves disease (see later). This common genetic predisposition to thyroid disease also extends to other conditions (Box 8.7).

In autoimmune hypothyroidism, an extensive lymphocytic infiltration is accompanied by autoantibodies directed against thyroglobulin and thyroid peroxidase. Some additional antibodies may block the TSH receptor. Progressive destruction of thyroid follicular tissue results in hypothyroidism. Riedel thyroiditis is rare and due to progressive fibrosis that causes a hard goitre.

Congenital disorders of the thyroid (~1/4000 births), more likely to present to the paediatric endocrinologist, include failure of thyroid gland formation, migration or hormone biosynthesis. Causes

> **BOX 8.7 Examples of organ-specific autoimmune diseases — risk is increased for some individuals**
>
> - Graves disease
> - Autoimmune hypothyroidism
> - Pernicious anaemia
>   - pernicious anaemia arises from autoimmune destruction of the parietal cell, loss of intrinsic factor secretion and consequently, vitamin B_{12} deficiency
> - Addison disease (Chapter 6)
> - Autoimmune atrophic gastritis
> - Type 1 diabetes mellitus (Chapter 12)

> **BOX 8.8 Causes of hypothyroidism**
>
> Goitre
> - Autoimmune thyroiditis (possibly no goitre)
> - Iodine deficiency (see earlier)
>   - 'cretinism'
> - Drugs (e.g. lithium)
>
> No goitre
> - Postradioiodine ablation or surgery (see treatment of hyperthyroidism)
> - Post-thyroiditis (transient)
> - Congenital hypothyroidism
> - Hypothalamic or pituitary hypothyroidism

of the latter, collectively called 'thyroid dyshormonogenesis', usually present with goitrous hypothyroidism early in life.

It is important to recognize and exclude transient causes of thyroid upset. Excessive iodine intake, such as from radiocontrast dyes, can transiently block synthesis and hormone release. Lithium, used in the treatment of manic depression/bipolar disorders, can do the same. Indeed, lithium and Lugol's iodine can be used to control hyperthyroidism in certain circumstances (see next section). Viral infection, for instance by Echo or Coxsackie virus, can cause painful inflammation and release of stored hormone. A brief thyrotoxicosis is followed by transient hypothyroidism and is known as 'De Quervain's subacute thyroiditis'.

Symptoms and signs. The effects of hypothyroidism in adults are largely the result of a lowered metabolic rate. The classic symptoms and signs are listed in Box 8.9. The facial appearance and the potential for carpal tunnel syndrome are due to the deposition of glycosaminoglycans in the skin. Children tend to present with obesity and short stature (Fig. 8.7). The distinction between permanent (treatment needed) and transient (treatment not needed) disorders is important. Short-lived symptoms (less than a few months) preceded by a sore throat or upper respiratory tract infection may indicate transient hypothyroidism. Permanent hypothyroidism is more likely if other family members have thyroid disease. A drug history should be taken.

Investigation and diagnosis. A diagnosis of primary hypothyroidism should not be made without biochemical evidence. A thyroid function test (serum TSH, ideally accompanied by free thyroid hormone levels) is needed (Table 8.1). Four scenarios are commonly encountered.
1. Raised TSH at least twice normal upper limit (can be more than 10-fold increased) plus thyroid hormone levels clearly below the normal range. This diagnosis of primary hypothyroidism is clear-cut.

BOX 8.9 Symptoms, signs and features of hypothyroidism

- Weight gain
- Cold intolerance, particularly at extremities
- Fatigue, lethargy
- Depression
- Coarse skin and puffy appearance (possible carpal tunnel syndrome)
- Dry hair
- Hoarse voice
- Constipation
- Menstrual irregularities (altered LH/FSH secretion)
- Possible goitre
- 'Slow' reflexes, muscles contract normally, but relax slowly
- Generalized muscle weakness and paraesthesias
- Bradycardia (with reduced cardiac output)
- Cardiomegaly (with possible pericardial effusion)

When accompanied by long-standing symptoms, underactivity will be permanent.
2. Raised TSH at least twice normal upper limit with normal thyroid hormone levels. This implies biochemical compensation. With significant symptoms, treatment is worthwhile; as subclinical hypothyroidism, treatment with thyroxine can still be justified, as ultimately the gland is likely to fail and produce frank hypothyroidism, especially if autoantibodies are detected.
3. TSH is only moderately raised and thyroid hormone levels are normal. This scenario is more difficult. These patients have an increased progression to frank hypothyroidism and, in the presence of significant symptoms, a therapeutic trial of thyroxine is one option. If the results are an incidental finding, repeat testing over the following months is an alternative, especially if there is concern over a transient viral hypothyroidism.
4. Thyroid function tests are unequivocally normal. **Do not treat with thyroxine, regardless of symptoms, as the patient is not hypothyroid.**

Other investigations are commonly not needed; however, if measured, a raised titre of thyroid antibodies may be detected. Creatinine kinase may be elevated. Dyslipidaemia is common with raised LDL-cholesterol. Prolactin may be elevated (stimulated by increased TRH secretion, see Chapter 5).

Treatment. Hypothyroidism is treated by oral thyroxine (i.e. T_4, therefore a hormone replacement rather than drug treatment); $100\,\mu g/day$ is the standard adult replacement dose ($\sim100\,\mu g/m^2$ per day in children). The goal of replacement is to normalize TSH. The correct dose is determined by repeat serum analysis after 6 weeks as the pituitary responds sluggishly to acute changes in thyroid hormones. In primary hypothyroidism, replacement will be for life. In patients with long-standing hypothyroidism and coexisting ischaemic heart disease, graded introduction of replacement therapy over several weeks is frequently used. A final caveat to initiating treatment is to be confident of excluding Addison disease (review Chapter 6), a clue to which might be hyperkalaemia. Increasing basal metabolic rate with thyroxine only increases the body's demand for an already inadequate cortisol supply and can send a patient into Addisonian crisis. The rare, yet high

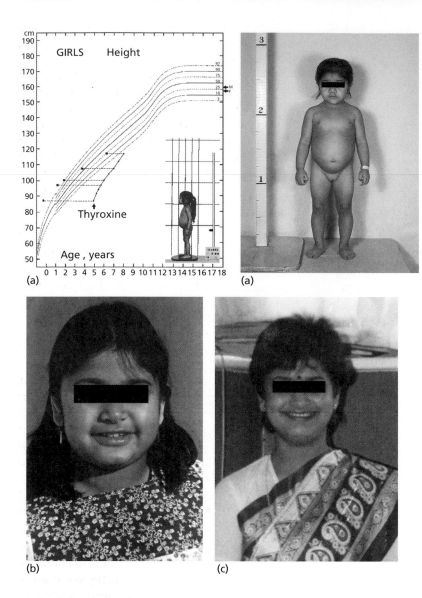

Figure 8.7 Hypothyroidism. At the age of 6 years, this girl (a, upper panels) presented with short stature and extremely delayed skeletal maturation. Circulating thyroid hormone levels were very low and TSH grossly elevated, as were titres of thyroid autoantibodies. A diagnosis of primary hypothyroidism was made. The response to thyroxine treatment is shown by rapid catch-up growth. Learning problems were not evident, as the condition was not congenital but acquired after major development of the brain was complete. Three (b) and eight (c) years later, as a result of continued hormone replacement, she has now gained a normal appearance.

mortality clinical scenario of myxoedema coma is summarized in Box 8.10.

Monitoring. Once stable, thyroid function tests should be measured annually although replacement rarely changes. Compliance issues can be encountered where fT_4 is normal (patient took tablet prior to clinic) but TSH is raised (chronically, the patient is taking inadequate thyroid hormone). Despite large trials, no convincing evidence has ever been presented that treatment with T_3 is better than with

T_4. T_3 needs to be taken three times daily and usually only precipitates worse compliance.

Secondary hypothyroidism

If the anterior pituitary thyrotrophs are underactive, TSH-dependent processes in the thyroid gland will fail. This translates as thyroid hormone deficiency. The causes are covered in Chapter 5. The principles of thyroxine replacement therapy are similar, although TSH is no longer a reliable marker of adequate replacement. The easiest approach is to treat with sufficient thyroxine so that fT_4 is in the upper half of the normal range (and fT_3 is also within the normal range).

Hyperthyroidism

Hyperthyroidism is overactivity of the thyroid gland. This produces the clinical effects of increased circulating thyroid hormones, called thyrotoxicosis. Note the difference: release of stored hormone in viral infection or overdose of thyroxine will cause transient thyrotoxicosis but is not actually hyperthyroidism. Most commonly, true hyperthyroidism has an autoimmune origin, is 10-fold more common in women, and is named after its discoverer, Thomas Graves. Other causes are associated with amiodarone use and overproduction of hormone from an autonomous thyroid nodule. These are considered in turn. Overactivity from excess TSH is incredibly rare.

Graves disease

Autoimmune hyperthyroidism affects ~2% of women in the UK and is due to thyroid-stimulating IgG antibodies that activate the TSH receptor on the follicular cell surface. This results in all the consequences of cAMP generation (Box 8.5) and, in many cases, goitre formation.

Symptoms, signs and biochemical profile. The natural history of Graves disease is one of waxing and waning. However, identifying the disorder is important, as its symptoms are unpleasant, potentially serious and yet amenable to treatment. Many of the classic symptoms are due to an increased basal metabolic rate and enhanced β-adrenergic activity (Box 8.11 and Case History 8.2). Additional features are specific to Graves disease and represent the autoimmune disease process affecting other sites in the body. Thyroid acropachy and pretibial myxoedema are caused by cytokines that stimulate the deposition of glycosaminoglycans.

BOX 8.10 Myxoedema coma: very severe hypothyroidism, usually in the elderly

- Diminished mental function → confusion → coma
- Hypothermia
- Low cardiac output/cardiac failure
- Pericardial effusion
- Hyponatraemia and hypoglycaemia
- Hypoventilation

Even with treatment, it still carries a high mortality

- Identify any precipitating cause (e.g. infection)
- Gradual rewarming
- Supportive ITU management (protect airway in coma, oxygen, broad-spectrum antibiotics, cardiac monitoring, glucose, monitor urine output)
- Take blood for thyroid function tests
- Treat with hydrocortisone until hypoadrenalism excluded
- Thyroid hormone replacement—both oral and i.v. T_4 and T_3 have been advocated with no clear consensus

---

CASE HISTORY 8.1

A 45-year-old woman attended her doctor feeling 'not quite right' for the last 6 months. She was tired and her hair had been falling out. She had noticed her periods being heavy and rather erratic and wondered whether she was entering the menopause. She had put on 5 kg during the last 6 months. The doctor did some blood tests: Na^+ 134 mmol/L, K^+ 3.8 mmol/L, urea 4.2 mmol/L, creatinine 95 μmol/L, TSH 11.2 mU/L, fT_4 7.4 pmol/L, Hb 112 g/L, gonadotrophins were normal.

What is the endocrine diagnosis and why?
What is the treatment?
Is she menopausal?
What is the potential significance of the haemoglobin level?

Answers, see p. 145

BOX 8.11 Symptoms and signs of thyrotoxicosis plus features associated with Graves disease

- Weight loss despite full, possibly increased, appetite
- Tremor
- Heat intolerance and sweating
- Agitation and nervousness
- Palpitations, shortness of breath/tachycardia +/− atrial fibrillation
- Amenorrhoea/oligomenorrhoea and consequent subfertility
- Diarrhoea
- Hair loss
- Easy fatigability, muscle weakness and loss of muscle mass
- Rapid growth rate and accelerated bone maturation (children)
- Goitre—diffuse, reasonably firm +/− bruit in Graves disease (Fig. 8.8)

Specific features associated with Graves disease
- Thyroid eye disease, also called Graves orbitopathy (Fig. 8.8)
- Pretibial myxoedema—thickened skin over the lower tibia
- Thyroid acropachy (clubbing of the fingers)
- Other autoimmue features, e.g. vitiligo

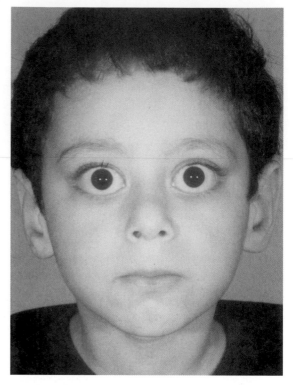

Figure 8.8 Hyperthyroidism. Graves disease in a 4-year-old. Note the goitre and eye signs.

Efficient clinical assessment of thyroid status is commonly required in the outpatient clinic (Box 8.12).

Diagnosis. Thyrotoxicosis requires biochemical proof of suppressed TSH and raised free thyroid hormone levels (Table 8.1). In the absence of extrathyroidal features, additional tests may help to distinguish between Graves disease and a toxic adenoma (the latter possibly part of a multinodular goitre). Antithyroglobulin and/or antithyroid peroxidase antibodies are easier to measure than anti-TSH receptor antibodies (the real 'pathogen') and may be elevated. Thyroid ultrasound has a characteristic appearance in Graves disease due to increased vascularity and blood flow in the overactive gland (the same features that cause the bruit on auscultation). Diffuse uptake on a radionuclide scan indicates Graves disease, while patchy uptake indicates toxic multinodular goitre; a single toxic nodule will show clearly as a 'hot' nodule. Transient hyperthyroidism will appear normal on ultrasound and have normal isotope uptake.

Treatment. There are three options to treatment:
1. *Antithyroid drugs* (Box 8.4). Since Graves disease waxes and wanes, a valid approach to treatment is to block the hyperthyroidism until remission. It is common to maintain patients on antithyroid drugs for 12 to 18 months and then to withdraw treatment to test for spontaneous remission. During this period, thyroid function tests are needed to ensure biochemical euthyroidism. The correct dose of drug, most commonly carbimazole, can be titrated or used at high dose (e.g. 40 mg) in combination with thyroxine (100 µg; 'block and replace'). Very rarely, antithyroid drugs can cause agranulocytosis and the patient must be warned to attend for a blood neutrophil

---

BOX 8.12 A 3-minute clinical assessment of thyroid status

- General inspection
  - Is there an obvious goitre or thyroid eye disease?
  - Is the patient appropriately dressed for the temperature?
  - Is the patient underweight, normal or overweight?
- Start with the hands
  - Are they warm and sweaty? Is there onycholysis or palmar erythema?
  - Is there thyroid acropachy?
  - Place sheet of paper on outstretched hands to assess tremor
  - Assess rate and rhythm of the radial pulse
  - Briefly assess character of pulse at the brachial artery
- Inspect front of neck, ask patient to swallow with the aid of a sip of water; is the neck painful?
- Move behind patient to palpate neck — is there a goitre? If so:
  - Assess size and movement on swallowing
  - Can the lower edge be felt (if not, it may extend retrosternally)?
  - Assess quality (e.g. firm, soft, hard)
  - Is it symmetrical?
  - Palpate for lymphadenopathy, especially if there is a goitre in a euthyroid patient
- Percuss for retrosternal extension
- Auscultate for a bruit
- Examine for other features of Graves disease (thyroid eye disease, pretibial myxoedema)

---

thyroidectomy can be used so long as the patient is adequately blocked preoperatively. Failure to achieve this runs the risk of 'thyroid storm' when handling the gland at operation can release huge stores of hormone and cause raging, life-threatening thyrotoxicosis. Carbimazole can be used to achieve biochemical euthyroidism or Lugol's iodine/potassium iodide can acutely block thyroid hormone release. Subtotal thyroidectomy leaves a small amount of tissue to try and minimize the risk of postoperative hypothyroidism (Box 8.8). Complications include: damage to the recurrent laryngeal nerve controlling the laryngeal muscles and voice; transient or permanent hypoparathyroidism due to damage or removal of the parathyroids; and bleeding. The scar, parallel to natural skin creases, is usually neat.

3. *Radioiodine.* Iodine-131 (I^{131}) can be used to treat thyroid overactivity in the absence of thyroid eye disease, which it aggravates, and pregnancy, where it is contraindicated. It requires the same preparation as surgery to avoid thyroid storm. In the UK, I^{131} has tended to be reserved for women who have completed their family, although evidence of increased tumour risk or diminished fertility is poor. It is used more liberally in Europe, except in children. It carries no risk to surrounding structures but it is highly likely to induce permanent hypothyroidism, for which the patient needs preoperative counselling, postoperative monitoring and, in all likelihood, lifelong replacement therapy.

For all of these approaches, beta-blockers, most commonly propanolol can be used to moderate the symptoms of adrenergic excess, especially as antithyroid drugs take 2 weeks to have much effect.

count in the event of sore throat or fever. Rash is a common side-effect and may settle with hydrocortisone cream. The success of this approach can be broken down into three categories: one-third of patients remits and remains well; one-third remits but relapses at some future time; and one-third relapses soon after stopping the drug and requires further treatment. The risk of falling into the last group is increased for males, having a high fT4 or large goitre at diagnosis and for those in whom TSH remains suppressed during treatment.

2. *Surgery.* If drugs fail or if a prompt definitive outcome is required (e.g. in pregnancy), subtotal

Graves disease in pregnancy. Autoimmune disorders, including Graves disease, tend to ameliorate during pregnancy. A common scenario is one of relative subfertility while hyperthyroidism is undiagnosed, followed by pregnancy once treatment becomes effective. Antithyroid drugs cross the placenta more efficiently than thyroxine and block the fetal thyroid. The minimum dose possible should be used and 'block and replace' avoided. Carbimazole increases the risk of aplasia cutis (a congenital scalp defect) and other abnormalities, so propylthiouracil (PTU) is preferred. In ~1% of mothers with Graves disease, past or present, high levels of thyroid-stimulating antibodies cross the placenta and cause fetal thyrotoxicosis, which is easy to forget when the mother has been treated by previous thyroidectomy. Fetal heart rate is a useful guide to its thyroid status. If needed, treatment is with antithyroid drugs. After birth, the symptoms recede with a time course that reflects the clearance of the maternal antibodies. If surgery is required during pregnancy, it is best planned for the second trimester. Postpartum, the mother is no longer 'protected' from Graves disease and may relapse. Monitoring with thyroid function tests is warranted.

Thyroid eye disease (Graves orbitopathy)

The same autoimmune infiltration that affects the thyroid can also affect the extraocular muscles of the orbit (Table 8.2). Although most commonly timed close to the thyroid disease process, it is possible for thyroid eye disease to run an entirely separate course. However, its presence with thyrotoxicosis confirms the diagnosis of Graves disease. For reasons that are unclear, thyroid eye disease is much worse in smokers.

Some symptoms of 'grittiness' are common, for which liquid teardrops are effective. All but minor thyroid eye disease warrants referral to an ophthalmologist. Detecting patients who can no longer close the eye due to proptosis is important because the cornea becomes at risk of ulceration. Taping the eyelids closed may be necessary at night. Although cosmetically undesirable, proptosis acts as a safeguard, relieving the retro-orbital pressure from swollen muscles. A relatively normal external appearance associated with retro-orbital pain or visual disturbance is far more concerning; there is risk of pressure on the optic nerve that can cause loss of vision.

The degree of retro-orbital inflammation and compression is assessed by magnetic resonance imaging (so-called 'stir' sequence MRI). If needed, treatment begins with cessation of smoking. Carbimazole probably possesses immunosuppressive qualities, so block and replace (see earlier) may be useful if there is coexisting thyroid disease. Radioiodine is contraindicated during active orbitopathy. Glucocorticoids are certainly immunosuppressive and can be used with steroid-sparing agents (e.g. azathioprine). The efficacy of orbital radiotherapy is contentious. Surgery can relieve sight-threatening compression. The natural history is for the disease to 'burn out'. Diplopia may remain from fibrosed mus-

Table 8.2 Symptoms, signs and examination of thyroid eye disease

Symptoms and signs	Gritty, weepy, painful eyes
	Retro-orbital pain
	Difficulty reading
	Diplopia
	Loss of vision
	'Staring' appearance
	Periorbital oedema and chemosis (redness) of the conjunctiva
	Injection over the insertion point of lateral rectus
	Lid retraction
	Proptosis (forward displacement of the orbit)
Examination	Inspect from the front for signs of inflammation and lid retraction
	Is the sclera visible around the entire eye (Fig. 8.8)
	Inspect from the side for proptosis
	Assess eye movements from the front asking the patient to report double vision
	Assess visual fields
	Ask the patient to look away while retracting the lateral portion of each eyelid in turn. The insertion point of lateral rectus is visible. Is it inflamed?
	Assess whether the patient can close the eyelids completely

cles, however, at this late stage, corrective surgery is highly effective.

Amiodarone-associated thyroid disease

Amiodarone is frequently used in cardiology to treat arrhythmias. It contains a lot of iodine and has a half-life longer than 1 month. It causes disordered thyroid function tests in up to half of patients as well as frank hyperthyroidism and hypothyroidism in up to 20% (Box 8.13).

Toxic adenoma

Hyperthyroidism, which is not autoimmune in origin, is usually due to thyroid autonomy associated with either a single adenoma (a 'toxic nodule') or a dominant nodule within a multinodular goitre (see below). Both are virtually always benign. Occasionally, adenomas secrete a predominant excess of T_3 to cause 'T_3-toxicosis' with normal fT_4 levels. This may require a special request to the laboratory to ensure that fT_3 is assayed.

BOX 8.13 Amiodarone can affect the thyroid gland and the thyroid function test

D1 and D2 are Types 1 and 2 selenodeiodinase respectively (review Fig. 8.6)
Effects on peripheral hormone metabolism and thyroid function tests:

- fT_3 slightly decreased
- fT_4 slightly increased } inhibition of D1 and D2 activity
- rT_3 formation increased
- Transient TSH increase

Amiodarone-associated hypothyroidism:
- Iodine content may inhibit hormone synthesis and release

Amiodarone-associated hyperthyroidism:
- Amiodarone may be directly toxic to the thyroid
- Iodine excess may stimulate overactivity in susceptible individuals

Inflammation may provoke transient thyrotoxicosis followed by hypothyroidism
Treatment:
- Uptake can be difficult as the thyroid is already loaded with iodine
- Try carbimazole
- If drugs fail, surgery can be considered

Such patients will not have the diffuse and symmetrical goitre characteristic of Graves disease, nor will they have signs of Graves eye disease. Ultrasound and uptake scans will demonstrate the lesion. Unlike Graves disease, spontaneous remission does not occur and definitive treatment with surgery or radioiodine is indicated. With thyroid lobectomy or with radioiodine (when most of the gland is quiescent and will not take up the I^{131}), the risk of post-treatment hypothyroidism is low.

Multinodular goitre

The pathogenesis of multinodular goitre, where many colloid-filled follicular nodules develop, is unclear. Frequency is increased in females, with age and with iodine deficiency. The case for treatment is pressed if autonomous functioning of a dominant nodule causes thyrotoxicosis, if local compressive symptoms occur (e.g. on the trachea) or if cosmetic disfigurement prevails. Surgery is best for cosmetic improvement of the largest goitres; otherwise I^{131} is effective, especially in the frail. As with toxic adenoma, the risk of hypothyroidism post-I^{131} treatment is relatively low.

As a sign of autonomy in multinodular goitres, TSH is often suppressed, yet fT_4 and fT_3 are in the normal range. Long-term, this subclinical overactivity increases mortality from cardiovascular disease. Treatment may also benefit seemingly minor symptoms. If treatment is decided against, annual progression to frank thyrotoxicosis in such patients is ~1% and occurs particularly in goitres with a dominant nodule greater than 2 cm diameter. In this scenario, annual monitoring of thyroid function is indicated.

Thyroid cancer

There are various types of thyroid cancer with quite different prognoses. Details here are restricted to clinically significant disease; it is relatively common to find small foci of papillary cancer ('microcarcinoma'), of dubious significance, upon histological examination of multinodular goitre. A general approach to the patient is given in Box 8.14.

In a patient with a goitre, diagnosing hyperthyroidism reduces the likelihood of thyroid malignancy. Fine needle aspiration is the investigation of choice for investigating 'cold' nodules and is ideally

CASE HISTORY 8.2

A 32-year-old man attended his doctor having lost 10 kg in weight and with poor sleep. He felt on edge and had had difficulty concentrating at work. He smokes five cigarettes per day. Colleagues had commented that he always looks like he is staring or glowering at them. The doctor completes the history and examination and takes a blood test. He knew the likely diagnosis beforehand, however the results provided proof: TSH <0.01 mU/L, fT_4 82.7 pmol/L, fT_3 14.2 pmol/L.

What is the biochemical diagnosis and why?
What features of the examination could have suggested the diagnosis for the doctor without the blood test?
What is the most likely treatment plan and with what advice?
What definitive treatment is not appropriate at present?

Answers, see p. 145

BOX 8.14 Approach to diagnosing thyroid malignancy

Although there is a female predominance, given the much-increased incidence of all thyroid disease in women, goitre in a male increases the relative risk of malignancy.

Suspicious features in the history:
- Rapid growth
- Alteration of the voice or dysphagia
- Previous irradiation of the neck
- Familial tumour predisposition syndrome (e.g. multiple endocrine neoplasia; see Chapter 10)

Suspicious features on examination:
- Firm, irregularly shaped goitre with euthyroidism
- Tethering to other structures
- Local lymphadenopathy

Investigation:
- 'Cold' nodule (decreased uptake in comparison to normal tissue) on radioiodine scanning
- Fine needle aspiration or biopsy
- Histological diagnosis

performed under ultrasound guidance; ~12% of cold nodules prove to be malignant. It tends to produce four results: clear malignancy, suspicion, normality, or 'nondiagnostic'. Endocrinologists vary in how follow-up is conducted of normal results. Clear malignancy requires total thyroidectomy. Suspicious results in high-risk individuals are probably best managed by local resection to provide a clear tissue diagnosis—malignancy then proceeding to total thyroidectomy. Repeated nondiagnostic aspirations and biopsies are relatively common and, if clinical suspicion is high, local surgery is probably the best option (as for suspicious biopsies). Despite the link to familial syndromes (Table 8.3), most medullary carcinoma is sporadic. Calcitonin serves as a circulatory marker. It is covered in greater detail in Chapter 10.

Papillary cell thyroid cancer carries a good prognosis. Spread is characteristically by the lymphatic system. Following thyroidectomy, doses of replacement thyroxine are given that suppress TSH. Thyroglobulin acts as a very sensitive marker of persisting or recurrent disease, to which radioactive

Table 8.3 Some characteristics of thyroid malignancies

Type	% of thyroid malignancies	Groups affected	Outcome
Follicular cell origin			
Papillary carcinoma	70–75	Young women	Good
Follicular carcinoma	15–20	Middle-aged women	Good
Anaplastic	5	Older people	Very poor
C-cell origin			
Medullary carcinoma	<10	Can be part of MEN	Poor
Others			
e.g. lymphoma, sarcoma	<10		Can be good

iodine ablation can be administered. Follicular carcinoma also carries a good prognosis. It consists of a mixture of neoplastic colloid-containing follicles, empty acini and alveoli of neoplastic cells. Intriguingly, follicular carcinomas predominate in geographical areas with low dietary iodine. Treatment and postoperative follow-up are similar to papillary carcinoma. In contrast, anaplastic carcinoma is almost always fatal and represents a fast-growing, poorly differentiated tumour, for which there is a mean survival from diagnosis of only 6 months.

Answers to case histories

Case history 8.1

The woman has primary hypothyroidism, which probably accounts for the tiredness and the hair loss. TSH is more than twice the upper limit of normal and fT_4 levels are below the normal range. fT_3 has not been measured but is unnecessary in this instance. The slightly low serum sodium is probably associated with the hypothyroidism. Treatment should be with oral thyroxine. The dose required is the one that normalizes the TSH on repeat thyroid function tests, which should be performed 6 weeks to 2 months after starting treatment. It is most likely to be a single daily tablet of 100 μg, which in the UK does not currently attract a prescription charge. Treatment is lifelong. She could start on this dose straightaway.

She is highly unlikely to be menopausal as gonadotrophins are normal. She has mild anaemia, possibly due to iron deficiency from the menorrhagia, which might also contribute to the hair loss. Alternatively, hypothyroidism can cause anaemia,

most probably normochromic normocytic, but possibly associated with mild macrocytosis. A finding of macrocytosis should also raise concern over pernicious anaemia, of which this patient is at increased risk. The mean cell volume should be measured and the anaemia should be investigated further by examining iron stores. If low, then a course of ferrous sulphate would be appropriate. The full blood count should be reinvestigated with the future thyroid function test.

Finally, the patient should be advised that restoring euthyroidism by itself will not necessarily cause loss of the weight gain. However, alongside careful diet and exercise, this should be attainable.

Case history 8.2

The thyroid function tests reveal thyrotoxicosis. TSH is undetectable and both free thyroid hormones are ~threefold the normal upper limit.

The scale of these blood results is very unlikely to be due to transient hyperthyroidism and the history contains no clues of recent viral infection. The diagnosis is clinched by the presence of thyroid eye disease. The staring appearance is due to the entire sclera being visible because of lid retraction and possible proptosis. In combination with the thyrotoxicosis, this diagnoses primary hyperthyroidism due to Graves disease. The other relevant feature of the examination could have been the detection of a thyroid bruit on auscultation over each lobe of the gland. A characteristic goitre is strongly suggestive of Graves disease; however, the bruit, indicative of diffusely increased vascularity, confirms the diagnosis. Although rare, pretibial myxoedema would also indicate that the thyrotoxicosis is due to Graves disease. Less specifically, a positive family history for autoimmune thyroid disease would be supportive.

The patient should be referred to an endocrinologist. However, treatment could be initiated with antithyroid drugs to attain biochemical euthyroidism. The most likely treatment plan is their use for 12 to 18 months, followed by withdrawal. In the UK, the most common agent is carbimazole at a starting dose of ~40 mg once daily. The prescription should be issued with a warning over the rare side-effect, agranulocytosis, and the need for urgent consultation in the event of sore throat or fever. Rash is a more common side-effect and may settle after a few days. Propranolol 40 mg three times daily could be prescribed to control symptoms, certainly during the 2 weeks or so that the carbimazole takes to begin its effect. Endocrinologists vary in their follow-up strategy, by either titrating the dose of carbimazole or using 'block-and-replace' (see earlier text in this chapter). By either approach, TSH would most likely remain undetectable at first; however, in time, it would be anticipated to rise back towards the normal range. Biochemical hypothyroidism should be avoided.

As a male with high levels of free thyroid hormones at diagnosis, he is already at higher risk of failure to remit and the need for definitive treatment with surgery. Persistently undetectable TSH during treatment and a large goitre would increase this risk further.

Further assessment of the thyroid eye disease is needed. The patient should be advised to stop smoking. If symptoms are limited to minor 'grittiness', the patient can close his eyes completely, and the remainder of the eye examination is largely unremarkable (e.g. vision normal, no retro-orbital pain), then observation would suffice. However, if the disease is any more significant, then referral should be made to an ophthalmologist.

Radioiodine would be contraindicated for definitive treatment of the thyroid disease, as, especially in an active smoker, it would be likely to exacerbate the eye disease.

CHAPTER 9

9 Calcium and metabolic bone disease

LEARNING OBJECTIVES

- To understand the importance of calcium metabolism:
  - appreciate normal calcium homeostasis and its principal regulators
  - understand the causes, clinical features and treatments of both hypocalcaemia and hypercalcaemia

- To gain a broad understanding of metabolic bone disease:
  - understand the aetiology, clinical features and treatments of osteoporosis
  - understand the aetiology, clinical features and treatments of rickets and osteomalacia

This chapter is divided into two halves in which we will examine calcium metabolism and metabolic bone disease

Calcium metabolism

Calcium is vital to many physiological processes (Box 9.1), and has a role in both intra and extracellular functions. The circulating concentrations are maintained within narrow limits (2.25–2.55 mmol/L) to allow these functions to occur. Within the cell, the concentration of calcium is much lower, ranging from 0.1 to 1 μM, while in the interstitial compartment, the values are intermediate (1.5 mM).

Calcium is a major constituent of all cell types and there is approximately 1.2 kg of calcium in the adult human body. The vast majority (1 kg) of this is stored with bone as hydroxyapatite $(3Ca_3(PO_4)_2.Ca(OH)_2)$. Within the plasma there is approximately 350 mg, around a half of which is unbound and biologically active. Most of the remainder is bound to plasma proteins, mainly albumin, while around 10% is complexed with citrate. When interpreting calcium concentrations, the values must always be corrected for the serum albumin. An erroneous diagnosis of hypocalcaemia may otherwise be made if albumin concentrations are low and similarly an erroneous diagnosis of hypercalcaemia can be made if albumin concentrations are increased.

There is a continuous exchange of calcium between different 'pools' in the body yet a balance between these various sites is usually maintained (Fig. 9.1). During childhood, calcium balance is positive as new bone is laid down. During young adulthood, the daily uptake of calcium from the gut is equivalent to daily losses from the urine and sweat while in older age, particularly in postmenopausal women, the output is greater and calcium is in negative balance.

Regulation of calcium balance is closely associated with that of phosphate, although the control of the latter is less precise. The normal range of

BOX 9.1 Key facts about calcium

It plays an important role in:
- Bone mineralization
- Blood clotting
- Muscle contraction
- Enzymatic action
- Release of hormones and neurotransmitters
- Nerve function
- Cell division and proliferation

Its concentrations are tightly regulated by PTH, vitamin D and calcitonin
- Serum concentration: 2.25–2.55 mmol/L
- Interstitial space concentration: 1.5 mM
- Intracellular concentration: 0.1–1 μM

There is ~1.2 kg of calcium in the adult human body
- 1 kg is stored in bone as hydroxyapatite
- 50% of plasma calcium is bound to either plasma proteins, mainly albumin, or complexed with citrate

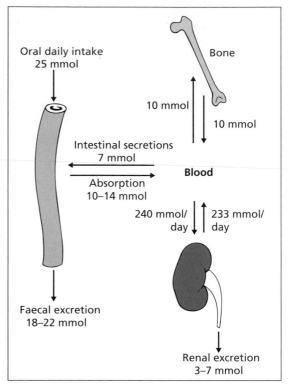

Figure 9.1 A schematic representation of calcium exchange in an adult who is in calcium balance. The daily net absorption from the gut (total absorption less intestinal secretion) equals urinary loss. In contrast, in a growing child, net absorption exceeds renal excretions, to allow for retention of calcium in the skeleton, and so the child is in positive calcium balance.

phosphate lies between 0.6 and 1.3 mmol/L but it is higher in children. A higher proportion of dietary phosphate is absorbed than calcium and so correspondingly more phosphate is excreted in the urine. Phosphate absorption and excretion is increased with high meat intake. A gene on the short arm of the X chromosome, *PHEX*, is important in the renal regulation of phosphate excretion. Mutations in this gene cause X-linked hypophosphataemia.

Dietary calcium

The recommended daily allowance for calcium is around 1 g per day. Calcium is abundant in many foods, especially dairy products such as cheese and milk. Absorption from the gut is inefficient such that only around 30% of ingested calcium is absorbed. This process is highly regulated and is one of the means by which serum calcium is controlled. Calcium absorption increases in childhood and during pregnancy and lactation but decreases with age and if calcium intake is high.

A number of dietary factors also affect calcium absorption. Basic amino acids and lactose in the gut enhance calcium absorption and so milk supplementation is a particularly effective way of providing calcium supplementation to children. In contrast,

phytic acid, which is present in unleavened or brown bread, inhibits calcium absorption because the phytic acid chelates the calcium in the gut. During the Second World War, bread was fortified with calcium in the UK and this practice continues to this day.

Regulation of calcium homeostasis

The body has three hormonal mechanisms to regulate calcium:
- Vitamin D
- Parathyroid hormone (PTH)
- Calcitonin

Vitamin D and PTH act to increase calcium while calcitonin lowers calcium concentrations.

Vitamin D

Although vitamin D is classed as a vitamin, it has many attributes that suggest it would be better classified as a hormone (Box 9.2). It is derived from cholesterol and has a structure that is similar to other steroid hormones (review Chapter 2). Although at least 10% of vitamin D is acquired from the diet in the form of vitamin D_2, the remainder is formed as vitamin D_3 in the skin under the action of ultraviolet light (Fig. 9.2).

Vitamin D_2 has an identical structure to vitamin D_3 except for a double bond between C22 and C23 in the side chain. The main sources of dietary vitamin D_2 (ergocalciferol) are fish and eggs and so strict vegans are at increased risk of vitamin D deficiency. Several food sources, including margarine, are fortified with vitamin D_2. Vitamin D_3 (cholecalciferol), which accounts for 90% of total vitamin D, is synthesized in the skin by photoisomerization under the influence of ultraviolet light. 7-dehydrocholesterol

---

BOX 9.2 Why vitamin D is not a vitamin but a hormone

- A vitamin is a compound that must be provided in the diet—although 10% of vitamin D is acquired in the diet, the vast majority is synthesized in the skin
- The active form of vitamin D is produced in the kidney and secreted in the bloodstream to act on a distant tissue

---

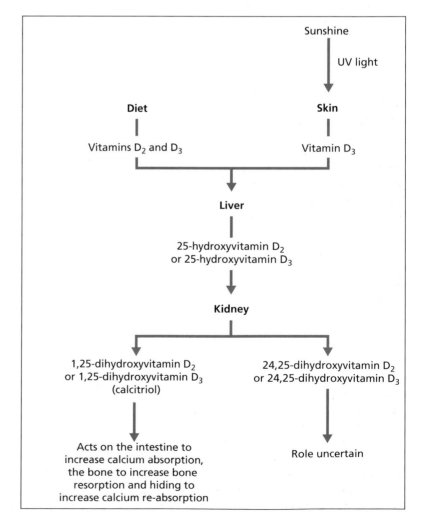

Figure 9.2 The sources and metabolism of vitamin D. The term vitamin D is used when it is not necessary to differentiate between vitamin D_2 and D_3.

is converted to previtamin D by opening the B ring of the cholesterol backbone. Subsequent rotation of the A ring produces mature vitamin D_3 (Fig. 9.3).

Vitamin D is activated by undergoing two important enzymatic additions of hydroxyl groups. The first step occurs in the liver where inactive vitamin D is converted to 25-hydroxy vitamin D. This is then converted in the kidney to the active 1,25 dihydrovit-

amin D (Fig. 9.4). 1,25 dihydrovitamin D_3 is also known as calcitriol.

Other metabolites of vitamin D include 24,25-dihydroxy vitamin D which is made by 24-hydroxylation of 25-hydroxy vitamin D in the kidney. The role of this compound is unknown but is probably biologically inert. Vitamin D is inactivated in the kidney by 24-hydroxylase to 1,24,25 tri-hydroxy vitamin D. The activity of

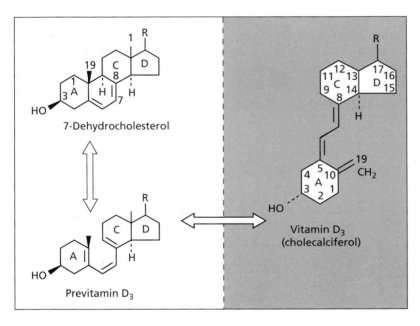

Figure 9.3 The formation of vitamin D_3. Ultraviolet irradiation, for example on skin, opens the B ring of 7-dehydrocholesterol to give previtamin D_3; rotation of the A ring then gives vitamin D_3 (cholecalciferol). In this illustration, R is the side-chain of cholesterol, 7-dehydrocholesterol and vitamin D_3 (see Fig. 9.4). Projection of groups relative to the plane of the rings: (▼), forwards; (¦), backwards.

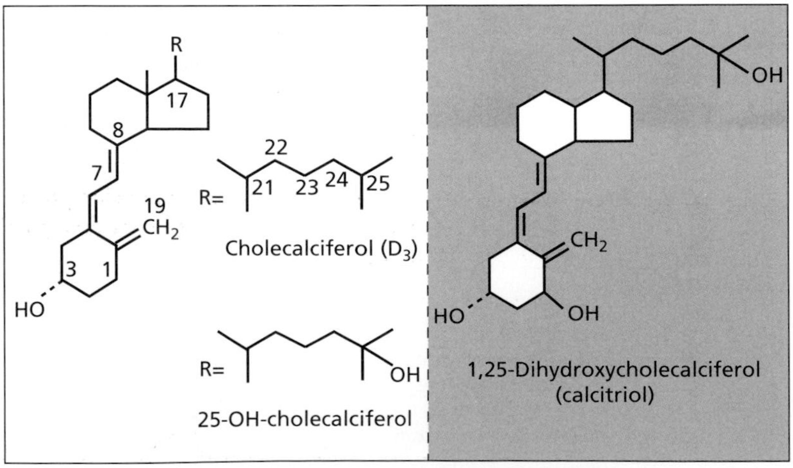

Figure 9.4 The formation of calcitriol. Cholecalciferol (vitamin D_3) is first hydroxylated in the liver to 25-OH-cholecalciferol. The latter is then hydroxylated at C-1 to 1,25-dihydroxycholecalciferol, which is also known as calcitriol. The hydroxyl group is in the alpha orientation, and so the renal enzyme responsible is known as 1α-hydroxylase.

24-hydroxylase is increased by high calcium concentrations (Fig. 9.5).

The production of active vitamin D is tightly regulated and subject to feedback control. While the concentration of 25-hydroxycholecaliferol in the circulation is quite high (3–30 μg/L), the concentration of calcitriol is very low (20–60 ng/L). Furthermore, there is a circulating vitamin D binding protein that has a high affinity for 25-hydroxy vitamin D and 24,25-dihydroxy vitamin D but low affinity for calcitriol.

The conversion of 25-hydroxy vitamin D to 1,25-dihydroxy vitamin D in the kidney occurs through the action of the enzyme 1α-hydroxylase. Low calcium or phosphate stimulates the 1α-hydroxylase enzyme while high calcium activates 24-hydroxylase leading to the production of increased 24,25-dihydroxy vitamin D and inactive 1,24,25 trihydroxy vitamin D. The synthesis of 1α-hydroxylase is increased by parathyroid hormone (PTH) whose secretion is regulated in part by vitamin D. This provides a means of co-ordinating the various controls of calcium homeostasis. The synthesis of 1α-hydroxylase is also increased by several other hormones including growth hormone, cortisol, oestrogens and prolactin.

The actions of vitamin D

Like steroid and thyroid hormones, vitamin D binds to specific nuclear receptors in a wide variety of cell types and promotes the synthesis of proteins involved in calcium absorption (Table 9.1). Within the gut, vitamin D increases the absorption of dietary

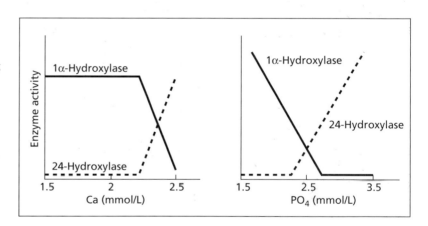

Figure 9.5 The effects of changing calcium and phosphate on the activity of renal hydroxylation of 25-hydroxycholecalciferol. Low calcium and low phosphate stimulate 1α-hydroxylation, which yields calcitriol, while high calcium and high phosphate increase 24-hydroxylation, which yields 24,25-dihydroxycholecalciferol.

Table 9.1 Comparison of actions of vitamin D, PTH and calcitonin

Site of action	Vitamin D	PTH	Calcitonin
Bone	↑ osteoclast activity ↑ bone resorption	↓ osteoblast activity ↑ bone resorption	↓ osteoclast activity ↓ bone resorption
Kidney	↑ Calcium reabsorption ↑ Phosphate reabsorption	↑ 1α-hydroxylase synthesis ↑ Calcium reabsorption ↓ Phosphate reabsorption	↓ Calcium reabsorption ↓ Phosphate reabsorption
Gut	↑ Calcium absorption ↑ Phosphate absorption	↑ Calcium absorption ↑ Phosphate absorption Indirect action only	
Blood	↑ Calcium ↑ Phosphate	↑ Calcium ↓ Phosphate	↓ Calcium ↓ Phosphate

calcium and phosphate by an unknown mechanism. In bone, vitamin D increases the release of calcium and phosphate by activating osteoclast activity to a small extent. The roles of osteoclast and osteoblast in bone turnover will be described in more detail in the section on metabolic bone disease later. Finally, in the kidney, vitamin D increases calcium and phosphate reabsorption. Vitamin D also has a number of actions outside calcium metabolism including effects on insulin sensitivity and cell differentiation in haematopoietic and epidermal cells.

Parathyroid hormone

There are usually four parathyroid glands but there may be additional accessory glands. They are small, lentil-sized glands and each weighs 40 to 60 mg, although they are larger in women than men. The parathyroid glands usually lie behind each of the lobes of the thyroid gland.

The parathyroid glands develop from the third and fourth embryological pharyngeal pouches (Fig. 9.6). These pouches are formed at the upper end of the foregut during weeks 4 and 5 of gestation. The pouches become separated from the gut and migrate downwards and by week 7 are in their final position in the neck. Interestingly, the two uppermost embryonic parathyroid glands cross the other two glands and end up as the most inferior glands. The migration may not always go to plan and this can explain why ectopic parathyroid glands may be found in the neck or mediastinum. This is of relevance to a surgeon seeking to remove overactive parathyroid tissue.

The parathyroid glands have a rich blood supply, derived mainly from the inferior thyroid arteries. The venous drainage is via the thyroid veins. The parathyroid glands are composed of two cells types—the chief cells which secrete parathyroid hormone (PTH) and oxyphil cells whose function is unknown. PTH is synthesized as a larger precursor molecule which is cleaved to the mature single chain 84 amino acid peptide hormone prior to storage in vesicles in the chief cells (Fig. 9.7 and review Figs 2.2 and 2.4). Release from these cells is controlled by low unbound serum calcium concentrations in a classical negative feedback mechanism (Fig. 9.8). The actions of PTH increase serum calcium and as calcium increases, so PTH secretion falls. Rapid changes in the

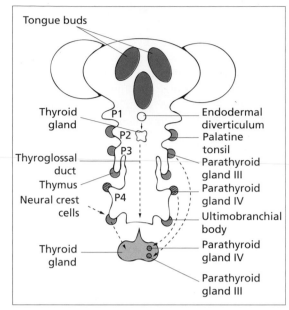

Figure 9.6 A horizontal section of a human fetal pharynx, looking down on its floor, and showing the origin of the thyroid and parathyroid glands. The thyroid originates in the floor of the pharynx at the level of the first pharyngeal pouch (P1). As the thyroid moves caudally, paired cell masses detach themselves from the third (P3) and fourth (P4) pharyngeal pouches, respectively, become positioned on the thyroid's posterior surface, and form the parathyroid glands III and IV. The origins of the thymus, palatine tonsils and tongue buds are also shown. (After K. L. Moore, *The Developing Human*, W.B. Saunders, Philadelphia).

secretion of PTH can occur, indicating that secretion is not dependent on *de novo* synthesis.

The actions of parathyroid hormone

The whole sequence of the parathyroid hormone is not necessary for full biological activity. The amino terminal is the important part and a synthetic peptide comprising the first 34 residues is fully active. PTH binds to a specific G-protein coupled cell surface receptor which is found on the renal tubule cells, osteoblast and gut epithelial cells (review Chapter 3). In the kidney, as well as activating 1α-hydroxylase,

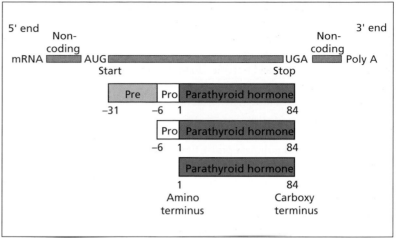

Figure 9.7 Messenger ribonucleic acid (mRNA) codes for the synthesis of parathyroid hormone (PTH), which begins with creation of a signal peptide with 25 amino acids, −31 to −6, of prepro-PTH. The signal peptide is normally removed before synthesis of the hormone is completed. Pro-PTH has 90 amino acids, the first six of which are removed before the 1–84 hormone is secreted.

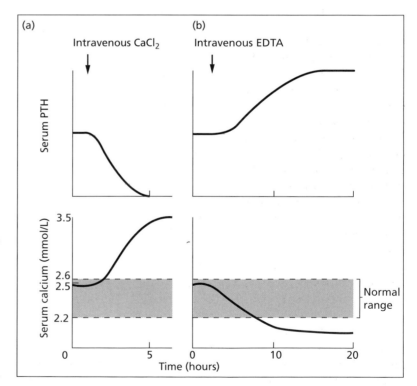

Figure 9.8 Changes in parathyroid hormone (PTH) secretion in response to alterations in serum calcium. (a) Rise in serum calcium reduces the secretion of PTH; this can be produced by infusion of calcium. (b) Conversely, a fall in serum calcium, produced by infusing ethylenediamine tetra-acetic acid (EDTA), which complexes calcium, stimulates PTH secretion.

PTH increases calcium and hydrogen absorption in the distal tubules but, unlike vitamin D, decreases phosphate and bicarbonate reabsorption. In the bone, PTH inhibits the bone-forming osteoblasts, leading to a release of calcium and phosphate through the unopposed action of the osteoclasts. It appears that PTH has no direct effect on calcium uptake from the gut but nevertheless calcium uptake is increased by the indirect action of PTH on vitamin D. It can be seen from this that PTH has diverging actions on phosphate but, overall, PTH lowers serum phosphate concentrations because the magnitude of the effect on kidney loss is greater than the release from bone.

Calcitonin

Calcitonin is secreted from the parafollicular or C-cells of the thyroid gland in response to a rise in calcium levels and acts to reduce calcium (see Chapter 8). It acts by binding to specific G-protein coupled cell surface receptors that are present on renal tubule cells and osteoclasts (review Chapter 3). In the kidney, calcitonin inhibits calcium and phosphate reabsorption while in bone it suppresses the release of calcium and phosphate.

The physiological relevance of calcitonin is unknown because no clinical syndrome develops during either its deficiency, for example following a thyroidectomy, or in excess, for example in medullary cell carcinoma of the thyroid (see Chapter 8). It may be important in growing children and pregnant women, contributing to growth or preservation of the skeleton. In nonmammalian species, its role may be more significant, as in birds it can modulate eggshell formation. Calcitonin may have a role in the treatment of several metabolic bone diseases.

The C-cells possess a number of cytochemical characteristics that are common to endocrine cells derived from the neural crest, such as the adrenal medulla cells that synthesize catecholamines (see Chapter 6), and other cell types such as those that secrete the gut and pancreatic islet hormones. The clinical significance is that they may give rise to a wide spectrum of neoplasia, the multiple endocrine neoplasia syndromes, which maintain many of the phenotypic characteristics of their normal progenitor cells. These are described in more detail in Chapter 10.

Medullary cell carcinoma of the thyroid may be a familial inherited condition or it may occur sporadically (see Tables 8.3 and 10.3). It may occur alone or as part of MEN-2. Patients with medullary cell carcinoma of the thyroid usually present with goitre, owing to enlargement of the thyroid (see Chapter 8). The calcitonin concentrations are very high but the calcium concentrations remain normal. Treatment is primarily by surgery.

Hypocalcaemia and hypercalcaemia

When calcium concentrations deviate from the normal range, the patients develop specific constellations of symptoms which will be described in the next section together with the causes and treatment.

Hypocalcaemia
Aetiology
The commonest cause of hypocalcaemia is a failure of the parathyroid gland to secrete sufficient PTH to meet the body's needs. There are a number of causes of hypoparathyroidism which are listed in approximate order of frequency:

- Iatrogenic—the parathyroid glands may be damaged or inadvertently removed during thyroid surgery. Surgical treatment of hyperparathyroidism may lead to hypoparathyroidism.
- Autoimmune—destruction of the parathyroid glands by specific autoantibodies. The parathyroid gland is one of the many endocrine glands affected by tissue specific autoimmune disorders (Box 8.7), e.g. Graves disease.
- Congenital (DiGeorge syndrome)—this rare syndrome occurs sporadically when the third and fourth pharyngeal pouches fail to develop in the embryo, resulting in the absence of the thymus and parathyroid glands. It is associated with congenital heart disease (see Fig. 4.4).
- Neonatal—suppression of the fetal parathyroid glands can occur if there is maternal hypercalcaemia.
- Renal failure—occurs because of a failure to hydroxylate vitamin D in the kidney.

Hypocalcaemia may also occur if there is magnesium deficiency because magnesium is a cofactor for some of the actions of PTH. PTH levels remain normal or even elevated but there is resistance to the action of PTH.

Tissue resistance to the action of PTH also occurs in the rare congenital condition pseudohypoparathyroidism. Despite raised PTH concentrations, the individuals have hypocalcaemia and hyperphosphataemia because the PTH fails to generate cAMP in bone and kidney. This occurs because of reduced G-protein coupling with the PTH receptor due to multitions in the $G_s\alpha$ subuint (review Box 3.8). In addition to the hypocalcaemia, these individuals have a characteristic phenotype of short round face, short neck and short metacarpals (Fig. 9.9). There may also be paradoxical ectopic calcification in muscle and brain.

Clinical features of hypocalcaemia

Unless hypocalcaemia occurs in the immediate postoperative period, its onset is usually insidious and causes remarkably few symptoms as the body is able to adapt to the changing calcium concentrations (Box 9.3). Corrected calcium values of less than 1.5 mmol/L, however, are incompatible with life.

Management

The aim of treatment is to normalize the calcium values to prevent the symptoms and signs. Although

---

BOX 9.3 Symptoms and signs of hypocalcaemia

Symptoms of hypocalcaemia
- Muscle cramps
- Numbness
- Paraesthesiae
- Mood swings and depression

Signs of hypocalcaemia
- Tetany
- Carpopedal spasm—this can be induced by applying a blood pressure cuff to the arm and is known as Trousseau's sign
- Neuromuscular excitability—tapping over the facial nerve causes the facial muscles to twitch (Chvostek's sign)
- Convulsions
- Cardiac arrythmias (long Q–T interval on ECG)
- Cataract

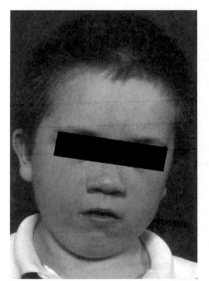

(a)

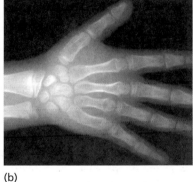

(b)

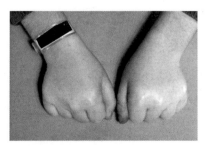

(c)

Figure 9.9 Clinical features of pseudohypoparathyroidism: (a) round face; (b) and (c) short fourth metacarpals.

CASE HISTORY 9.1

A 30-year-old woman underwent a difficult subtotal thyroidectomy for the treatment of Graves disease. She is anxious about the outcome of her operation and 2 days postoperatively, she complains of tingling in her fingers and mouth.

What are the possible explanations of her symptoms?
What would be your management?

Answers, see p. 167

BOX 9.4   Causes of hypercalcaemia

- Common
  - primary or tertiary hyperparathyroidism
  - malignancy
  - drugs and dietary causes
- Rare
  - immobilization
  - thyrotoxicosis
  - sarcoidosis
  - hypoadrenalism
  - acromegaly
  - familial benign hypercalcaemia

PTH is available, it must be given parenterally and is very expensive. Furthermore supplementation with calcium and vitamin D is sufficient to maintain calcium values in the normal range. PTH is important for 1α-hydroxylation during the conversion of inactive to active Vitamin D. Therefore, in hypoparathyroidism, supplementation should be with Vitamin D that has already been modified to 1α-calcidol (Case history 9.1).

Hypercalcaemia

Aetiology

Although hyperparathyroidism and malignancy are the commonest cause of hypercalcaemia, there are several other important causes that should be considered to prevent the patient from being subjected to unnecessary and potentially harmful investigations and treatment (Box 9.4). It is important to measure the calcium in a fasting state and without the application of a tourniquet as both of these can cause spurious rises in calcium. It is important to take a drug history as several drugs, including thiazide diuretics, antacids and vitamin A and D preparation, may cause hypercalcaemia.

Primary hyperparathyroidism. Hyperparathyroidism occurs when one or more of the parathyroid glands autonomously secretes excess parathyroid hormone. In around 80% of cases, the cause is a single parathyroid adenoma with the remainder caused by parathyroid hyperplasia. Parathyroid malignancy is extremely rare. Parathyroid adenomas can occur alone or as part of the multiple endocrine neoplasia syndromes (Chapter 10). Primary hyperparathyroidism has an incidence of around 1 in 1000 and occurs more commonly after the age of 45 years, where there is a female predominance of 2 : 1.

Secondary and tertiary hyperparathyroidism usually occur in renal failure although can occasionally result from calcium malabsorption. Renal impairment causes hypocalcaemia through a failure of vitamin D hydroxylation in the kidney and PTH increases in an attempt to normalize calcium. This is at the expense of normal bone health and a typical osteodystrophy occurs. With prolonged high secretion of PTH, the parathyroid glands may become autonomous and continue to hypersecrete PTH even after calcium concentrations are 'normalized'. This leads to hypercalcaemia.

Malignancy. Hypercalcaemia is frequently seen in malignant disease. This may occur because of direct metastatic destruction of the bone or by the secretion of an osteoclast-activating factor, such as prostaglandin, by metastases (Box 9.5). Haemopoietic tumours, such as multiple myeloma, are also frequently associated with hypercalcaemia because of osteoclast activation by tumour lymphokines. Tumours which have no bony involvement may also cause hypercalcaemia by secreting parathyroid-hormone-related peptide (PTHrP). The genes encoding PTH and PTHrP are separate yet very similar and probably arose from an ancient duplication event during human evolution. Thus, PTHrP is structurally related to PTH but is larger. As it does not cross-react with many PTH assays, the measured PTH concentration is low as the parathyroid switches off its own PTH secretion in response to the hypercalcaemia. PTHrP can also be synthesized by the placenta and lactating breast tissue and is important in the fetus for bone development.

Drugs and dietary causes. Several drugs, including thaizide diuretics, may cause hypercalcaemia. Overdose of vitamin D may also cause hypercalcaemia. Although this may occur from the over-treatment of hypocalcaemia, it may also occur in the unwary who take large doses of multivitamins. Rarely, ingestion of large amounts of milk and calcium-containing antacids for peptic ulceration can cause hypercalcaemia. This is much less common now that H_2 antagonists and proton pump inhibitors can effectively treat peptic ulceration.

Thyrotoxicosis. Hypercalcaemia may occur in thyrotoxicosis because of increased bone turnover as thyroid hormones increase osteoclast activity.

Sarcoidosis. Hypercalcaemia occurs in around 1 to 2% of patients with sarcoidosis because of the over-production of 1,25 dihydroxyvitamin D in the granulomatous cells of the sarcoid lesion.

Acromegaly. Hypercalcaemia may rarely occur in acromegaly because of stimulation of 1α-hydroxylase in the kidney by growth hormone.

Familial benign hypercalcaemia

Also known as familial hypocalciuric hypercalcaemia, this autosomal dominant condition forms part of the differential diagnosis especially in hypercalcaemia presenting to the paediatric endocrinologist. It is caused by inactivating mutations in the calcium sensing receptor leading to reduced negative feedback of the parathyroid glands and consequently increased PTH and mild hypercalcaemia. It is important to recognise as no treatment is necessary.

BOX 9.5 Sites of primary tumours that most commonly metastasize to bone

- Lung
- Breast
- Prostate
- Kidney
- Thyroid

BOX 9.6 Symptoms and signs of hypercalcaemia 'Bones, moans, groans and stones'

Symptoms of hypercalcaemia
- Bony pain
- Abdominal pain from peptic ulceration, acute pancreatitis or constipation
- Anorexia and nausea
- Thirst and polyuria
- Muscle weakness
- Headache and confusion
- Palpitations through cardiac arrythmias
- Tiredness and fatigue

Signs of hypercalcaemia
- Renal stones
- Bone fractures
- Convulsions and coma if severe
- Corneal calcification
- Hypertension

CASE HISTORY 9.2

An overweight, 50-year-old woman with a history of hypertension was found to have a calcium concentration of 2.86 mmol/L with albumin of 36 g/L. She believes strongly in self-help and had regularly attended a health food shop. Her mother died from breast cancer and our patient is concerned that she may have breast cancer too.

What is her corrected calcium?

What are the possible explanations for her hypercalcaemia?

Answers, see p. 167

Clinical features of hypercalcaemia

The wide availability of automated biochemistry testing has meant that a large proportion of patients are picked up by routine clinical testing with mild hypercalcaemia that is frequently asymptomatic (Case history 9.2). Patients with more severe degrees of hypercalcaemia may present several symptoms or signs shown in Box 9.6. Persistent hypercalcaemia can lead to ectopic calcification which can be seen on plain radiographs of the heart, joints and kidney. Hepatic and pancreatic calcification may rarely be seen.

Investigations of hypercalcaemia

The investigations are predominantly designed to determine the cause of the raised calcium. They include:
- Serum PTH
  - in the presence of hypercalcaemia, PTH concentrations should be suppressed and therefore even a PTH in the normal range is indicative of hyperparathyroidism
  - the samples should be handled with care as proteolytic degradation of the hormone may occur if the assay is not completed within a few hours
- 24 hr urinary calcium
  - this defines the severity of PTH overactivity in primary hyperparathyridion as calcuim is ultimately lost from the body
- Serum ACE
  - serum ACE is increased in active sarcoidosis
- Vitamin D
  - both 25-hydroxycalciferol and calctriol can be measured
  - 25-hydroxycalciferol is the most reliable index of vitamin D status
  - may indicate vitamin D toxicity
- Investigations of malignancy—this may include:
  - CXR—carcinoma of the bronchus
  - bone scan—bony metastasis
  - prostatic-specific antigen
  - mammogram
  - urinary Bence–Jones protein and serum protein electophoresis—multiple myeloma
- Hand X-rays
  - characteristic bone resorption with hyperparathyroidism—not frequently seen today as most cases diagnosed earlier

> **BOX 9.7 Emergency management of hypercalcaemia**
> - Intravenous rehydration
> - Loop diuretics may be of limited value
> - Steroids if vitamin D toxicity or haematological malignancy
> - Bisphosphonates

Management

Hypercalcaemia may present as a medical emergency (Box 9.7). Under these circumstances, the treatment is different from that for patients presenting asymptomatically. Most emergency patients are dehydrated and require fluids. Dietary calcium intake should be restricted. Several drugs are effective in lowering calcium. The treatments of choice are the bisphosphonates which inhibit bone resorption and lead to a rapid reduction in calcium. These may be administered orally or intravenously in cases of emergency. Corticosteroids are effective in cases of haematological malignancy or sarcoidosis.

It is important to treat the underlying cause, as even asymptomatic individuals may feel better once their calcium has fallen to normal. Surgery is the treatment of choice for hyperparathyroidism. In the case of an adenoma, parathyroidectomy of the affected gland is indicated although the other glands should be identified as multiple tumours may be present. All four glands are removed to treat parathyroid hyperplasia. In the past a gland has been reimplanted in the forearm to prevent the patient from becoming hypoparathyroid. The reason for the reimplantation is that repeat neck surgery is technically difficult and it is easier to conduct a repeat operation on the arm if the patient remains hypercalcaemic postoperatively. Location of the tumour can be difficult because of the subtle variations in embryological migration of the parathyroid glands. The surgeon may be helped by nuclear medicine scanning or selective venous sampling (Fig. 9.10) as well as standard imaging techniques such as ultrasound and CT/MRI scanning. Intraoperative histology using frozen samples with or without the use of dye improves the likelihood that the surgeon has successfully removed the tumour.

While it is relatively simple to decide that a

symptomatic patient with hyperparathyroidism should undergo surgery, the decision is less clear for an elderly asymptomatic individual whose hyperparathyroidism was discovered by routine biochemistry (Box 9.8). An analysis of these individuals has suggested that even mild hypercalcaemia is associated with excess morbidity, including depression, malaise, renal stones, hypertension and osteoporosis. Elevated 24-h urinary calcium excretion ('hypercalciuria') is associated with an increased risk of stones and a bone mineral density scan will detect asymptomatic osteoporosis. For many individuals, a watching brief is all that is needed. Presentation at less than 40 years of age should raise suspicion of potential multiple endocrine neoplasia (see Chapter 10) (Case history 9.3).

Metabolic bone disease

Bone and the skeleton support the body and protect its vital organs, including the brain and bone marrow. However, far from being an inert substance, bone is constantly being remodelled as it contributes to calcium and phosphate turnover. Bone is the largest store of calcium in the body and also contains 90% of the body's phosphate, 50% of its magnesium and 33% of its sodium. Bone mass increases during childhood and reaches a peak in early adulthood. Thereafter, there is a progressive loss of bone, which is accelerated at the time of the menopause in women (Fig. 9.11).

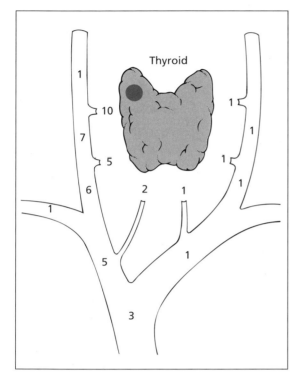

Figure 9.10 Localization of parathyroid tumours by assaying parathyroid hormone. Blood samples are taken after cannulation of the great veins of the neck and also the small thyroid veins. The numbers indicate the relative concentration of hormone in a patient with a tumour of the right upper parathyroid gland. The peak concentrations are in the right superior thyroid vein and the right internal jugular vein. The concentrations (shown in arbitrary numbers) are lower in the other veins such as the inferior thyroid veins and superior vena cava, thus pointing to the probable location of the tumour in the upper right parathyroid.

BOX 9.8 Indications for parathyroidectomy

Definite complications of disease:
- Renal stones
- Bone disease
- Symptomatic muscle disease
- Age <50 years irrespective of symptoms
- Moderate to severe hypercalcaemia (>3.0 mmol/L)

Other possible indications should be considered carefully but may include:
- Hypertension
- Psychiatric morbidity

CASE HISTORY 9.3

A 30-year-old man attends following a routine medical which showed hypercalcaemia. He is anxious about this because his father needed an operation on his neck but this was not successful. His uncle also had high calcium levels. Nevertheless both men are still well in their late 50s.

What are the possible familial causes of hypercalcaemia?

Answers, see p. 167

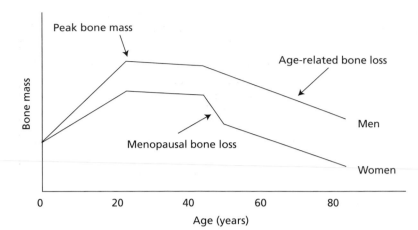

Figure 9.11 Changes in bone mass during a lifetime in men and women.

BOX 9.9 Characteristics of the two main types of bone

- Lamellar or compact bone
  - found in the cortex of adult long bones
  - consist of concentric lamellae around a central blood vessel
  - is relatively inert metabolically
- Cancellous or spongy bone
  - found in young subjects, at fracture sites and at the end of long bones
  - collagen fibres are in the form of loosely woven bundles
  - increases in hyperparathyroidism
  - high rates of bone turnover
  - large numbers of osteocytes are present

BOX 9.10 What is collagen?

- It is a protein rich in the amino acids glycine, proline and hydroxyproline
- It has the general formula $(glycine–proline.X)_{333}$ where X is another amino acid
- Its molecular weight is ~300 000 kDa, its length is 300 nm and diameter is 1.5 nm
- It is a semirigid, rod-like molecule
- It readily polymerizes to form microfibrils and fibrils
- It is involved in the initiation of hydroxyapatite crystallization

Bone growth and remodelling

Bone comprises a hard, calcified extracellular matrix and connective tissue, consisting of the osteoprogenitor cells, osteoblasts, osteocytes and osteoclasts (Box 9.9). Although the constituents of bone varies with age and gender, the inorganic or mineral component accounts for around 65% of the bone's mass while the remainder is organic constituents such as collagen.

Collagen is the most abundant constituent, accounting for 90 to 95% of the organic matrix of bone. The rest is made of proteoglycans, glycoproteins, sialoproteins and a small amount of lipid. Collagen is synthesized on the rough endoplasmic reticulum of osteoblasts as procollagen, which is subsequently cleaved to form the smaller, mature collagen in the extracellular space (Box 9.10).

During childhood new bone is being formed to meet the requirements of the child's growth, with both the length and diameter of the bone increasing. In adulthood, although the overall size of the bone does not change there is turnover of existing bone. The exact function of this is not fully understood but probably reflects the need to repair microtrauma and the need to contribute to calcium and phosphate metabolism. Bone turnover is tightly regulated by a number of local and humoral factors to ensure that bone resorption is coupled with new bone formation (Box 9.11; Fig. 9.12). There is, however, a small mismatch, particularly at the time of the menopause, whereby resorption exceeds new bone formation and consequently with time bone mass falls.

Bone turnover occurs as a result of the actions of osteoclasts and osteoblasts (Box 9.12). Osteoclasts

BOX 9.11 Factors regulating bone turnover

- Local factors
  - trauma
  - growth factors
    - IGF1
- Hormonal factors
  - PTH
  - vitamin D
  - sex hormones
  - growth hormone
  - corticosteroids

BOX 9.12 Comparison of osteoclasts and osteoblasts

- Osteoclasts
  - break down bone
  - stimulated by PTH and vitamin D
  - inhibited by calcitonin
- Osteoblasts
  - synthesize new bone
  - involved in calcium homeostasis

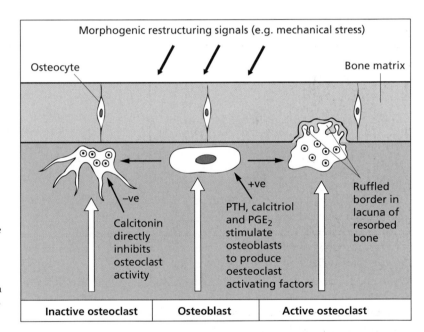

Figure 9.12 Factors that affect the remodelling of bone. Morphogenic restructuring signals such as mechanical stress can influence bone remodelling, while hormone factors control osteoblast activity. Calcitonin has an inhibitory action, with formation of an inactive osteoclast. Parathyroid hormone (PTH), calcitriol and prostaglandin E_2 (PGE_2) act on the osteoblast to produce osteoclast-activating factors that stimulate bone-matrix resorption by osteoclasts. Other hormones, such as thyroid hormones, can increase osteoclast activity.

are large, multinucleated cells formed by the fusion of mononuclear phagocytes from bone marrow. Osteoclasts appear on the surfaces of bone, which is subsequently resorbed as the osteoclasts break down components of bone through the action of lysosomal enzymes.

Osteoblasts are derived from fibroblast-like cells and enter the area of bone turnover after the osteoclast activity. Osteoblasts stimulate new bone formation by synthesizing the organic constituents of bone (osteoid) and are subsequently involved with its mineralization. Although formation of osteoid is relatively rapid and can occur within 6 to 12h of initiation, the secondary mineralization takes much longer (1–2months). After bone formation is complete, the osteoblasts become surrounded by the new bone matrix and differentiate into relatively inactive cells called osteocytes.

Osteoporosis

Osteoporosis is a skeletal disorder characterized by low bone mass and microarchitectural deterioration of bone tissue with a consequent increase in the risk of fracture—mainly at the hip, spine and wrist (Fig. 9.13). These fractures are a major cause of

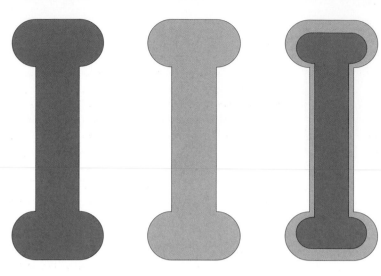

Normal bone | Osteoporotic bone showing loss of bone mass | Osteomalacia bone showing demineralized osteoid on the bone surface

Figure 9.13 Representation of normal, osteoporotic and osteomalacia bone.

morbidity and mortality in the elderly. In the UK, approximately 60 000 hip fractures, 50 000 distal radial fractures and 40 000 vertebral fractures occur annually, although many vertebral fractures may not come to clinical attention. Recent epidemiological data based on a UK sample suggest that 1.2 million women have osteoporosis.

Although bone formation exceeds bone resorption in youth, after the third to fifth decade of life there is a gradual loss of bone mass. Age is therefore the major risk factor for primary osteoporosis. While osteoporosis can affect both sexes, postmenopausal women are at the greatest risk, because bone loss is accelerated, to varying degrees, after the menopause due to loss of oestrogen production. Around one in six women over the age of 50 develops an osteoporotic fracture at some point during her lifetime. The calculated lifetime risk of an osteoporotic fracture in men is 13.5% at the age of 50 years and 25.6% at the age of 60.

Hip fracture is the most devastating manifestation of osteoporosis. Up to 20% of patients will die within 1 year of the fracture event and up to 50% lose their independence, often requiring institutionalization. The total cost of managing osteoporosis is staggering; the annual cost to the NHS of the acute management of osteoporotic fractures is £942 million, with hip fracture patients occupying 20% of all orthopaedic beds.

BOX 9.13 Diagnostic criteria for osteoporosis

Normal:	T score above −1
Osteopaenia:	T score −1 to −2.5
Osteoporosis:	T score below −2.5
Severe osteoporosis:	T score below −2.5 plus one or more fractures

Osteoporosis is diagnosed on the basis of bone mineral density. In recent years, several techniques have been developed to measure of bone mass accurately and precisely, of which dual energy X-ray absorptiometry (DEXA) is the method of choice. Following the measurement of absolute bone density at the hip and spine, patients are given a T score, which represents the number of standard deviations above or below the mean reference value for healthy young individuals. This T-score is used to define the diagnosis (Box 9.13).

There are a number of risk factors that increase the likelihood of age-related osteoporosis (Box 9.14). Furthermore, osteoporosis may occur secondary to a number of other causes (Box 9.15).

Clinical features

The most common clinical presentation of osteoporosis is fracture or bone pain. However, many patients will be found to be osteoporotic as a result of bone mineral density scanning that is performed in high-risk individuals, such as those receiving corticosteroid therapy (Case history 9.4).

BOX 9.14 Major risk factors for osteoporosis

- Caucasian or Asian race
- Female sex
- Age
- Low body mass index
- Family history of fracture
- Premature menopause
- Corticosteroid therapy

BOX 9.15 Secondary causes of osteoporosis

- Endocrine
  - primary and secondary hypogonadism
  - thyrotoxicosis
  - hyperparathyroidism
  - Cushing syndrome
  - hyperprolactinaemia
- Malignancy
- Drug-related
  - glucocorticoids
  - heparin
  - alcohol
- Connective tissue disorders
- Malabsorption or bowel disease
- Chronic liver disease
- Chronic renal failure
- Post-transplantation
- Rheumatoid arthritis

Treatment

As immobilization is associated with bone loss, patients should be encouraged to undertake weight bearing exercise. This should not become so excessive as to cause oestrogen deficiency through hypothalamic hypogonadism, as is frequently seen in elite female athletes and ballet dancers (see Chapter 7). A dietary supplementation with calcium and vitamin D has been shown to reduce fracture rates in the elderly.

It has been estimated that in the UK 10 to 20% of women with osteoporosis receive drug treatment for the condition. The choice of interventions is influenced by factors such as bone mineral density, stage of disease progression, nature and site of fracture, patient age, underlying comorbidities and side-effects. Agents that are used in the prevention and treatment of osteoporosis are generally classified as either antiresorptive or anabolic (Table 9.2). Drugs in the antiresorptive category preserve bone mass, while anabolic agents lead to an increase in cancellous bone mass which is sustained throughout the duration of therapy.

Table 9.2 Drugs used in the treatment of osteoporosis

Inhibitors of resorption	Stimulators of bone formation
Hormone replacement therapy	Sodium fluoride
Selective oestrogen receptor modulators	Parathyroid hormone
Bisphosphonates	Strontium ranelate
Calcitonin	
Calcium and vitamin D	
Anabolic hormones	

CASE HISTORY 9.4

A 51-year-old woman with long-standing, severe asthma tripped while coming down the last four stairs. She now complains of a pain in her back and a radiograph shows osteoporotic bone and a wedge fracture of her L3 vertebra.

Why has this woman had a fracture?
What are the possible treatments?

Answers, see p. 167

Hormone replacement therapy has been used extensively in the treatment of postmenopausal osteoporosis. It is undoubtedly effective at reducing fracture rates during the period in which it is taken. However, after cessation of treatment rapid bone loss occurs and it is unlikely that 5 to 10 years of hormone replacement therapy at the time of the menopause will provide significant protection against the development of hip fracture two to three decades later. There is an increasing anxiety that long-term hormone replacement therapy is associated with an increase in the risk of cardiovascular disease and stroke and therefore this form of treatment is now largely discouraged (see Box 7.17).

Selective oestrogen receptor modulators (SERMs), such as raloxifene, are a class of drugs with selective activity in various organ systems, acting as weak oestrogen receptor agonists in some systems and as oestrogen antagonists in others. Studies have shown that treatment with SERMs results in significant reductions in vertebral fracture risk whilst minimizing many of the side-effects of hormone replacement therapy.

The fall in the use of hormone replacement therapy has largely followed the introduction of the bisphosphonates, such as alendronate and risedronate. These drugs are associated with the most robust fracture risk reductions—approximately 40 to 50% reduction in vertebral fracture risk, 30 to 40% in nonvertebral fracture risk and 40 to 60% in hip fracture risk. Bisphosphonates are synthetic analogues of pyrophosphate that become incorporated into bone where they have a very long half-life. They inhibit both osteoclast activation and function.

Salmon calcitonin nasal spray is associated with a reduced fracture risk but is not routinely used. Newer therapies, such as the synthetic parathyroid hormone, celled teriparatide and strontium ranelate, also reduce vertebral and nonvertebral fracture risk.

Treatment can be monitored by serial bone mineral density scans every 2 years or so. A number of biochemical markers of bone resorption and formation have been identified. These provide indices of whole-body bone turnover during relatively short periods of time. The large inter- and intraindividual variability in these markers, however, restricts their value in clinical practice, although serial measurements may be useful in monitoring short-term responses to therapy.

Osteomalacia and rickets

Although vitamin D is intimately involved in the regulation of calcium metabolism, the effects of vitamin D deficiency are not usually manifested by hypocalcaemia but by the bony diseases osteomalacia and rickets. These are both characterized by failure of calcification of osteoid (Fig. 9.13). The effect on bone depends on whether the bone is growing or not and so rickets is seen in children and osteomalacia in adults.

Vitamin D deficiency in children was a major public health problem in industrialized nations in the northern hemisphere until the 1920s when it was found that cod liver oil could cure rickets. This led to widespread fortification of the milk supply, which was effective in virtually eliminating rickets. More recently, the cessation of the provision of free school milk in the UK has led to a resurgence of vitamin D deficiency. Although only 15 min per day of head and neck exposure to the sun in Western Europe during the summer months is sufficient to meet a white European person's requirement for vitamin D, the liberal use of sun creams to prevent skin cancer has also led to the re-emergence of vitamin D deficiency in Western Europe and Australasia. There are also a number of groups that are at particularly high risk of developing vitamin D deficiency (Box 9.16).

Although vitamin D deficiency is the commonest cause of osteomalacia and rickets, they may also be caused by several other conditions (Box 9.17).

Pathological and clinical features of osteomalacia
In the mature skeleton, osteomalacia leads to the production of wide layers of osteoid which eventually cover the majority of the available bone surfaces.

BOX 9.16 Groups at risk of vitamin D deficiency

- The elderly, particularly in residential care
- Babies of vitamin D deficient mothers
- Those with skin conditions where avoidance of sunlight is advised
- Dark skinned people, particularly if veiled
- Patients with malabsorption.

The main clinical feature is bony pain which may occur because of partial fracture leading to the X-ray appearance of a 'Looser zone' or pseudofracture. In addition, there may be a proximal myopathy causing profound weakness of the hip and shoulder girdle. Hypocalcaemia may occur with the symptoms described above.

Pathological and clinical features of rickets

Rickets is characterized by elongation and distortion of the normal columnar arrangement of chondrocytes in the zone of hypertrophy of cartilaginous growth (Fig. 9.14). In the zone of maturation, provisional calcification is delayed or absent. Vascularization via defective or obliterated channels is impaired and irregular while the primary spongiosa is grossly abnormal.

The main clinical features of rickets are bone pain, skeletal deformity and muscle weakness. Many of the physical and radiological signs are found at areas where bone growth is most rapid, usually in the metaphyseal region of long bones. At birth, the skull is growing most rapidly and therefore neonatal rickets may show craniotabes, where the cranial vaults have the consistency of a ping-pong ball. From the first year of life rickets becomes manifest in the swollen epiphyses of the wrist and in swelling of the costochondral junction, the so-called rickety rosary.

Treatment of osteomalacia and rickets

Vitamin D deficiency can be treated with small doses such as 3000 units/day or 0.5 μg/day of calcitriol. Improvement occurs within weeks but it may take as long as a year before the skeleton returns to normal. Although vitamin D replacement leads to rapid normalization of 25-hydroxycholecalciferol concentrations, calcitriol levels become and remain supraphysiological for many months. This occurs because of the increased 1α-hydroxylase activity and is, in part, a consequence of persistent secondary hyperparathyroidism.

Other causes of rickets and osteomalacia will also respond to vitamin D replacement, although much higher doses may be required in the case of hypophosphataemic rickets. As in primary hypoparathyroidism, where there is a lack of 1α-hydroxylase activity, the active calcitriol should be given.

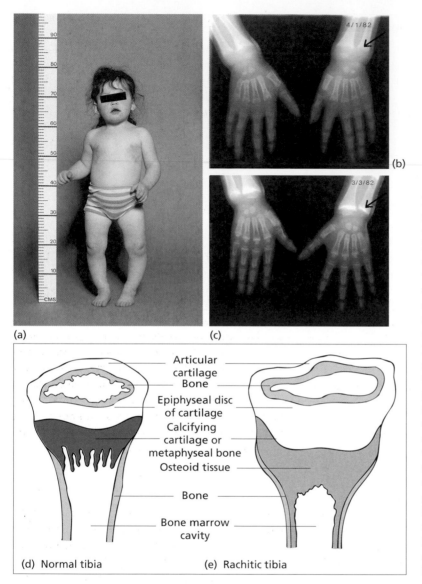

(a)

(b)

(c)

(d) Normal tibia

(e) Rachitic tibia

Articular cartilage
Bone
Epiphyseal disc of cartilage
Calcifying cartilage or metaphyseal bone
Osteoid tissue
Bone
Bone marrow cavity

Figure 9.14 Rickets. (a) Clinical appearance in a 3-year-old. Note the bowing of the tibiae. (b) Radiological features showing expansion, irregularity and 'cupping' of the metaphyses (arrow). (c) Radiological features of healing rickets: note the increased density and definition of the same metaphysis (arrow). Note also the reduction in the radial epiphyseal cartilage thickness from (b) to (c). The growing tibial head in (d) is normal and that in (e) is rachitic. (d) A normally growing epiphyseal disc of cartilage is seen, with the underlying zone of calcifying cartilage. (e) The epiphyseal disc of cartilage is greatly enlarged, and underneath it there is a thick zone of osteoid tissue, i.e. uncalcified bone matrix. Note also the generally thickened epiphyseal region in the rachitic bone, as shown in (b).

Answers to case histories

Case history 9.1

The most likely explanation of her tingling is hypocalcaemia because of inadvertent removal or damage of the parathyroid glands or hyperventilation because of her anxiety. The symptoms are the same because overbreathing may induce a fall in the ionized calcium concentration in serum. This results from the disturbance of the following equilibria:

$$CO_2 + H_2O \rightleftharpoons H_2CO_3^-$$
$$H_2CO_3^- \rightleftharpoons H^+ + HCO_3^-$$
$$Protein\text{-}H \rightleftharpoons Protein^- + H^+$$
$$Protein^- + Ca^{2+} \rightleftharpoons Protein\text{-}Ca$$

As the woman overbreathes, the partial pressure of carbon dioxide falls. This leads to an alkalosis as the production of H^+ from $H_2CO_3^-$ falls. Hydrogen ions consequently dissociate from albumin to compensate. This leads to increased binding of calcium ions to the protein, so that the ionized calcium concentration is decreased. This can be sufficient to induce clinical features of hypocalcaemia, such as tetany or parasthesisiae.

The two causes can be easily distinguished because there will be no change in the total calcium concentration in the overbreathing woman while calcium concentrations will fall if there is parathyroid dysfunction.

Hypoparathyroidism is treated by supplementation with calcium and vitamin D, usually α-calcidol, to maintain calcium values in the normal range. It is worth checking that normal parathyroid function has not returned several months after the operation. Hyperventilation may be treated with rebreathing into a paper bag.

Case history 9.2

An approximate correction is to add or substract 0.02 mmol/L for every g/L by which the albumin lies above or below a standard figure of 40 g/L. Our patient's calcium is 2.86 mmol/L and albumin 36 g/L. Therefore her corrected calcium is approximately:

$$2.86 + 0.02 \times (40 - 36) = 2.94 \, mmol/L$$

The history gives us some clues about the possible causes of her hypercalcaemia but these may be red herrings. Her love of health food shops may suggest vitamin supplementation. Her obesity may have suggested difficulties in obtaining a blood sample and prolonged tourniquet application. She may be taking a thiazide for her hypertension. She may have a familial form of breast cancer. Each of these must be looked for systematically as well as other causes of hypercalcaemia such as primary hyperparathyriodion.

Case history 9.3

There are several causes of familial hypercalcaemia including multiple endocrine neoplasia type I and II. These are discussed in more detail in Chapter 10. The fact that both men are well and the neck operation was unsuccessful suggests that this might not be the cause of the hypercalcaemia. Another possibility is familial benign hypercalcaemia. This is a dominantly inherited condition in which hypercalcaemia is present from birth. It results from a genetic abnormality of the calcium sensing receptor which causes calcium concentrations to be maintained at abnormally high values. It is benign in most situations but is important to recognize to prevent unnecessary parathyroidectomies.

Case history 9.4

Although we do not know the force with which she fell, it is not usual to break a bone falling down four stairs. This suggests that she has a pathological fracture. Given the X-ray finding of osteopaenia, the most likely cause is osteoporosis although due consideration should be given to other pathological causes such as metastatic deposits. The contributing factors to her osteoporosis are her menopausal age and her asthma. She has severe asthma and is likely to have received systemic glucocorticoid therapy, a side-effect of which is osteoporosis.

Most patients taking long-term glucocorticoids will receive therapy to prevent steroid-induced bone loss. As well as calcium and vitamin D supplementation, the most commonly used agent would be a bisphosphonate.

10 Endocrine neoplasia

LEARNING OBJECTIVES

- To understand the clinical consequences of gut hormone tumours
- To understand how endocrine tumours can be inherited
- To appreciate ways in which endocrinology may interact with oncology:

— To understand the clinical implications of how hormones can affect other solid tissue tumours
— To understand the clinical manifestations of ectopic hormone production

In this chapter we will review the endocrine tumours and their clinical presentation and management

Introduction

Endocrine tumours are fascinating. Furthermore, caring for patients with endocrine tumours is also rewarding, as they are frequently cured. Functioning endocrine tumours result in syndromes with wide-ranging symptoms and signs that reflect the hormones secreted either inappropriately or in excess by the tumour. Even nonfunctioning tumours, such as pituitary nonfunctioning tumours, may cause endocrine syndromes by preventing the normal function of surrounding endocrine tissues. Some tumours have been considered in the chapter that specifically relates to the particular endocrine gland. This chapter will concentrate on the endocrine tumours that occur in nonclassical endocrine tissues, such as the gastrointestinal tract, or where endocrine tumours occur in multiple glands simultaneously, such as the multiple endocrine neoplasia (MEN) syndromes.

A number of solid tumours are affected by or lead to hormonal action and these will also be considered in the second half of the chapter.

Gut hormone tumours

The gastrointestinal system secretes a large number of hormones (Fig. 10.1). Some of these hormones lead to distinct endocrine syndromes when secreted in excess by tumours of the gastrointestinal tract (Box 10.1). Gastrointestinal hormones are difficult to study because for the most part they are not secreted by well-defined endocrine glands but by single cells scattered along the digestive tract. Several of the gastrointestinal 'hormones' are also found in neurones and nerve terminals and so it is difficult to establish whether the effects represent endocrine or neurotransmitter activity or both (review Fig. 1.1).

Two of the earliest identified gastrointestinal hormones, secretin and cholecystokinin, do not appear

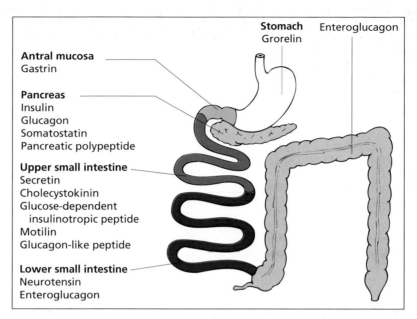

Stomach Enteroglucagon
Grorelin

Antral mucosa
Gastrin

Pancreas
Insulin
Glucagon
Somatostatin
Pancreatic polypeptide

Upper small intestine
Secretin
Cholecystokinin
Glucose-dependent
  insulinotropic peptide
Motilin
Glucagon-like peptide

Lower small intestine
Neurotensin
Enteroglucagon

Figure 10.1 The distribution of the hormones of the pancreas and gastrointestinal tract. The approximate location of hormones is shown by shaded areas. Insulin, glucagon and somatostatin are synthesized in cells of the pancreatic islets of Langerhans. Gastrin is located in the antral mucosa of the stomach, while the other peptide hormones are found in the endocrine cells in the upper or lower small intestine, as shown in the diagram. Enteroglucagon is quite widely distributed throughout the small intestine, as well as in the mucosa of the colon and rectum.

BOX 10.1 Clinical features of major gastrointestinal hormone tumours

- Gastrinoma
  - presents with profound reduction in gastric pH leading to severe ulceration of the stomach and duodenum
  - treated by proton pump inhibitors or surgery
- Insulinoma
  - presents with hypoglycaemia
  - treated by surgery
  - hypoglycaemia may be improved with diazoxide or somatostatin analogues
- Glucagonoma
  - presents with secondary diabetes and a typical skin rash
  - may be identified through villous hypertrophy during gastroscopy
  - treated by surgery
- Somatostatinoma
  - presents with secondary diabetes, reduced gastric acid secretion, gall stones, steatorrhoea and weight loss
  - treated by surgery
- VIPoma and the Verner–Morrison syndrome
  - presents with severe watery diarrhoea, hypokalaemia and flushing of the skin
  - treated by surgery or somatostatin analogues
- Carcinoid tumour
  - presents with flushing, diarrhoea, abdominal pain, bronchoconstriction, heart disease or rash
  - treated by somatostatin analogues, surgery, chemotherapy, or, potentially, interferon α

to be associated with syndromes of excess secretion but nevertheless are important for normal gut function. Secretin is released by the proximal small intestine in response to acid in the duodenum. It causes the pancreas to secrete a fluid that is rich in bicarbonate. Cholecystokinin is also released from the proximal small intestine but in response to fat and protein in a meal. It increases gall bladder contraction and stimulates the pancreas to secrete a fluid that is rich in enzymes such as amylase and trypsinogen.

Gastrin and the Zollinger–Ellison syndrome

Gastrin is secreted from specialized endocrine G-cells which are located in the antral part of the gastric mucosa following distension of the stomach by food or by the presence of small peptides or amino acids within the stomach. Anticipation of eating also increases gastrin secretion through the action of the vagus nerve. The main action of gastrin is to increase gastric acid secretion but it also increases blood flow to the gastric mucosa. Once the pH of the stomach falls below 2.5, the release of gastrin is inhibited by the direct action of acid on the G-cells. Gastrin is also thought to play a role in gastric motility and controls gastric peristalsis.

Tumours of the G-cells, first described by Zollinger and Ellison, are functional and lead to an uncontrolled hypersecretion of gastrin. The profound reduction in gastric pH causes severe ulceration of the stomach and duodenum. The treatment of choice remains the discrete surgical removal of the tumour or, if this is not possible, gastrectomy. However, proton pump inhibitors, such as omeprazole, are effective in controlling the acid secretion.

Islet cell tumours

Tumours may rarely occur in any of three major cell types within the pancreatic islet leading to insulinomas, glucagonomas and somatostatinomas.

Insulinoma

Insulinomas result from tumours of the β-cell of the islet and secrete insulin in excess and in an unregulated fashion. The tumours are usually benign but occasionally they are malignant and may metastasize.

They may lead to prolonged and severe hypoglycaemia (the clinical features and management are given in Chapter 12). As these tumours are rare, clinicians need a high index of suspicion to make the diagnosis. Outside of MEN (see later), the median age of presentation is approximately 50 years. Often the patients have vague symptoms that are precipitated by fasting or extreme exercise and are relieved by eating. The diagnosis is made by the finding of hypoglycaemia with inappropriately elevated serum insulin levels during a prolonged 72-h fast. During the fast, the plasma glucose is measured regularly and, if hypoglycaemia occurs, a simultaneous sample is taken for the analysis of insulin. Lack of suppressed insulin, as would be expected in a normal individual, is diagnostic (see Table 4.1).

Once a biochemical diagnosis has been made, the tumour needs to be identified. Insulinomas are more frequently found in the tail of the pancreas, corresponding to the location of the majority of the β-cells. Ideally the tumour should be identified prior to surgery by arteriography, CT scanning or ultrasound but this can be challenging because the tumours may be small and may be multiple.

Treatment is by surgery but where this is impossible, diazoxide may ameliorate the hypoglycaemia. Somatostatin analogues, such as octreotide, may also be useful in preventing hypoglycaemia by inhibiting the secretion of insulin.

One of the differential diagnoses is factitious hypoglycaemia where a patient surreptitiously gives themselves insulin or a sulphonylurea to induce hypoglycaemia (Box 10.2). The former can be assessed by measuring a C-peptide concentration at the same time as the insulin. As exogenous insulin does not contain C-peptide, factitious insulin administration is associated with low C-peptide values while insulinomas are associated with high values. Sulphonylureas can be detected by measuring the drug directly (Case history 10.1).

Glucagonoma

Glucagonomas are tumours of the pancreatic α-cells which secrete excess glucagon. The physiology of glucagon is described in more detail in Chapter 11. As would be expected as glucagon antagonizes insulin, glucagonomas lead to secondary diabetes but, in addition, can cause a typical skin rash. They may also lead to hypertrophy of the intestinal villi and mucosal thickening which may be noted during gastroscopy or CT scanning of the abdomen. Treatment is by surgery.

Somatostatinoma

Somatostatinomas are tumours of the pancreatic δ-cells. Somatostatin is also released from both the hypothalamus and gastrointestinal tract where it has multiple inhibitory effects on gastrointestinal motility and exocrine secretion as well as endocrine function (see Fig. 5.4). Within the pancreas, it inhibits the secretion of insulin and glucagon. The presentation of somatostatinomas is unpredictable, depending on the relative effects of somatostatin on different tissues. In general, these tumours cause diabetes, reduced gastric acid secretion, gall stones, steatorrhoea and weight loss. Treatment is by surgery.

VIPomas and the Verner–Morrison syndrome

VIPomas occur from the overproduction of vasoactive intestinal peptide (VIP) from neural gangliomas. VIP was originally found in the gut but was subsequently isolated in greater quantities from the central nervous system. In the gut as well as the CNS, VIP is found in neurones and their synapses. At pharmacological doses, VIP increases hepatic glucose release, insulin secretion and pancreatic bicarbonate production while inhibiting gastric acid production, partly through relaxation of blood vessels and smooth muscle. These actions are similar to the actions of glucagon, secretin and gastric inhibitory peptide (GIP) and it has been suggested that these hormones may have evolved from a single gene.

Excess VIP causes severe watery diarrhoea and flushing of the skin. The diarrhoea may be associated with a life-threatening hypokalaemia. This presentation was first described by Verner and Morrison. While resection of tumour cures the syndrome, somatostatin or its analogues can also be used to treat the symptoms.

Carcinoid tumour

Neuroendocrine tumours of the gastrointestinal tract are also called 'carcinoids'. These tumours can be categorized according to their clinical behaviour.

BOX 10.2 Differential diagnosis of hypoglycaemia

- High insulin, low C-peptide
  - insulin overdose—accidental or deliberate; common in patients with diabetes (Chapter 12)
- High insulin, high C-peptide
  - reactive hypoglycaemia
  - sulphonylurea overdose
  - insulinoma
  - persistent hyperinsulinaemic hypoglycaemia of infancy—a rare autosomal recessive trait resulting in constitutively active ATP-sensitive potassium channels leading to severe hypoglycaemia in infancy
- Low insulin
  - nonislet cell tumour hypoglycaemia
  - hypoadrenalism

CASE HISTORY 10.1

An overweight, 37-year-old woman complained to her doctor that she had noticed that around 2 to 3 h after a meal she became light-headed, sweaty and felt faint. Her symptoms improve with a piece of cake. She has a family history of type 2 diabetes and her mother is taking gliclazide tablets. She mentioned that once when she felt unwell she borrowed her mother's blood glucose meter and found that the reading was only 2.3 mmol/L.

What is the most likely diagnosis?
How would you investigate the cause of her symptoms?

Answers, see p. 180

While most tumours are nonfunctioning, functioning tumours are responsible for the carcinoid syndrome. Carcinoid syndrome, first described in 1888, refers to the clinical manifestation of tumours that secrete excess biogenic amines, especially serotonin, and other factors into the circulation.

Carcinoid tumours may also be classified into foregut, midgut and hindgut tumours based on their location and the embryological derivatives of the different parts of the gastrointestinal tract. This classification aims to gather tumours with common features into distinct groups. The foregut carcinoid tumours arise in the lung, stomach, duodenum and pancreas and also include those in the thymus. Midgut tumours occur in the jejunum, ileum and ascending colon and hindgut tumours originate in the distal colon and rectum. Around 85% of carcinoid tumours develop in the gastrointestinal tract with 10% in the lung (Table 10.1).

Carcinoid tumours constitute around a third of all tumours in the small intestine but only 1% of neoplasms occurring in the stomach, colon or rectum. In total, carcinoid tumours constitute around 2% of all malignant tumours. The incidence is approximately one in 100 000 and may occur at all ages, including children. In young patients, the appendix is the commonest location and tumours are frequently found incidentally during operations for appendicitis. In older patients, carcinoids are more frequently found in the ileum and jejunum.

Carcinoid tumours may metastasize, with lymph nodes and liver being the commonest metastatic sites. Colonic and ileal carcinoids are more prone to produce metastases, with approximately 70% of all colonic tumours giving rise to metastasis compared with only 2 to 5% of appendiceal carcinoids. The risk of metastasis increases with the size of the tumour.

Clinical features

The majority of all carcinoids are only detected during post-mortem examination and therefore did not give rise to any clinical symptoms. Nevertheless, carcinoid tumours may lead to the development of a constellation of symptoms known as the carcinoid syndrome (Box 10.3). Almost all patients with the carcinoid syndrome and gastrointestinal carcinoid tumours have metastatic disease, although some

Table 10.1 Distribution of carcinoid tumours

Site	Frequency (%)
Foregut	
Thymus	<1
Lung	10
Stomach	2
Duodenum	2
Midgut	
Ileum	11
Jejunum	1
Appendix	44
Caecum	3
Hindgut	
Colon	5
Rectum	15

BOX 10.3 Clinical features of carcinoid syndrome

- Flushing
- Diarrhoea
- Abdominal pain
- Bronchoconstriction and asthma-like episodes
- Tricuspid or pulmonary valve abnormalities
  - occur in 60–70%
  - may be complicated by right heart failure
  - consists microscopically of fibrous tissue superimposed on mural and valvular endocardium
  - the aetiology remains obscure but is unrelated to tumour mass or disease duration
  - the extent of the cardiac disease seems related to circulating tumour products such as serotonin and tachykinins
- Pellagra-like skin lesions
  - pellagra is a nutritional disorder caused by combined deficiency of tryptophan and niacin (nicotinic acid)
  - carcinoid is associated with a depletion of tryptophan as this is consumed by the tumour for serotonin synthesis
  - may be associated with psychosis

CASE HISTORY 10.2

A 65-year-old man presents with breathlessness, rash, flushing, abdominal pain and diarrhoea. Examination revealed a wheeze and his peak flow rate was reduced. A chest X-ray is unremarkable but an ultrasound of his abdomen showed a single mass in his liver. A barium meal and follow through demonstrated an ileal mass. Urinary 5-HIAA was markedly raised upon 24-h collection.

What is the diagnosis?
What are the treatment options?
What factors are likely to affect his prognosis?

Answers, see p. 180

bronchial carcinoid tumours may present without metastasis.

Diagnosis

Carcinoid tumours synthesize and secrete serotonin in excess (Case history 10.2). Serotonin is synthesized from tryptophan in two stages. It is first 5-hydroxylated to form 5-hydroxytryptophan (5-HT) which is then decarboxylated to form serotonin. Many tumours have a relative lack of the 5-HT decarboxylase enzyme and so the tumour may secrete a combination of 5-HT, serotonin and 5-hydroxyindoleacetic acid (5-HIAA). The measurement of urinary 5-HIAA is one of the most important tumour markers for patients with the carcinoid syndrome, both for diagnosis and follow-up. It has a sensitivity of around 70% and specificity of 100% for patients with the carcinoid syndrome. In addition, chromogranin A, a constituent of secretory granules that is released along with hormone upon stimulation, can also be used as a serum marker of carcinoid in diagnosis and follow-up.

After a biochemical diagnosis, tumour localization is determined by different techniques including gastrointestinal endoscopy, barium enema, chest radiograph, ultrasound, computed tomography, magnetic resonance imaging, angiography, selective venous sampling and radionucleotide scanning.

Surgical treatment should be considered in every patient with carcinoid tumours as this may be curative where there is only local disease. Even in patients with 'bulky' disease and metastasis, an aggressive surgical approach may be of clinical benefit in reducing symptoms. As carcinoid tumours express large numbers of high-affinity somatostatin receptors, medical treatment with somatostatin analogues is usually employed. Other treatment includes chemotherapy and interferon alpha.

Carcinoid tumours are reported to have a benign clinical cause and patients may live for 10 to 15 years after the occurrence of metastatic disease. The 5-year survival rates, when liver metastases are present, however, are 18 to 38% with a median survival time of around 23 months. Around a third of patients die from carcinoid heart disease and heart valve replacement is important to prevent this.

Inherited endocrine neoplasia

Endocrine neoplasms, like any tumour, can occur sporadically or as inherited tumours. In either case the frequency and age of presentation can be influenced by environmental factors. Inherited endocrine tumours are notable for a number of well-defined syndromes. In some of these, the genetic cause has been identified and the mechanism is now understood while in others the gene remains unknown. The endocrine tumours can be divided into four loose categories (Table 10.2).

There are many genes involved in the control of cell growth and a single mutation rarely leads directly to neoplasia. Tumours arise through the sequential acquisition of mutations which give rise to a clone of cells with a growth or survival advantage. These mutations tend to affect four broad classes of genes:
- Proto-oncogenes—mutation confers a positive growth advantage on the cell involved
- Tumour suppressor genes—mutation derestricts the expansion of the clone of cells

Table 10.2 Categories of endocrine tumours

Group	Primarily endocrine	Description	Example
Classical MEN	Yes	Well-defined syndrome resulting from multiple tumours in multiple endocrine glands	MEN-1
Single endocrine syndrome	Yes	Well-defined syndrome resulting from multiple tumours in one endocrine glands	Familial parathyroid tumours
Nonendocrine tumour with minor endocrine component	No	Well-defined syndrome but only a minority develop endocrine tumours	Neurofibromatosis
Other	No	Diverse dysfunction from fundamental genetic abnormality	McCune–Albright syndrome (review Fig. 3.14)

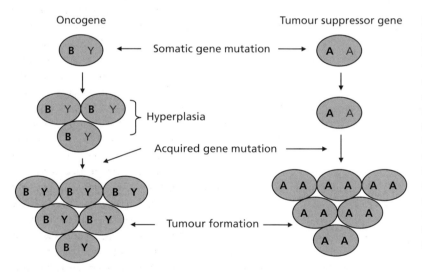

Figure 10.2 Inheritance of a mutated oncogene (B) usually leads to hyperplasia of all cells where the gene is normally expressed. Subsequent tumour development occurs at varying rates, depending on the chance acquisition of further mutations (Y). In contrast, the inheritance of a single mutated tumour suppressor gene (A) is silent until a further somatic mutation in the normal allele occurs. This leads to the loss of function of the tumour suppressor gene and the development of a tumour.

- DNA repair genes—mutation increases the likelihood of further mutations
- Invasion and metastasis genes—mutation increases the likelihood of spread of the tumour

Inheritance of a mutated proto-oncogene usually leads to hyperplasia of all cells where the gene is normally expressed (Fig. 10.2). Subsequent tumour development occurs at varying rates, depending on the chance acquisition of further mutations. An example is the *RET* oncogene, mutation of which causes MEN-2.

Inheritance of a single mutated tumour suppressor gene would not be expected to show any direct effect other than the liability to form multiple tumours. A further somatic mutation leading to the loss-of-function of the second, normal allele is needed for tumour development. As such, hyperplasia is not normally seen prior to the tumour development as the unaffected gene maintains normal function. Neurofibromatosis is an example of a tumour that results from the inheritance of a mutated tumour suppressor gene.

Neither repair genes nor genes for invasion or metastasis have yet been shown to be responsible for inducing inherited endocrine tumour syndromes, although the function of some genes associated with endocrine neoplasia remain incompletely understood.

Most of these tumour predisposition syndromes are inherited in a dominant manner (i.e. mutation in only one of the two alleles is sufficient to predispose to tumour formation). By inheriting one of these tumour-promoting mutations in every cell in the body, the tumours also tend to be multiple and to occur at an earlier age than in individuals without the inherited defects. Therefore, these syndromes should be considered in any patient with multiple endocrine tumours, in patients in whom an endocrine tumour is found at a particularly early age, or in those with a positive family history of tumour formation.

Multiple endocrine neoplasia (MEN)

MEN syndromes are rare genetic conditions that lead to tumours in multiple endocrine glands. MEN may occur in a familial inherited fashion or as a result of new mutations, in which case they present sporadically. Liaison with colleagues in the specialty of clinical genetics is important for effective tracing of relatives and screening. There are two main types of MEN, although MEN type 2 is further subdivided into type 2a and type 2b (Table 10.3).

MEN-1

Multiple endocrine neoplasia type 1 (MEN-1) is characterized by tumours in the parathyroid, pancreas and pituitary glands. Rarely carcinoid tumours, lipomas and tumours of the adrenal cortex have been described. MEN-1 is inherited in an autosomal dom-

Table 10.3 Features of MEN

Type	Endocrine glands affected
Type 1	'The 3 P' tumours Parathyroid, pancreatic tumours and pituitary adenomas
Type 2a	The 'ATP' tumours Phaeochromocytoma (adrenal), medullary carcinoma of the thyroid and parathyroid adenomas
Type 2b	Medullary carcinoma of the thyroid, phaeochromocytoma, and mucosal neurofibromas

inant or sporadic manner but it may not always be possible to differentiate these if a parent has died before the patient developed symptoms. Molecular genetic studies have identified the gene causing MEN-1 and have named it *MENIN*. It is a tumour suppressor gene.

The clinical features and treatment of the MEN-1 are related to the sites of the tumours and to their secreted hormones (see above and other relevant chapters). It is important to screen asymptomatic members of families with MEN-1 biochemically, as early diagnosis and treatment of these tumours reduces mortality and morbidity. Screening in MEN-1 is not straightforward because the clinical and biochemical manifestations within any one family are not always the same and the age at which individuals develop tumours can differ quite dramatically. At present, it is suggested that individuals at high risk, such as first-degree relatives, should be screened annually. The screening should commence in early childhood as the disease has developed in some individuals by the age of 5 years and should continue for life as some individuals have not developed the disease until the eighth decade. History and examination should be directed towards eliciting the symptoms of hypercalcaemia, pituitary dysfunction and subcutaneous lipomata. Serum concentrations of calcium, gastrointestinal hormones and prolactin should also be measured. Mutations in *MENIN* are not identified in all cases, which makes genetic screening of relatives difficult. Conversely, in families where the mutation is known, biochemical screening can be reserved for those known to have inherited the mutated allele. Unaffected relatives can be reassured and discharged.

MEN-2

MEN-2 is characterized by medullary carcinoma of the thyroid (MTC) in combination with phaeochromocytoma and parathyroid adenomas (MEN-2a) or in combination with phaeochromocytoma, neurofibromata and Marfanoid habitus (arm span being greater than height) (MEN-2b). Medullary carcinoma of the thyroid may be inherited in isolation when it is known as familial MTC.

MEN-2 is inherited as an autosomal dominant trait with a high degree of penetrance. MEN-2 is caused by mutations in the *RET* proto-oncogene, which

---

CASE HISTORY 10.3

A 35-year-old fireman was referred with hypercalcaemia and hypertension. He had been well previously and there was no family history of any endocrine disease. Investigations confirmed that calcium was elevated in conjunction with a raised PTH. The doctor who saw the patient referred him to the endocrine surgeon but asked his GP to treat the hypertension with a β-blocker. Five days later, the man was admitted collapsed with a blood pressure of 230/110.

What diagnosis did the doctor pick up?
What diagnosis was missed?
Why was he admitted?
After treatment of the two diagnosed conditions, what else should be considered for him and for his family?

Answers, see p. 180

---

encodes a cell surface receptor with tyrosine kinase activity (review Chapter 3), and leads to potent growth stimulation, hyperplasia and tumour formation of both the thyroid gland and adrenal medulla. The clinical features and treatment of MEN-2 are related to the sites of the tumours and to the hormones secreted by the tumours (Case history 10.3).

Genetic screening for MEN-2 is also important but is simpler than for MEN-1 because, in most cases, the causative mutation can be identified within the coding region of the *RET* gene (review Fig. 2.2). It is therefore possible, in the great majority of families, to detect which individuals have inherited the mutated allele. Those without the mutation can be reassured, while in affected individuals a definitive diagnosis can be made in early childhood and biochemical monitoring commenced. For medullary carcinoma of the thyroid or its preceding C-cell hyperplasia (see Chapter 8), this is done by annual measurement of calcitonin either without stimulation or during a pentagastrin stimulation test. Screening for phaeochromocytoma is most commonly achieved by annual measurement of urinary catecholamines (see Chapter 6). Periodic measurement of serum calcium is probably adequate for screening for parathyroid adenomas.

Once over the age of 5 to 6 years, prophylactic thyroidectomy should be considered as the tumour almost inevitably develops in affected individuals (>90% by 30 years). In contrast, and highlighting the future value of advancing molecular genetics, not all affected individuals require adrenalectomy be cause some mutations have been identified that to date have never been associated with phaeochromocytoma.

BOX 10.4 Hormone-responsive tumours

- Prostate cancer
- Breast cancer
- Testicular cancer
- Ovarian cancer
- Endometrial cancer

Hormonally sensitive solid tumours

Human tumours consist of cells that lack the normal negative feedback of growth control. Cell growth is regulated by both internal controls as well as external growth factors that elicit a variety of intracellular signals and actions following binding to cell surface receptors. Polypeptide growth factors activate two main receptor subclasses—those with and those without intrinsic tyrosine kinase activity (review Chapter 3). These similarities in intracellular signalling indicate significant functional overlap with hormones, although growth factors perhaps tend to act in a more paracrine or autocrine fashion. Several solid tumours respond to these stimuli and their manipulation can provide a valuable therapeutic option. In particular, hormone-responsive tumours constitute approximately 20% of all cancers prevalent in the western world (Box 10.4).

Prostate cancer

Prostate cancer accounts for 8.3% of all cancers in men and is the fourth commonest cause of death from malignant disease in men in England and Wales. Carcinoma of the prostate becomes increasingly common with ageing such that by 80 years,

80% of men have malignant foci within the glands although most of these appear to be clinically insignificant. Androgenic hormones play an important role in the aetiology and progression of the tumour and consequently endocrine manipulation is an important part of treatment (Box 10.5).

Surgical removal by prostatectomy is the first line of therapy but endocrine manipulation is needed if metastases are present. The aim of therapy is to reduce or inhibit the action of androgens and is achieved by bilateral orchidectomy or endocrine modulation.

The commonest hormone therapies used against prostate cancer are continuous gonadotrophin-releasing hormone (GnRH) analogues, such as leuprorelin or goserelin, which effectively produce a medical castration (review Chapter 5). Approximately 30% of tumours respond to this therapy. Initially, therapy is also combined with the androgen receptor antagonist, cyproterone acetate, although more efficacious 'antiandrogens' are currently being developed for the treatment of this condition. As testosterone is converted to its active metabolite dihydrotestosterone, inhibition of the enzyme 5α-reductase is a further potential therapeutic treatment (see Fig. 7.7). The first drug to do this is finasteride and this is already used clinically to control prostatic hypertrophy and its related urinary symptoms. Clinical trials are under way to examine its effectiveness in prostatic cancer.

Breast cancer

Breast cancer is the commonest tumour in women. Its incidence has increased in recent years and affects 54 per 100 000 women per year. There have been spectacular advances in the treatment of breast cancer over the last decade of which endocrine treatments have played an important part. The aims of endocrine treatment of breast cancer are to decrease the production of oestrogen or to block its actions via the oestrogen receptor at the breast. In women with breast cancer, the most important determinant of whether they will respond to hormonal therapy is the presence or absence of the oestrogen receptor in the tumour. If the tumour is oestrogen receptor positive, there is a 60% chance that it will respond to hormonal therapy while if the tumour is oestrogen receptor negative, the likelihood falls to only 10%. Overall, around 60% of breast cancers are oestrogen receptor positive and so approximately 30% of all breast tumours will respond to hormone therapy (Box 10.6).

The most commonly prescribed hormone therapy is tamoxifen, which acts as an oestrogen antagonist in breast cancer cells while acting as a weak agonist in other tissues. Tamoxifen has a low incidence of side-effects, is effective in both pre- and postmenopausal women and can be used as treatment for metastatic disease as well as adjuvant therapy.

Progestins, such as medroxyprogesterone acetate or megestrol acetate, help to diminish oestrogen action in breast cancers and are effective in both pre- and postmenopausal women. They are considered as second-line agents and are helpful in approximately half of women who have previously responded to endocrine therapy.

In premenopausal women, oestrogens are produced mainly from the ovary and therefore drugs that block the ovarian production of oestrogen, such

---

BOX 10.5 Endocrine treatments of prostate cancer

- Continuous gonadotrophin-releasing hormone (GnRH) analogues (see Chapter 7) — leuprorelin or goserelin
- Androgen receptor antagonists — cyproterone acetate
- Bilateral orchidectomy

BOX 10.6 Endocrine treatments of breast cancer

- Oestrogen antagonists
  - e.g. tamoxifen
  - effective in both pre- and postmenopausal women
- Blockade of oestrogen production
  - continuous GnRH analogues or bilateral oophorectomy — both induce a premature menopause
  - aromatase (CYP19) inhibitors — anastrozole or letrozole; used in postmenopausal women
- Progestins
  - e.g. medroxyprogesterone acetate or megestrol acetate
  - effective in both pre- and postmenopausal women
  - second-line therapy

as continuous GnRH analogues, lead to a significant fall in oestrogen concentrations by silencing the hypothalamic–anterior pituitary–ovarian axis (see Chapter 7). The unavoidable 'side-effect' (actually the desired effect) of these drugs is that they induce a premature menopause. An alternative is bilateral oophorectomy (surgical removal of the ovaries).

In postmenopausal women, oestrogens are mainly formed through the peripheral conversion of androgens by the action of aromatase (CYP19; Fig. 7.11). Inhibition of this enzyme with drugs such as anastrozole or letrozole leads to a significant fall in oestrogen levels. In recent trials, these drugs have appeared more effective in treating postmenopausal breast cancer than tamoxifen.

Most recently, there has been much interest in monoclonal antibodies that block the epidermal growth factor receptor and limit signalling through tyrosine kinase linked pathways. These agents are entering clinical use in pre-menopausal women with more advanced disease.

Ovarian cancer

Excluding the breast, ovarian cancer is the commonest endocrine malignancy, accounting for 4 to 6% of all cancers in women. There are three types of ovarian neoplasm: epithelial, germ cell and sex cord stromal tumours, with the vast majority of malignant tumours being epithelial. Ovarian cancer is generally more common in developed countries with incidence rates in North Europe and North America of between 8 and 12/100000 per year. The lowest rates are seen in Japan and the developing world.

The cause of ovarian cancer remains unclear, but hormonal factors appear to be important as the lifetime number of ovulations is related to risk. Nulliparity and low parity increase risk, while use of oral contraceptive pill is protective. An older age at menopause also increases the risk. From these findings, it appears that total oestrogen exposure is important to some degree.

Although some data suggest that hormonal therapies may have some effect on ovarian cancer in palliative settings, no hormonal therapy has been approved and further studies are needed in this area.

Testicular cancer

Testicular cancer is uncommon, with incidence rates of between 3 and 9/100000 per year in white men and much lower rates in Africans and Asians. The majority of testicular cancer is of germ cell origin and can be divided into seminoma and nonseminomatous tumours. Testicular cancer has a distinct pattern with age, with most presenting before the age of 40 years old. The incidence then increases modestly after the age of 65 years old (see Box 7.12).

A major, established risk factor for testicular cancer is maldescent of the testis. The mechanism is unknown but it appears that the risk is only raised in the maldescended testis and not in the opposite one. Increased exposure to environmentally oestrogens has also been proposed as a possible cause but as yet there is no definite evidence to support this hypothesis.

At present, hormonal treatments are not available for testicular cancer but measurement of hormonal markers, such as human chorionic gonadotrophin, are important in monitoring the treatment of nonseminomatous germ cell tumours.

Endometrial cancer

Endometrial cancer has an annual incidence of about 142000 women worldwide, and an estimated 42000 women die from this cancer. Most cases are diagnosed after the menopause, with the highest incidence around the seventh decade of life. The early appearance of symptoms, such as postmenopausal bleeding, explains why most women with endometrial cancer have early-stage disease at presentation. Overall, the 5-year survival is around 80%.

There is, however, a significant prognostic difference between the histological types of endometrial cancers. The most common lesions are typically hormone sensitive and low grade and have an excellent prognosis, whereas other tumours are high grade with a tendency to recur, even in early stage.

The first-line treatment for endometrial cancer is surgery, which not only is important for staging purposes but also enables appropriate tailoring of adjuvant treatment modalities to benefit high-risk patients. Currently, there is no proof that adjuvant hormone therapy leads to a better outcome in early cancers but progestagens may have a place in the treatment of metastatic endometrial cancer. The response rate ranges from 15 to 20% and is related to the presence of steroid-hormone receptors. Tamoxifen also has a small benefit in this setting. Progesterone is certainly important in preventing endometrial carcinoma, as chronic unopposed oestrogen increases the risk approximately sixfold. Hence, there is a need for a withdrawal bleed every four months or so in polycystic ovarian syndrome (see Chapter 7).

Acromegaly and cancer

Patients with acromegaly may have higher rates of cancer, possibly because of increased plasma levels of insulin-like growth factor 1 (IGF1), which is known to promote cellular growth. In particular, there may be an increased risk of colorectal neoplasia, but the exact extent of this remains controversial. This issue is discussed in more detail in Chapter 5.

Ectopic hormone syndromes

Some solid tumours secrete peptide hormones or analogues of hormones in an uncontrolled manner which may cause the patient to present with features of hormone excess. Ectopic means 'out of place' and refers to the fact that many of the tissues from which the tumours were derived do not normally secrete these hormones. This may be a slight misnomer because in some cases the tumours may have developed from specialized neuroendocrine cells within the tissue. An alternative explanation may be that as the cells become malignant, they become dedifferentiated and begin to express genes that encode for the secreted hormone. A final hypothesis is that specific oncogenes activate the hormone production. Examples of syndromes caused by ectopic hormone secretion are shown in Table 10.4.

Nonislet cell tumour hypoglycaemia (NICTH)

NICTH occurs when solid mesenchymal tumours secrete big IGF-2. This fails to bind to the IGF binding proteins and leads to hypoglycaemia. The

Table 10.4 Examples of ectopic hormone secretion

Endocrine abnormality	Hormone secreted by tumour	Tumour
Cushing syndrome Sometimes hypokalaemia alone	ACTH or ACTH-like peptides	Small cell carcinoma of the lung, medullary carcinoma of the thyroid, thymic carcinoma, islet cell tumours
Hyponatraemia	Antidiuretic hormone	Small cell carcinoma of the lung, gastrointestional tumour
Gynaecomastia (ultimately due to oestrogen activity)	Human placental lactogen, oestrogen, testosterone	Carcinoma of the bronchus, liver or kidney
Hypoglycaemia	Insulin or 'big-IGF2'	Hepatomas, large mesenchymal tumours
Galactorrhoea	Prolactin	Carcinoma of the bronchus or kidney
Hypercalcaemia	Parathyroid hormone related peptide (PTHrP)	Squamous cell carcinoma of the bronchus and breast carcinoma
Polycythaemia	Erythropoietin	Carcinoma of the kidney and uterus

KEY POINTS

- Endocrine tumours may arise in classical endocrine glands and from endocrine cells within nonclassical endocrine tissues such as the gastrointestinal tract
- Endocrine neoplasms can occur sporadically or as inherited tumours
- Inherited endocrine tumours are notable for a number of well-defined syndromes
- In some of these, the genetic cause has been identified and the mechanism is now understood
- Inherited neoplasms should be considered in those with multiple endocrine tumours or in patients in whom an endocrine tumour is found at a particularly early age, or in patients with a positive history
- Endocrine-responsive tumours constitute approximately 20% of all cancers occurring in the western world

presentation is similar to that of an insulinoma but, in contrast to the latter, the insulin concentrations are undetectable. Surgical removal of the tumour is the treatment of choice but if this is impossible, medical treatment with corticosteroids or growth hormone can prevent the hypoglycaemia.

Answers to case histories

Case history 10.1

She presents with symptoms of hypoglycaemia that are relieved by food. When she measured her blood glucose, this was low. The differential diagnosis is given in Box 10.2.

It is important to admit her to hospital for a prolonged fast. In this case, she did not become hypoglycaemic, which excludes the possibility of an insulinoma or nonislet cell tumour hypoglycaemia. Given her family history, the most likely diagnosis is reactive hypoglycaemia or sulphonylurea overdose using her mother's tablets.

The next investigation is to perform a prolonged 75 g oral glucose tolerance test. After 3 h she became hypoglycaemic (2.9 mmol/L). Insulin and C-peptide concentrations were elevated and sulphonylureas were undetectable.

Her diagnosis was reactive hypoglycaemia. Treatment is through dietary advice. Weight loss is beneficial as is the use of low glycaemic index, high fibre foods.

Case history 10.2

The diagnosis is likely to be a carcinoid tumour with hepatic metastasis.

The primary treatment is surgical. Unlike many other intra-abdominal tumours, the presence of hepatic spread is not a contraindication to surgery. Indeed surgical removal of the hepatic tumour may be curative. If he is unfit for surgery, treatment with somatostatin analogues, interferon alpha and chemotherapy should be considered.

His prognosis is reduced by the metastasis but nevertheless he may live a considerable time after his diagnosis. Although it would appear that bronchoconstriction is the cause of his breathlessness, it is important to consider carcinoid heart disease, which has a poorer prognosis. High levels of tumour markers, particularly postsurgery, would worsen his prognosis.

Case history 10.3

The presence of high levels of PTH in association with hypercalcaemia indicates hyperparathyroidism. The lack of any past medical history suggests this was primary hyperparathyroidism.

A phaeochromocytoma was missed. One has to have sympathy with the doctor. This is a rare diagnosis but hypertension in a fit young man is unusual.

The unopposed action of the raised catecholamines on α-receptors after the β-receptors were blocked led to a hypertensive crisis (see Chapter 6).

The combination of a parathyroid adenoma and a phaeochromocytoma should suggest MEN-2a. He requires thorough investigation for medullary carcinoma of the thyroid, which, if the patient does have a mutation in the *RET* proto-oncogene, is highly likely to be present by the age of 35 years. Calcitonin should be measured either unstimulated or during a pentagastrin stimulation test.

The patient should be referred to a clinical geneticist and the *RET* proto-oncogene should be sequenced. If a mutation is found, the genetic screening should be offered to his family members. This may be a sporadic case, however, if the causative mutation becomes known, unaffected family members gain great reassurance and can be discharged. Those carrying the mutation, or, if the mutation remains cryptic, all first-degree relatives should be encouraged to undertake annual biochemical screening as described in the chapter text.

Unfortunately, this man had a malignant phaeochromocytoma and died 18 months later.

PART 3

3 Clinical Diabetes and Obesity

11 Overview of diabetes

LEARNING OBJECTIVES

- To understand what diabetes is and how it is diagnosed and classified
- To understand physiology of the actions of insulin

In this chapter, we will gain an overview of the commonest of all endocrine disorders—diabetes mellitus

Introduction

Diabetes mellitus is a complex metabolic disorder characterized by persistent hyperglycaemia (higher than normal blood glucose levels) resulting from defects in insulin secretion, insulin action or both. The two main types of diabetes are type 1 (formerly known as insulin-dependent diabetes), and type 2 (formerly known as noninsulin-dependent diabetes). Type 1 diabetes is caused by the autoimmune destruction of the insulin-producing β-cells of the pancreatic islets, while type 2 diabetes results from both impaired insulin secretion and resistance to the action of insulin. Diabetes currently affects 2 million, or around 3%, of the adult UK population and is predicted to affect 3 million people by 2010 as the prevalence of diabetes has doubled in the UK every 20 years since the end of the Second World War (Fig. 11.1). Type 2 diabetes has a slow and gradual onset and the diagnosis is frequently delayed by up to 10 years. As the prevalence increases with age, the lifetime risk of developing diabetes is around 10%. It is estimated that there are a further 750,000 people in the UK with undiagnosed diabetes (Case history 11.1). Worldwide, the number of adults with diabetes was estimated to be 177 million in 2000 and will almost double to 370 million by 2030 (Fig. 11.2).

Diabetes was first described in ancient Egyptian times and has a long history (Box 11.1).

Diabetes is associated with premature mortality, predominantly as a result of atherosclerotic vascular disease. Microvascular complications, which affect the small blood vessels in the eye, kidney and nerves, are associated with considerable morbidity. The economic and social costs of diabetes are enormous, both for healthcare services and through loss of productivity. In developed countries, 10% or more of the total health budget is spent on the management of diabetes and its complications.

Diagnosis of diabetes

A diagnosis of diabetes is made if the fasting plasma glucose is ≥7.0 mmol/L or the random or 2-h glucose tolerance test plasma glucose is ≥11.1 mmol/L (Table 11.1). The WHO diagnostic criteria also recognize two further categories of abnormal glucose concentrations: impaired fasting glycaemia (IFG) and impaired glucose tolerance (IGT); the latter can only be diagnosed following a 75-g oral glucose test.

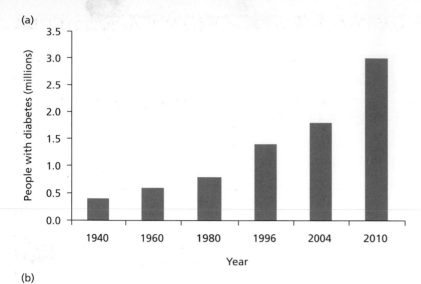

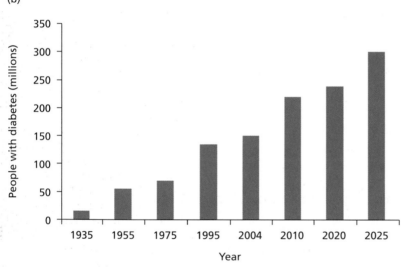

Figure 11.1 (a) Prevalence of diabetes in the UK since 1940. (b) Worldwide prevalence of diabetes since 1935. Source Diabetes UK: Diabetes in the UK in 2004. http://www.diabetes.org.uk/ infocentre/reports/in_the_UK_ 2004.doc.

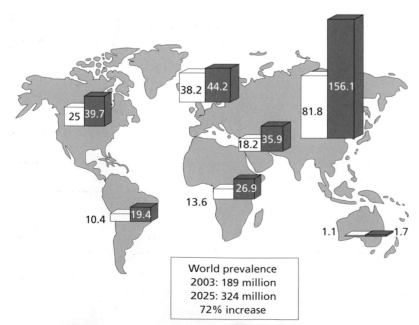

World prevalence
2003: 189 million
2025: 324 million
72% increase

Figure 11.2 Worldwide prevalence of diabetes in 2003 with projected figures in 2025. Diabetes is increasing in every continent. Figures given are number of people with diabetes in millions. Source: Zimmet *et al.*, *Diabetic Medicine*, 2003, **20**, 693–702.

CASE HISTORY 11.1

The local Public Health Consultant would like to know the prevalence of diabetes in your region and would like to know if it differs from the national average.

What are the difficulties they may encounter?
How might these be overcome?

Answers, see p. 196

BOX 11.1 A brief history of diabetes

1550 BC: The oldest description of diabetes as a polyuric state in ancient Egypt.

2nd century AD: Aretaeus of Cappadocia first used the term 'diabetes', coming from Greek meaning 'siphon' or 'pass through'.

5th/ 6th century AD: Indian physicians, such as Susrata, recognized the sweet, honey-like taste of urine from polyuric patients, which attracted ants and insects. The descriptions of diabetes also recognized the distinction between two forms of diabetes, one in older, fatter people, and the other in thin people who rapidly succumbed to their illness.

17th century AD: Thomas Willis, physician to King Charles II, rediscovered sweetness in urine. He noted the importance of lifestyle when he remarked that the prevalence of diabetes was increasing because of 'good fellowship and gusling down chiefly of unalloyed wine'.

1776: Matthew Dobson showed that urinary sweetness was caused by sugar and was associated with a rise in blood sugar.

End of 18th century: John Rollo first used the term 'diabetes mellitus' (honey) to distinguish the condition from 'diabetes insipidus' (tasteless).

19th century: Claude Bernard, a French physiologist, discovered that:

- sugar was stored as glycogen in the liver
- transfixation of the medulla in conscious rabbits caused hyperglycaemia (piqure diabetes).

1869: Paul Langerhans discovered the pancreatic islets.

1889: Oskar Minkowski removed the pancreas from a dog and discovered that the animal developed diabetes.

1893: Edouard Laguesse showed islets were the endocrine tissue of the pancreas.

1921: Frederick Banting, Charles Best, James Collip and J.J.R. Macleod, in Toronto, discovered insulin.

1920s: First patients treated with insulin by physicians such as Elliot P. Joslin, who introduced systematic education in the US and Robin D. Lawrence who had diabetes himself and founded the British Diabetic Association (now Diabetes UK).

1955: Primary structure of insulin elucidated by Frederick Sanger.

1969: Dorothy Hodgkin described the three dimensional structure of insulin using X-ray crytallography.

2000: James Shapiro and colleagues establish the 'Edmonton protocol' revitalizing efforts to cure type 1 diabetes by transplantation.

Table 11.1 The 1999 World Health Organization diagnostic criteria for diabetes

2-h plasma glucose following a 75-g oral glucose test (mmol/L)	Diagnosis		
	Fasting plasma glucose (mmol/L)		
	<6.1	≥6.1–6.9	≥7.0
<7.8	Normal	Impaired fasting glycaemia	Diabetes
≥7.8–11.0	Impaired glucose tolerance	Impaired fasting glycaemia and impaired glucose tolerance	Diabetes
≥11.1	Diabetes	Diabetes	Diabetes

Only one test is required in a patient with classical diabetic symptoms but a supplementary test is required in asymptomatic individuals (Case history 11.2). The gold standard test for diabetes, endorsed by World Health Organization (WHO), is the oral glucose tolerance test which requires an overnight fast followed by a 75-g glucose drink, with blood samples taken to test for glucose concentrations before the drink and 2 h afterwards (Box 11.2).

The criteria for the diagnosis of diabetes have only recently been updated and it is instructive to consider why there has been so much debate about this diagnosis. Plasma glucose concentrations show a skewed normal distribution in the general population and, as such, the delineation of abnormal from normal is arbitrary (Fig. 11.3). An analogy to this would be height within the population. Height is normally distributed and so any definition between short, normal and tall is somewhat subjective. For example, many would suggest a tall man is someone over 6 foot tall (~180 cm) but in reality there is little difference in height between this man and another man who is 5′ 11″ (178 cm). The same is true for glucose and so it is an important to consider why the WHO chose the particular cut-off values. The reason is that the diagnostic criteria reflect the concentration of plasma glucose at which there is an increased risk of developing microvascular complications, particularly retinopathy. Although the

---

BOX 11.2　How a glucose tolerance test is performed

- The patient should fast overnight although water may be drunk
- The patient should refrain from smoking for 12 h prior to the test
- After collection of the fasting blood sample, the patients should drink 75 g of anhydrous glucose in 250–300 ml of water over 5 min
- A second blood sample should be collected 2 h after the glucose challenge

---

CASE HISTORY 11.2

An asymptomatic, 80-year-old, frail woman is found to have a random blood glucose of 11.3 mmol/L.

Does she have diabetes?

Answers, see p. 196

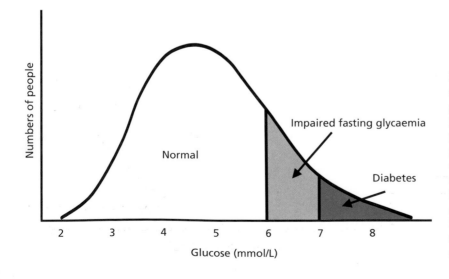

Figure 11.3 Representative distribution of fasting plasma glucose within the general population. It can be seen that people with impaired fasting glycaemia and diabetes are not discretely different from the rest of the population. As such, the diagnostics cut-off limits are somewhat arbitrary but are largely based on the risk of developing microvascular complications.

relationship between the exposure to hyperglycaemia and microvascular complications is exponential—allowing for a diagnostic cut-off at the inflection of the curve—the relationship between hyperglycaemia and macrovascular complications is more linear, suggesting that there is no threshold for the development of cardiovascular disease (Fig. 11.4). This implies that cardiovascular risk will also increase with increases in blood glucose across the normal population.

Impaired fasting glycaemia (IFG) and impaired glucose tolerance (IGT) are not distinct clinical entities, but rather risk factors for future diabetes and cardiovascular disease. Indeed, the American Diabetes Association has recently suggested that the new term 'prediabetes' is used to describe IGT and IFG.

A diagnosis of diabetes has important social, legal and medical implications for the patient and it is therefore essential that any diagnosis is secure. The diagnosis of diabetes should not be made on the basis of glycosuria, and the glucose concentration should be measured on a venous plasma sample in an accredited laboratory.

Classification of diabetes

The original WHO classification of diabetes (1980 and revised in 1985) was based on clinical characteristics. The two commonest types of diabetes were insulin-dependent diabetes mellitus (IDDM) and noninsulin dependent diabetes mellitus (NIDDM) and were a reflection of the need for insulin treatment to survive. The WHO classification also recognized malnutrition-related diabetes mellitus, other types of diabetes mellitus associated with specific conditions and gestational diabetes, which is diabetes diagnosed for the first time during pregnancy. In 1997, the American Diabetes Association proposed a classification, subsequently adapted by the WHO, that distinguished the types of diabetes according to aetiology (Box 11.3).

The terms IDDM and NIDDM were considered to be confusing, with many clinicians wrongly categorizing insulin-treated patients with NIDDM as having IDDM. The preferred terminology is now type 1 diabetes, which is equivalent to IDDM, and type 2 diabetes, which is equivalent to NIDDM. Malnutrition-related diabetes was omitted from the new classification because its aetiology is uncertain and it is unclear whether it is a separate type of diabetes.

Insulin

Insulin is a 51 amino acid peptide hormone comprising two polypeptide chains, the A and B chains, which are linked by disulphide bridges (Fig. 11.5). Insulin is synthesized in the β-cells of the islets of Langerhans in the pancreas (Fig. 11.6). The main cell types of the islet are the β-cells producing insulin, the α-cells producing glucagon, the δ-cells producing

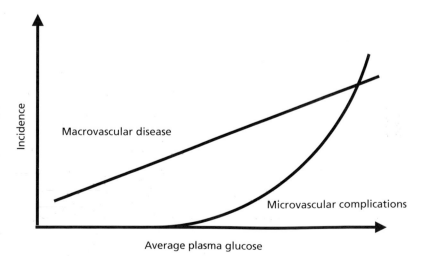

Figure 11.4 Relationship between plasma glucose and microvascular and macrovascular complications. Note how the incidence of macrovascular disease increases in a linear fashion with increasing plasma glucose. In contrast, there is a threshold for the development of microvascular complications and this has been used to define diabetes.

BOX 11.3   1999 WHO classification of diabetes

Type 1 diabetes
— immune mediated
— idiopathic
Type 2 diabetes
— Equivalent to noninsulin dependent diabetes
Secondary diabetes (also known as type 3 diabetes)
(a) Diabetes secondary to pancreatic disease
— chronic pancreatitis
— haemochromatosis
— pancreatic surgery
(b) Diabetes secondary to endocrine disease
— acromegaly
— Cushing syndrome
— phaeochromocytoma
(c) Diabetes secondary to drugs and chemicals
— glucocorticoids
— diuretics
— neuroleptics
— β-blockers
(d) Diabetes secondary to genetic abnormalities
— MODY (maturity onset diabetes of the young)—glucokinase mutations, hepatic nuclear factor mutations, insulin promoter factor 1 mutations
— Insulin receptor mutation e.g. leprechaunisn
— Leprechaunism
— Cystic fibrosis
— DIDMOAD (Wolfram) syndrome
— Lipoatrophy
Gestational diabetes (also known as type 4 diabetes)

somatostatin and the PP cells producing pancreatic polypeptide. The β-cells are the most numerous and are mainly located at the centre of the islet while the other cells are located around the periphery.

Insulin is synthesized in the ribosomes of the rough endoplasmic reticulum (RER) as a single amino acid chain precursor molecule called pre-proinsulin (review Figs 2.3 and 2.4). After removal of the signal peptide, proinsulin is transferred from the RER to the Golgi apparatus, where soluble zinc-containing proinsulin hexamers are formed. The prohormone convertase enzyme finally acts outside the Golgi apparatus to produce the mature insulin and connecting peptide (C peptide). Both insulin and C peptide are released simultaneously in equimolar quantities by exocytosis in response to a number of stimuli, including glucose and amino acids.

Insulin secretion

Insulin is secreted in a co-ordinated, pulsatile fashion from the islet cells into the portal vein in a characteristic, biphasic pattern (Fig. 11.7); first there is an acute, rapid first phase release of insulin lasting for a few minutes followed by a less intense, more sustained second phase. Pancreatic β-cells secrete 0.25 to 1.5 units of insulin per hour during the fasting state and this accounts for over 50% of total daily insulin secretion. Meal-related insulin secretion accounts for the remaining fraction of the total daily output. Glucose is the principal stimulus for insulin secretion, though other macronutrients, hormonal and neuronal factors may alter this response (Table 11.2).

When glucose is taken up by the β-cell, it undergoes phosphorylation and metabolism by glycolysis to produce ATP (Fig. 11.8). The rise in ATP closes potassium channels leading to depolarization of the membrane. This is followed by an influx of calcium ions which triggers insulin granule translocation to the cell surface and exocytosis. The mechanism of action of sulphonylureas, a class of oral hypoglycaemic agents, is by binding to a receptor in close apposition to the potassium channels and results in their closure.

Insulin action

Insulin exerts its biological actions by binding to the insulin receptor on the target cell surface (review Fig. 3.6). The insulin receptor is a heterotetramer consisting of two α and two β glycoprotein subunits linked by disulphide bonds. Insulin binds to the extracellular α subunits, resulting in conformational change enabling ATP to bind to the intracellular component of the β subunit and triggers phosphorylation of the β subunit, conferring tyrosine kinase activity. This enables tyrosine phosphorylation of intracellular substrate proteins known as insulin responsive substrates (IRS), which can then bind other signalling molecules and so mediate further cellular actions of insulin (Fig. 11.9).

Between meals, insulin is secreted at a low basal

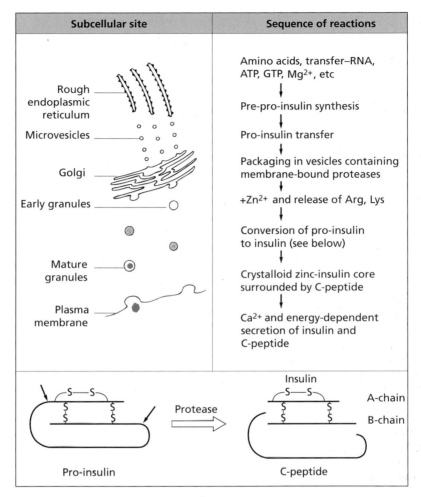

Subcellular site	Sequence of reactions
Rough endoplasmic reticulum	Amino acids, transfer–RNA, ATP, GTP, Mg^{2+}, etc ↓ Pre-pro-insulin synthesis ↓
Microvesicles	Pro-insulin transfer ↓
Golgi	Packaging in vesicles containing membrane-bound proteases ↓
Early granules	$+Zn^{2+}$ and release of Arg, Lys ↓ Conversion of pro-insulin to insulin (see below) ↓
Mature granules	Crystalloid zinc-insulin core surrounded by C-peptide ↓
Plasma membrane	Ca^{2+} and energy-dependent secretion of insulin and C-peptide

Figure 11.5 Insulin synthesis and secretion from the β-cells of pancreatic islets of Langerhans. Protein synthesis on the rough endoplasmic reticulum yields preproinsulin, which is transferred into the lumen of the endoplasmic reticulum. Hydrolysis yields proinsulin, which is then transferred to the Golgi apparatus, about 20 min after the initiation of protein synthesis. Proinsulin is enclosed in vesicles that carry specific proteases bound to the membrane. Over a period of about 30 min to 2 h, the specific proteases act on proinsulin to release the C-peptide and insulin within the granule. Progressive maturation and crystallization of zinc insulin takes place to yield a dense crystalloid region surrounded by a clear space containing C-peptide. When the cells are stimulated, e.g. by a rise in blood glucose, an energy-dependent and calcium ion-dependent fusion of the granules with the plasma membrane of the cell releases the contents into the bloodstream. Insulin and C-peptide are released in approximately equimolar amounts. The lower portion of the illustration shows a schematic diagram of the structures of proinsulin and insulin. Proinsulin, on the left, is cleaved at two points (arrows) by a specific protease, pro-hormone corrertase, packaged into early β-cell granules. The C-peptide is cleaved from a single-chain peptide to form insulin, which then has two chains, A and B, linked by two disulphide bridges, with the A chain also carrying an intrachain disulphide bridge. Proinsulin contains 86 amino acids, while insulin has 21 amino acids in the A chain and 30 in the B chain.

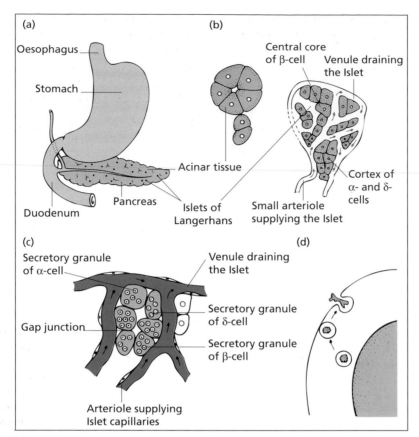

Figure 11.6 The endocrine pancreas. (a) This consists of small groups of cells, the islets of Langerhans, embedded in the exocrine acinar tissue. (b) Each islet consists of a core mainly of β-cells surrounded by a rim or cortex of α- and δ-cells. The islet is supplied with one or more small arterioles that penetrate to the centre of the islet and then break up into capillaries. These first supply the central β-cells and then flow to the periphery of the islet to supply the rim of α- and δ-cells. The capillaries leave the islet and form the draining venules. In this way, the circulation ensures that the β-rich core of islet cells is the first to be exposed to high glucose concentrations, and the peripheral α- and δ-cells are exposed to high insulin concentrations from the inner β-cells. (c) The three cell types of the islet have distinctive secretory granules, which enable them to be easily identified under the electron microscope. All three cell types have been shown to possess gap junctions, and thereby to be dye-coupled to one another. (d) Part of a β-cell, showing a secretory granule discharging its contents in the process of exocytosis, leading to the release of insulin.

level but concentrations rise rapidly following meals. As such, insulin may be considered as a hormone that signals the 'fed' state and as the pivotal hormone regulating cellular energy supply and macronutrient balance and directing anabolic processes of the fed state (Fig. 11.10). Insulin has major anabolic actions on intermediate metabolism, affecting glucose, lipid and protein metabolism. The major insulin-sensitive tissues are the liver, skeletal muscle and adipose tissue. Following secretion of insulin, 60% is subsequently removed by the liver; thus portal vein insulin concentrations reaching the liver are almost threefold higher than in the peripheral circulation. Insulin plays a major role in regulating hepatic glucose output by inhibiting gluconeogenesis and promoting glycogen storage. Similarly in muscle cells, insulin-mediated glucose uptake enables glycogen to be synthesized and stored, and for carbohydrates, rather than fatty acids or amino acids, to be utilized as the immediately available energy source for muscle contraction. Adipose tissue fat breakdown is suppressed and its synthesis promoted.

Intracellular actions of insulin

Glucose metabolism

Normally plasma glucose concentration is maintained within a narrow range despite wide fluctuations in nutrient supply and demand. Under normal physiological conditions, insulin, together with its principal counter-regulatory hormone glucagon, is the prime regulator of glucose metabolism.

Insulin is involved in the regulation of carbohydrate metabolism at many steps (Table 11.3). As already mentioned, insulin increases glucose uptake

into key insulin-sensitive tissues. Glucose is carried into cells across the cell membrane by a family of specialized transporter proteins called glucose transporters:

- GLUT-1 is involved in basal and noninsulin-mediated glucose uptake in cells

Table 11.2 Some factors regulating insulin release from the β-cells of the pancreatic islets

Factors increasing insulin release	Factors decreasing insulin release

Nutrients:
  raised glucose
  amino acids
	Nutrients:
	  low glucose

Hormones:
  glucagon
  gastrin, secretin
  cholecystokinin
  GIP, GLP-1
	Hormones:
	  somatostatin

Pancreatic innervation:
  sympathetic α receptors
  parasympathetic
	Pancreatic innervation:
	  sympathetic β receptors

	Stress:
	  exercise
	  hypoxia
	  hypothermia
	  surgery
	  severe burns

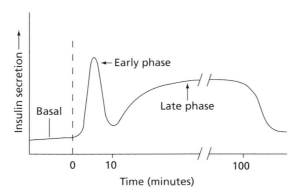

Figure 11.7 Characteristic biphasic release of insulin in responsive is continuous glucose perfusion.

GIP, glucose-dependent insulinotrophic peptide
GLP-1; glucagon like protein

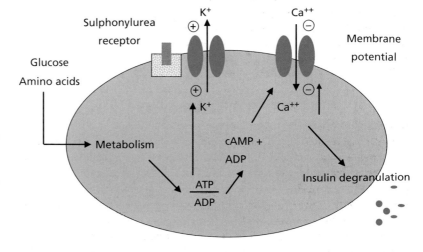

Figure 11.8 Mechanism of insulin release. Glucose is metabolized to increase ATP concentrations. This results in closure of the potassium channels which in turn leads to opening of calcium channels and release of intracellular calcium stores. The rise in intrcellular calcium leads to insulin secretion.

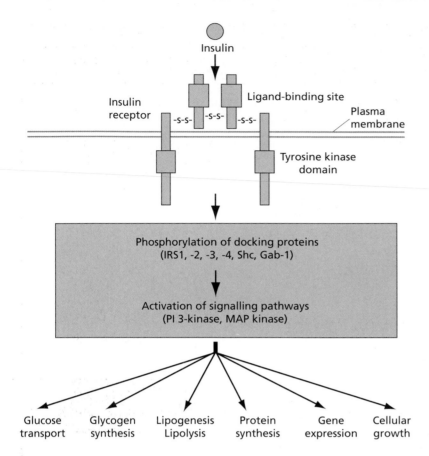

Insulin

Insulin receptor

Ligand-binding site

-s-s-   -s-s-   -s-s-

Plasma membrane

Tyrosine kinase domain

Phosphorylation of docking proteins
(IRS1, -2, -3, -4, Shc, Gab-1)

Activation of signalling pathways
(PI 3-kinase, MAP kinase)

Glucose transport | Glycogen synthesis | Lipogenesis Lipolysis | Protein synthesis | Gene expression | Cellular growth

Figure 11.9 Insulin signalling cascade.

- GLUT-2 is important in the β-cell for glucose sensing.
- GLUT-3 is involved in noninsulin-mediated glucose uptake into the brain.
- GLUT-4 is responsible for insulin-stimulated glucose uptake into muscle and adipose tissue.

GLUT-4 is normally located within the vesicles in the cytoplasm and following binding of insulin to its receptor, these transporters are translocated to the cell surface where they act as a pore for glucose entry.

Insulin acts to increase glycogen synthesis and inhibit glycogen breakdown. The control of glycogen metabolism is dependent on the phosphorylation and dephosphorylation of the enzymes controlling glycogenolysis to glycogen synthesis (Fig. 11.11); the rate-limiting enzymes are the catabolic enzyme phosphorylase and the anabolic enzyme glycogen synthase. Insulin increases glycogen synthesis through its action to activate glycogen synthase while inhibiting glycogenolysis by dephosphorylating glycogen phosphorylase kinase. Glycolysis is stimulated and gluconeogenesis inhibited by dephosphorylation of pyruvate kinase (PK) and 2,6 biphosphate kinase. Insulin also enhances the irreversible conversion of pyruvate to acetyl CoA by activation of the intramitochondrial enzyme complex pyruvate dehydrogenase. Acetyl CoA may then be directly oxidized via the Krebs' cycle, or used for fatty acid synthesis.

Lipid metabolism
Insulin increases the rate of lipogenesis in several ways in adipose tissue and liver, and controls the formation and storage of triglyceride. The critical step in lipogenesis is the activation of the insulin-sensitive lipoprotein lipase in the capillaries (Fig. 11.12). Fatty acids are then released from circulating chylomicrons or very low-density lipoproteins and taken

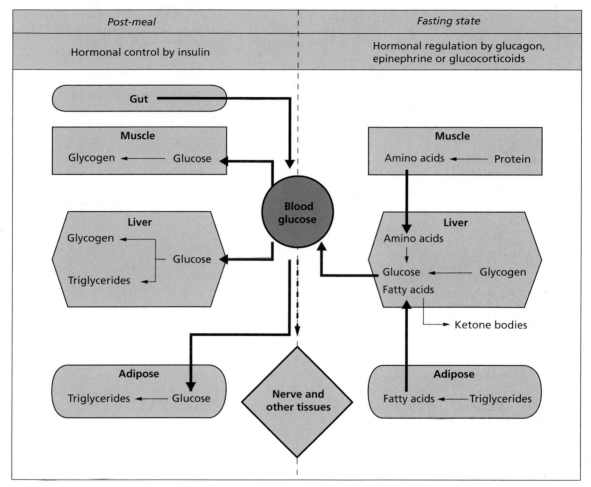

Figure 11.10 Regulation of blood-glucose concentration; tissue utilization of metabolites after a meal and in a fasting state are contrasted. Food is absorbed from the gut and increases the blood glucose concentration. Insulin facilitates absorption and the control of the synthesis of glycogen and triglyceride storage depots in liver and adipose tissues. Approximately 90% of stored glucose is in the form of lipids. In the fasting state, amino acids are mobilized from muscle proteins to yield pyruvate in the liver, where gluconeogenesis and glycogenolysis are capable of maintaining the blood-glucose concentration required for utilization by brain, nerves and other tissues. Various hormones, including epinephrine, glucagon and glucocorticoids, exert a regulatory action at different sites in these tissues. Fatty acids, mobilized from adipose tissues under the control of a number of hormones (epinephrine, glucocorticoids, glucagon, growth hormone), provide a substrate for liver and muscle metabolism. Ketone bodies produced in the liver provide an energy source for muscle and brain during long periods of fasting.

Table 11.3 Insulin actions on carbohydrate metabolism

Action	Mechanism
Increases glucose uptake into cells	Translocation of GLUT-4 glucose transporter to cell surface
Increases glycogen synthesis	Activates glycogen synthase
Inhibits glycogen breakdown	Inactivates glycogen phosphorylase kinase by dephosphorylation
Inhibits gluconeogenesis	Dephosphorylation of pyruvate kinase and 2,6 biphosphate kinase
Increases glycolysis	Dephosphorylation of pyruvate kinase and 2,6 biphosphate kinase
Converts pyruvate to acetyl CoA	Activates the mitochondrial enzyme complex pyruvate dehydrogenase

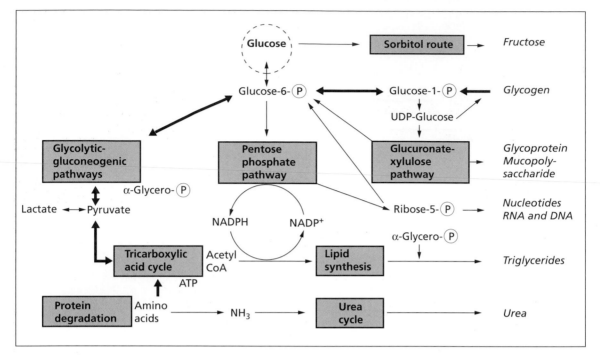

Figure 11.11 Interrelationships among alternative routes of glucose metabolism. The central role of glucose in carbohydrate, fat and protein metabolism is summarized. The principal metabolic pathways are shown enclosed in boxes in order to simplify the diagram; some key intermediates and products of metabolic interconversions are shown. The reversibility of certain reaction sequences implied by double-headed arrows is not necessarily intended to suggest that the same enzymes are involved in both the forward and reverse reactions. The principal reversible pathways that are activated during fasting are marked with heavy arrows.

up into the adipose tissue. Fatty acid synthesis is increased by activation and increased phosphorylation of acetyl CoA carboxylase, while fat oxidation is suppressed by inhibition of carnitine acyltransferase (Table 11.4). Lipogenesis is also facilitated by the uptake of glucose, because its metabolism by the pentose phosphate pathway provides reducing equivalents, such as NADPH, for fatty acid synthesis.

Triglyceride synthesis is stimulated by esterification of glycerol phosphate, while triglyceride breakdown is suppressed by dephosphorylation of hormone-sensitive lipase.

Cholesterol synthesis is increased by activation and dephosphorylation of HMGCoA reductase while cholesterol ester breakdown appears to be inhibited by dephosphorylation of cholesterol esterase. Phospholipid metabolism is also influenced by insulin.

Protein metabolism
Insulin stimulates the uptake of amino acid into cells and promotes protein synthesis in a range of tissue. There are effects on transcription of specific mRNA, as well as translation of mRNA into proteins in the ribosomes. Examples of enhanced mRNA transcription include the mRNA for glucokinase and fatty acid synthase, while insulin action decreases mRNA for liver enzymes such as carbamoyl phosphate synthetase, a key enzyme in the urea cycle. However the major action of insulin is to inhibit the breakdown of proteins (Fig. 11.13). In this way it acts synergistically with growth hormone and insulin like growth factor-1 to increase protein anabolism.

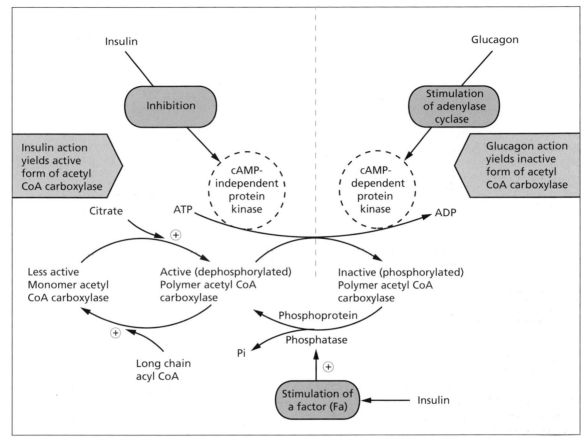

Figure 11.12 Regulation of acetyl coenzyme A (CoA) carboxylase by allosteric regulators and by phosphorylation–dephosphorylation mechanisms. Acetyl CoA carboxylase, which is involved in fatty-acid synthesis, exists as a monomer and in two polymeric forms, which are interconvertible by dephosphorylation. Citrate and long-chain acyl CoA control the relative proportions of the less active monomer and the active polymeric form of acetyl CoA carboxylase by allosteric mechanisms. As in the case of glycogen synthetase, two protein kinase enzymes are capable of regulating the conversion of active polymer acetyl CoA carboxylase to the inactive phosphorylated form of the enzyme. The cyclic adenosine 5′-monophosphate (cAMP)-dependent protein kinase may be activated by glucagon (top right of the illustration), while the cAMP-independent protein kinase is inhibited by insulin action on the target cell (top left of the illustration). Glucagon action on the cell hence decreases lipogenesis, while insulin stimulates fatty-acid synthesis.

Table 11.4 Insulin actions on fatty acid metabolism

Action	Mechanism
Increases fatty acid synthesis	Activation and increased phosphorylation of acetyl CoA carboxylase
Suppression of fatty acid oxidation	Inhibition of carnitine acyltransferase
Increases triglyceride synthesis	Stimulates esterification of glycerol phosphate
Inhibits triglyceride breakdown	Dephosphorylation of hormone sensitive lipase
Increases cholesterol synthesis	Activation and dephosphorylation of HMGCoA reductase
Inhibition of cholesterol ester breakdown	Dephosphorylation of cholesterol esterase

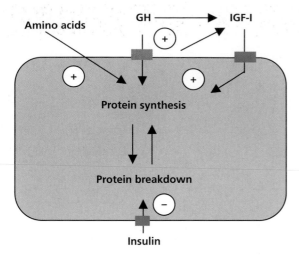

Figure 11.13 Growth hormone and insulin and their effect on protein synthesis.

Glucagon

Glucagon is a polypeptide with a molecular weight of around 3.5 kD. It is synthesized as a large precursor, preproglucagon, and is cleaved within the α-cells to the active hormone. Its secretion is stimulated by a fall in blood glucose and by amino acids. Release of glucagon is also under neurological control and sympathetic adrenergic activation increases glucagon release.

Glucagon plays an important part in preventing significant hypoglycaemia during fasting by antagonizing the actions of insulin. Its primary site of action is the liver where it binds to specific glucagon receptors that are linked to adenylate cyclase. It leads to the mobilization of glycogen and to the production of glucose from noncarbohydrate precursors by gluconeogenesis.

Answers to case histories

Case history 11.1

There is a large burden of undiagnosed diabetes in every community. It is estimated that for every patient with known diabetes, there may be another patient who does not know they have the disease. Diabetes prevalence varies from region to region according to the demographics of the region and therefore estimates from other regions may be inappropriate. As the prevalence is increasing sharply, comparing the current prevalence in year region with historical publications may be inappropriate as that would lead to an over estimate of the degree that your region differs from the national average.

Establishing registers of patients with diabetes is one way of obtaining a reasonable estimate of known cases of diabetes. Epidemiologists have produced models based on published studies that can be used to estimate the burden of diabetes locally.

Case history 11.2

We do not know. In order to make a diagnosis of diabetes in an asymptomatic person, two values above the international agreed criteria are required. A random blood glucose of 11.2 mmol/L is in the diabetic range but a second confirmatory test is required. The WHO recommends that the gold standard confirmatory test is a 75-g oral glucose tolerance test.

KEY POINTS

- Diabetes is the commonest endocrine condition and its prevalence is increasing rapidly

- The commonest forms are type 1 and type 2 diabetes

- It is defined by elevations in blood glucose

- Insulin is the pivotal hormone regulating cellular energy supply and macronutrient balance during the fed state

12 Type 1 diabetes

LEARNING OBJECTIVES

- To discuss the epidemiology, aetiology and pathology of type 1 diabetes
- To understand the clinical features of type 1 diabetes and in particular

   recognize the importance of diabetic ketoacidosis
- To understand the principles of insulin therapy and its pitfalls

In this chapter we will learn about type 1 diabetes

Introduction

Although not the commonest type of diabetes, its presentation and acute complications are the most dramatic. The discovery of insulin and treatment of patients with type 1 diabetes is one of the greatest advances in medicine in the 20th century. It has saved and transformed the lives of millions of people worldwide.

What is type 1 diabetes?

Type 1 diabetes is caused by an absolute deficiency of insulin, usually as the result of a T-cell mediated autoimmune destruction of the β-cells of the pancreas (Box 12.1).

Epidemiology of Type 1 diabetes

Type 1 diabetes represents around 10% of all cases of diabetes, affecting approximately 20 million people worldwide. Although type 1 diabetes affects all age groups, the majority of individuals are diagnosed either in the preschool years or in the teens and early adulthood.

The incidence of type 1 diabetes varies dramatically throughout the world. The highest incidence rates are in Northern Europe, in Finland and Sweden, where the rates are nearly 500 times greater than in China or Venezuela (Fig. 12.1). Worldwide, the incidence and prevalence of type 1 diabetes is increasing. Across Europe, the average annual increase in the incidence in children under 15 years of age is 3.4%, with the steepest rise in the under-5-year-old age group. In 1994, it was estimated that worldwide there were approximately 11.5 million people with type 1 diabetes and this figure is projected to rise to 23.7 million by 2010.

During the 1970s, diabetes was slightly commoner in European boys and in populations of European origin while, in contrast, in African or Asian populations, girls were more commonly affected. However, during the 1990s the sex-specific pattern changed and the male excess disappeared from many but not all populations.

Aetiology and pathogenesis of type 1 diabetes

The aetiology of type 1 diabetes remains poorly understood, but the most likely scenario is that an environmental factor triggers a selective autoimmune destruction of the β-cells of the pancreas in a genetically predisposed individual. The autoimmune basis for type 1 diabetes is suggested by its association with a number of other organ-specific autoimmune diseases such as autoimmune thyroid disease, coeliac disease, pernicious anaemia and Addison disease (Case history 12.1) (Box 8.7) .

The autoimmune nature is also suggested by the pathological finding of a chronic inflammatory mononuclear cell infiltrate of mainly T lymphocytes and macrophages in the islet cells (insulitis) of patients with newly diagnosed type 1 diabetes. The presence of circulating islet-related autoantibodies, including islet cell autoantibodies, insulin antibodies and glutamic acid decarboxylase autoantibodies, in patients with type 1 diabetes adds further evidence of an autoimmune process. These antibodies are present prior to the onset of diabetes and have been used to predict which individuals will develop the disease. Follow-up of individuals with these individuals has added considerably to our understanding of the natural history of type 1 diabetes. It was previously observed that the presentation of type 1 diabetes is usually fairly rapid, over a period of

---

BOX 12.1 What is autoimmunity?

Under normal circumstances, the body's immune system does not react against itself. This is known as immune tolerance. Autoimmunity is caused by a breakdown of this normal immune tolerance of self.

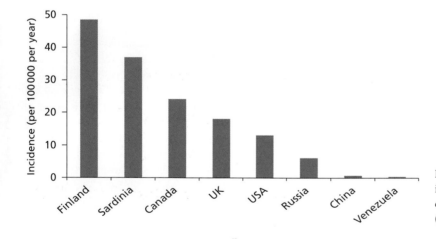

Figure 12.1 Age-standardized incidence of type 1 diabetes in children less than 15 years old (per 100 000 per year).

CASE HISTORY 12.1

A 24-year-old woman with previously well-controlled type 1 diabetes presents with tiredness and lethargy. She also remarks that she has had many more hypoglycaemic episodes than previously and has had to cut her insulin dose by 50%. She mentions that she often feels dizzy when she stands up and has noticed that she is more 'tanned' than usual.

What is the possible explanation for her symptoms?
How will you confirm your diagnosis?

Answers, see p. 214

several weeks. It is now known that β-cell loss can be slow and some individuals have not developed diabetes for several years after appearance of the autoantibodies (Fig. 12.2). Furthermore, not all individuals with autoantibodies develop diabetes, suggesting that insulitis itself does not necessarily progress to critical β-cell loss and diabetes.

Twin and family studies have suggested that genetic factors are important in the aetiology of type 1 diabetes. For example, if one monozygotic twin has type 1 diabetes, the risk of the other monozygotic twin developing diabetes is around 30 to 50% (Table 12.1).

The risk of diabetes is modified markedly by the genes in the class II region of the human leucocyte antigen (HLA) system (Box 12.2). Over 95% of white European patients with type 1 diabetes have HLA-DR-3 and or DR-4 class II HLA antigens as compared with only 50% of nondiabetic individuals while

Table 12.1 Risk of developing type 1 diabetes for relatives of people with diabetes

Family member	Risk (%)
Monozygotic twin	30–50 in other twin 65–70 if twin diagnosed before age of 5
Dizygotic twin	15
HLA identical sibling	16–20
One HLA identical sibling	9
HLA nonidentical sibling	3
Mother	2
Father	8
Both parents	30
General population	0.4

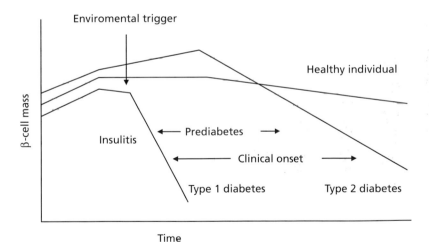

Figure 12.2 The natural history of diabetes. β-cell mass increases during childhood and reaches a peak in early adulthood. Thereafter there is a progressive loss of β-cell mass of approximately 1% per year. In type 2 diabetes, the rate of β-cell loss is accelerated to approximately 4%. One model for the natural history of type 1 diabetes is that certain individuals are genetically predisposed to develop diabetes. Environmental factors act as triggers or regulators of the autoimmune destructive process that then results in insulitis, β-cell injury and finally loss of β-cell mass. As β-cell function falls, first phase insulin secretion is lost, followed by the development of prediabetes and eventually overt diabetes. At the onset of diabetes, some β-cells will remain and their presence can be identified by the detection of circulating C-peptide. With time, however, these remaining cells will also be destroyed leading to absolute insulin deficiency. The differences between type 1 and type 2 diabetes appear to be one of tempo and there has been debate recently about whether the division into two types is wholly justified. An alternative view is that they are opposite ends of a spectrum of β-cell loss.

BOX 12.2 What are HLA molecules?

- HLA antigens are glycoproteins found on the cell surface that are involved in the immune process
- There are two classes, I and II, that differ in their structure
- Class I molecules are found on all nucleated cells while class II are only found on antigen-presenting cells such as macrophages
- Class II molecules bind foreign antigen peptides and are presented to T helper lymphocytes
- There are three types of class II molecule—DP, DQ and DR; each of these is subclassified by numbers

BOX 12.3 Putative but unproven environmental triggers of type 1 diabetes

- Chemicals
  - *N*-nitro compounds—streptozocin, nitrosamines, nitrosamides
- Viruses
  - mumps
  - rubella
  - cytomegalovirus
  - enteroviruses
  - retroviruses
- Bacteria
  - Streptomyces
- Vaccination
- Stress
- Perinatal factors
  - maternal rubella
  - blood group incompatibility
  - maternal age
  - pre-eclampsia
  - caesarean section
  - birth weight
  - gestational age
  - birth order
- Food components
  - milk protein
  - wheat protein
  - vitamin D deficiency

certain HLA haplotypes such as HLA DQ-6 may protect against diabetes. In Europe, around 5 to 6% of the siblings of children with type 1 diabetes will develop diabetes themselves by the age of 15 years. However, if their HLA genotype is identical to their diabetic sibling, the risk of developing diabetes increases to 20%, while siblings who share one HLA gene have a risk of 9%.

Although the genetic susceptibility to type 1 diabetes is inherited, only 12 to 15% of type 1 diabetes occurs in families. This indicates that genetic factors do not account entirely for the development of type 1 diabetes, and several environmental triggers, including viral infections, nutritional factors, parental age and low birth weight, have been suggested (Box 12.3). How these factors affect the autoimmune response is unclear but one potential mechanism is that the environmental trigger leads to an abnormal production of costimulatory molecules and up-regulation of the HLA antigens in susceptible people. This may lead to self-antigens being presented to T-helper cells triggering an immune response. Another potential mechanism is that self-antigens may be modified and become antigenic. A further possibility is that an immune response against a dietary or infective agent may cross-react with self-antigens, so called molecular mimicry.

Clinical features

Patients with type 1 diabetes usually present with a short duration of illness of 1 to 4 weeks. Although there is diversity in the clinical presentation, the effects of insulin on intermediate metabolism can explain the majority of the clinical features of diabetes (Box 12.4).

Many of the symptoms are linked to the osmotic effect of the hyperglycaemia or the inability to transport fuel substrates into the cells because of a lack of insulin. As the plasma glucose exceeds the renal threshold for reabsorption of glucose (approximately 10 mmol/L), glucose is excreted in the urine. It exerts an osmotic effect that can lead to profound dehydration and hypovolaemia as water leaves the cells along the osmotic gradient, only to be lost in the urine. Elevations in intraocular glucose concentration lead to a similar osmotic effect which distorts the lens and causes blurred vision. The most serious presenting feature is the development of diabetic ketoacidosis which will be discussed in more detail later in the chapter.

Prognosis

Patients with type 1 diabetes have premature mortality compared with the general population. It is said that on the day that a patient is diagnosed with diabetes their life expectancy is reduced by around one-third (Fig. 12.3). Consequently, the greatest burden of diabetes is placed on those who are diagnosed during childhood. Adults with diabetes have an annual mortality of about 5.4%, double the rate for nondiabetic adults. The commonest cause of death is cardiovascular disease, where the standardised mortality ratio is approximately three to five times greater than the general population. The risk of dying from a renal cause is approximately 100 times greater than the general population. Cardiovascular disease and diabetic nephropathy are discussed in Chapter 14.

Diagnosis

The diagnosis of diabetes is relatively straight forward once it is considered. As the patients have symptoms, only one plasma glucose concentration above the diagnostic cut-off is needed to confirm the diagnosis. While the clinical features are often clear cut, it is becoming increasingly difficult to distinguish patients with type 1 and type 2 diabetes as the latter is becoming more common in children. The detection of islet autoantibodies is indicative of type 1 diabetes.

A catch for the unwary is the patient with MODY (maturity-onset diabetes of the young). These are monogenic forms of diabetes that are highly penetrant within families. As they often present in childhood, they may be mistaken for type 1 diabetes. A family history of early-onset diabetes should alert the clinician to this possibility.

BOX 12.4 Presenting features of type 1 diabetes

- Symptoms relating to osmotic effect of the hyperglycaemia
  - increased thirst and polydipsia
  - polyuria and nocturia
  - blurred vision
  - drowsiness and dehydration
- Cutaneous candidal infection
  - vulva (pruritus vulvae)
  - foreskin (balanitis)
- Symptoms relate to the inability to transport fuel substrates
  - extreme fatigue
  - muscle wasting through protein breakdown
  - weight loss
- Diabetic ketoacidosis

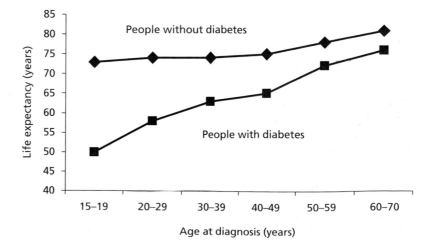

Figure 12.3 Life expectancy and diabetes. Adults with diabetes have an annual mortality of about 5.4%, double the rate for nondiabetic adults. Life expectancy is decreased by 5 to 10 years.

Management of type 1 diabetes

The aims of treatment for patients with diabetes are fourfold:
- Save life
- Alleviate symptoms
- Achieve good control to minimize long-term complications
- Avoid iatrogenic side-effects such as hypoglycaemia

In order to achieve these goals, it is important to provide insulin replacement to meet the physiological insulin requirements of the individual. The ability to achieve this can be assessed through home blood glucose monitoring and hospital laboratory tests of control. Patients require structured education to allow them to take control of their diabetes and to make an informed judgement about a healthy diet and exercise.

The discovery of insulin in 1922 transformed the management of patients with diabetes (Fig. 12.4). Prior to its introduction, patients with diabetes were left with a choice of death by diabetic ketoacidosis or death by 'inanition', the exhausted condition resulting from want or insufficiency of nourishment. Patients could survive for several years on diets of around 500 to 700 calories a day but inevitably lost weight until either the patient broke their diet or died from starvation.

In patients without diabetes, insulin is secreted at a slow basal rate throughout the day, which gives rise to low blood insulin concentrations between meals and during the night. Following a meal, there is a rapid rise and peak in blood insulin concentrations which fall back to baseline within 2 h (Fig. 12.5). The philosophy of managing the insulin replacement in patients with diabetes is to mimic this pattern as

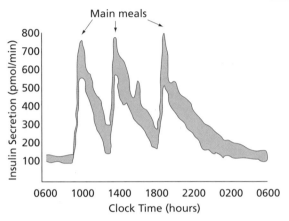

Figure 12.5 Normal insulin secretion throughout a 24-h period. There is a background insulin secretion throughout the day superimposed on which are meal-time-related peaks of insulin. Redrawn from O'Meara *et al. Am. J. Med.*, 1990, **89**, 11S–16S.

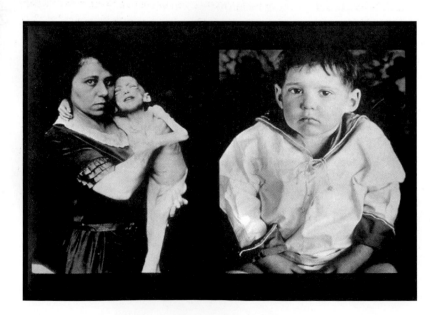

Figure 12.4 One of the first patients with diabetes to receive insulin in the 1920s, before and after treatment with insulin. Reproduced with kind permission of Eli Lilly and Co.

closely as possible (Box 12.5). Although the introduction of insulin transformed patients' lives, and in our view is one of the most significant advances in medicine, it became apparent that subcutaneous insulin delivery was not ideal and many developments have happened since the 1920s to allow the replacement of insulin in a more physiological pattern. The use of insulin has to be tailored to meet individual requirements in order to achieve the best possible control without the risk of disabling hypoglycaemia.

Types of insulin

There are three main types of insulin.

1. **Soluble insulin** was first introduced in 1922 and still plays an important part in the management of patients with type 1 diabetes. Usually it is administered subcutaneously but may also be given intravenously or intramuscularly whilst managing diabetic emergencies. Initially, insulin was isolated from pigs or cattle but since the 1980s, insulin has been produced biosynthetically using recombinant DNA technology and the insertion of cloned human insulin genes into *Escherichia coli*. This technology has allowed large amounts of insulin to be produced in a highly purified manner. Some patients are still treated with animal insulin but these patients are becoming rarer.

2. **Protamine insulin** and **insulin zinc** suspensions were introduced to form **isophane insulin** in the 1930s and 1950s respectively. These preparations prolong the action of insulin to provide a basal level of insulin.

3. Most recently, short-acting and long-acting **insulin analogues** have been introduced to mimic more closely the physiological changes of insulin concentration. When soluble insulin is injected subcutaneously it forms a hexamer which delays its absorption from the injection site. For this reason it is more slowly acting than endogenously secreted insulin. In order to meet this challenge, newer rapid-acting insulin analogues (insulin lispro, insulin aspart or insulin glulysine) that do not form hexamers, and are therefore more rapidly absorbed, have been introduced. Long-acting insulin analogues (insulin glargine or insulin detemir) have been introduced to provide a more predictable basal insulin with less variation in insulin concentrations.

Injection sites and technology

Insulin is given subcutaneously by intermittent injection or by continuous infusion. Although it can be injected almost anywhere if there is enough flesh, the best sites are the front and side of the thigh, lower abdominal wall, buttocks and upper arms (Fig. 12.6).

Intermittent insulin injections may be given by needle and syringes but more commonly patients now use insulin pen devices which deliver metered doses of insulin from an insulin cartridge (Fig. 12.7). These are portable, use a fine needle and have a simplified procedure for measuring the insulin. The

---

BOX 12.5 Disadvantages of subcutaneous insulin administration compared with endogenous insulin production

- Must be given by injection
- Insulin is delivered into the systemic rather than portal circulation
  - the liver is exposed to less insulin while peripheral tissues, such as adipose tissue, are exposed to higher concentrations
  - insulin has a number of actions in the liver that are not normalized, e.g. production of IGF-1
- Loss of normal feedback mechanism between glucose concentrations and insulin secretion
- The pharmacodynamics are altered making it difficult to match insulin supply to requirement

---

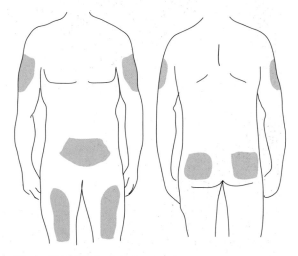

Figure 12.6 Sites for injection.

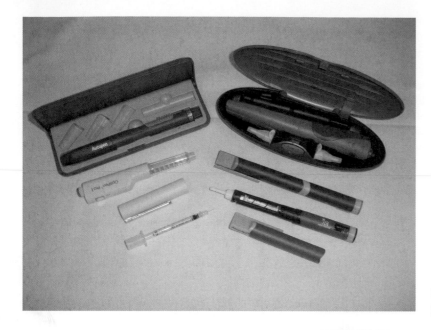

Figure 12.7 A variety of insulin pen devices and carrying cases.

pens allow the patient to dial up and dispense their required doses. The many advantages of insulin pens include convenience, easier injection and less pain.

Continuous subcutaneous insulin infusion or insulin pumps are alternative forms of insulin delivery that combine basal infusion rates with mealtime boluses (Fig. 12.8). These systems can be used by well-motivated patients and result in improved control with fewer episodes of hypoglycaemia.

Recently, inhaled insulin has became available although currently its use is limited to those who are unable to use subcutaneous insulin.

Insulin regimens

In theory, any combination of insulin can be used as long as the patients achieve good control. However, there are several regimens that are more commonly used (Fig. 12.9). One of the simplest in use for patients with type 1 diabetes is twice daily mixed insulin. The mixed insulin contains both short- and intermediate-acting insulin and is given at breakfast and with the evening meal. While the advantage of this regimen is that the patients only need two injections per day, there are several disadvantages, such as inflexibility and poorer control, that make basal–bolus regimens the treatment of choice for most individuals (Table 12.2) (Case history 12.2).

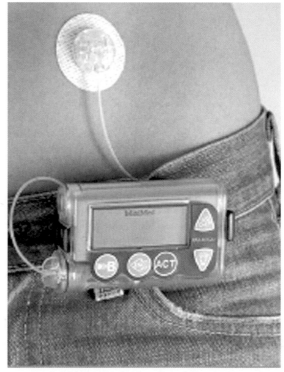

Figure 12.8 Patient with diabetes wearing a Medtronic Paradigm insulin pump.

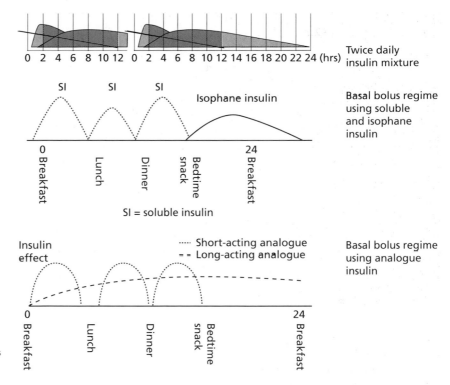

Figure 12.9 Insulin profiles with different regimens.

Table 12.2 Advantages and disadvantages of insulin regimens

Factor	Advantages and disadvantages		
	Twice daily insulin mixture	Basal–bolus using soluble insulin	Basal–bolus using analogue insulin
No of injections	2	Usually 4	Usually 4
Timing	20–30 min before breakfast and evening meal	20–30 min before each meal and prebed	5–10 min before each meal and prebed
Flexibility of mealtimes	No—patient must eat regularly at predetermined times	Yes—injection given before meal	Yes—injection given before meal; may also miss meals with long-acting analogues
Variable meal sizes	Lunch insulin is delivered at breakfast time therefore little flexibility	Yes—meal doses can be adjusted according to need	Yes—meal doses can be adjusted according to need
Need for between meal snack	Yes	Yes	No
Risk of hypoglycaemia	High	Lower	Lowest
Glycaemic control	Achievable	Better control than twice daily insulin mixture	Best control
Insulin allergy	Possible	Possible	Reduced risk

CASE HISTORY 12.2

A 35-year-old man who has type 1 diabetes attends the clinic complaining of late morning 'hypos'. He is currently treated with twice daily premixed insulin containing 30% soluble insulin and 70% isophane insulin. He mentions that work is hectic and he does not always know when he is going to eat lunch.

What possible changes to his insulin regimen could you make?

Answers, see p. 214

Complications of insulin therapy

Hypoglycaemia

Hypoglycaemia occurs when the blood glucose falls below 3.5 mmol/L. It is the most important side-effect of insulin therapy and a severe hypoglycaemic episode affects around 10% of patients with type 1 diabetes each year. It occurs more frequently in young children and those with tight glycaemic control. Hypoglycaemia is a serious side-effect because it may be associated with cardiac arrhythmias and sudden death. Hypoglycaemia may also be responsible for cognitive impairment and lowered academic achievement in children diagnosed with diabetes before the age of 5 years. It significantly affects the quality of life of patients with type 1 diabetes and is a major barrier to optimal glycaemic control.

Hypoglycaemia is caused by an inappropriately raised insulin concentration and may result from hyperinsulinaemia or an enhanced insulin effect. This may occur when there is poor matching of the patient's insulin requirement to their lifestyle (Case history 12.3) (Box 12.6).

The physiological response to a fall in blood glucose is to produce a range of symptoms and signs that are relieved by the restoration of circulating blood glucose concentration. These symptoms are also im-

---

BOX 12.6 Causes of hypoglycaemia

- Excessive insulin administration
  - patient, doctor or pharmacist error
  - deliberate overdose during a suicide or parasuicide attempt
- Unpredictable insulin absorption
  - insulin is absorbed more rapidly from the abdomen
  - lipohypertrophy
- Altered clearance of insulin
  - decreased insulin clearance in renal failure
- Decreased insulin requirement
  - missed, small or delayed meals
  - alcohol—inhibits hepatic glucose output
  - vomiting—may occur with gastroparesis, a long-term complication of diabetes
  - exercise—also increases rate of insulin absorption (Exercise here really means physical activity. Another common cause of hypoglycaemia is when a patient becomes more active during everyday life. For example, this may occur when the patient begins a new job.)
- Recurrent hypoglycaemia and unawareness

CASE HISTORY 12.3

A 35-year-old builder with well-controlled diabetes was admitted to hospital with diarrhoea and vomiting. He was initially treated with intravenous fluids and insulin but was subsequently changed back to his normal insulin regimen. The doctors noticed that his normal doses were not controlling his glucose concentrations adequately and so they increased his doses substantially. Two days after discharge, the man had a severe hypoglycaemic episode and was admitted back to hospital.

What is the most likely reason why this man became profoundly hypoglycaemic on discharge? Could this have been prevented?

Answers, see p. 214

portant as they alert the individuals to the presence of hypoglycaemia and prompt them to take corrective action. The symptoms can be divided into two main categories, autonomic and neuroglycopaenic, although patients may also experience nonspecific symptoms (Table 12.3). Autonomic symptoms occur because of activation of the autonomic nervous system while neuroglycopaenic symptoms result from inadequate glucose supply to the brain leading to neurological dysfunction.

The initial response to hypoglycaemia is the acute release of counter-regulatory hormones, in particular glucagon and norepinephrine, when the blood glucose concentration is between 3.6 and 3.8 mmol/L. As the concentration of these hormones rises, patients develop autonomic symptoms. Cognitive function usually starts to deteriorate when the blood glucose reaches approximately 3.0 mmol/L.

The development of autonomic symptoms before cognitive dysfunction is clinically relevant as the patient is able is take appropriate corrective action before cognitive impairment begins. However, with recurrent hypoglycaemia and longer duration of diabetes, the ability of patients to recognize symptoms falls because the magnitude of the counter-regulatory hormone response falls. Patients become unaware of their hypoglycaemia and severe hypoglycaemia becomes more common as the patients are no longer unable to respond (Fig. 12.10).

Treatment of hypoglycaemia

Suspected hypoglycaemia should be treated immediately with oral glucose if possible. If the patient is unconscious or unable to swallow safely, intramuscular or subcutaneous glucagon or intravenous glucose can be administered. Glucagon is an insulin antagonist that causes mobilization of the hepatic glycogen stores. When glucagon is used to treat hypoglycaemia, these stores are diminished and so it is important to administer longer-acting carbohydrate to replenish glycogen stores.

The patient usually recovers within minutes, after which it is important to ascertain the cause of the hypoglycaemic episode to try to prevent this from happening in the future. If the patient suffers from recurrent hypoglycaemia, it may be necessary to relax the glycaemic control to allow the patient to regain their awareness of hypoglycaemia (Case history 12.4).

Lipohypertrophy and lipoatrophy

When insulin is repeatedly injected into the same subcutaneous sites, it can lead to an accumulation of fat, lipohypertrophy, because of the local trophic effects of insulin. This can be unsightly and also

Table 12.3 Symptoms and signs of hypoglycaemia

Autonomic	Neuroglycopaenic	Nonspecific
Sweating	Difficulty in speaking	Nausea
Pins and needles	Loss of concentration	Hunger
Feeling hot	Drowsiness	Weakness
Shakiness	Dizziness	
Anxiety	Hemiplegia	
Palpitations	Fits	
	Coma	
	Death	

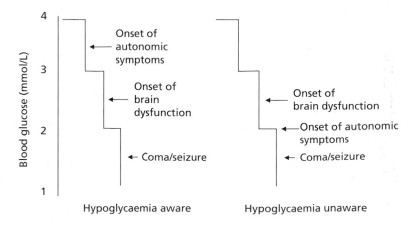

Figure 12.10 Hypoglycaemia unawareness—the threshold for activation of hypoglycaemic symptoms in hypoglycaemic aware and unaware. Note the threshold for the onset of brain dysfunction does not change.

CASE HISTORY 12.4

A 28-year-old woman has recently tried hard to improve her glycaemic control but unfortunately had a car accident when she was hypoglycaemic. She mentions that her usual warning has disappeared and when you look at her glucose monitoring records, you find she is having frequent 'hypos'.

How can you help her?

Answers, see p. 214

---

increases the variability of insulin absorption. The affected sites are often painless and therefore may be favoured by the patient. The best way to avoid hypertrophy is to rotate the site of injection within a given anatomical area.

Now that highly purified insulin is available, insulin allergy is rare. However, immunoglobulin G immune complexes against insulin can be formed and can produce local atrophy of fat tissue as well as affect insulin action.

Diabetic diet

Patients with type 1 diabetes require active dietary management to help achieve good glycaemic control. Patients with diabetes are at increased risk of vascular disease and therefore it is important to encourage patterns of healthy eating. Ideally, 60% of total caloric intake should be provided by carbohydrate with no more than 30% coming from fat. Saturated fats should be substituted with poly-unsaturated or monounsaturated fats where possible. Eating of complex carbohydrates such as bread, potatoes, pasta and rice in moderate amounts with each meal should be encouraged. Complex and low glycaemic index (GI) carbohydrates cause a slower rise in blood glucose concentration than simple sugars because of their slower rate of absorption. Simple sugars, such as sugar itself, nondiet soft drinks, jams, honey, cakes and biscuits should be replaced where possible with low sugar alternatives. Moderation of alcohol intake is important.

It should be recognized, however, that the real limitations of the diet are dictated by the inadequacy of the available insulin regimens rather than the nature of the disease itself. Historically, patients were taught to count carbohydrate intake so that the carbohydrate content in each meal or snack could be matched to the prescribed insulin dose. The rigidity of this ap-

proach became unpopular and was replaced by more general advice advocating healthy eating. The pendulum is now swinging back towards the use of carbohydrate counting. However, it is now being used to teach the patient to adjust their meal-related insulin according to their carbohydrate intake rather than *vice versa*. This approach has been used in Europe for several years and has recently been introduced into the UK through schemes such as the Dose Adjustment For Normal Eating (DAFNE) project. These structured education programmes aim to allow patients to achieve good glycaemic control while eating flexibly and have resulted in improved diabetic control and quality of life.

Monitoring diabetic control

In order to reduce the long-term complications of diabetes, it is important that the metabolism in the person with diabetes differs as little as possible from that of a person without diabetes. Traditionally, diabetic control has focused on blood glucose, with 'good glycaemic control' referring to the maintenance of near-normal blood glucose concentrations throughout the day. In some circumstances monitoring of ketone bodies, usually in the urine, may also be useful as an early indicator of the development of diabetic ketoacidosis.

The measurements of blood glucose control can be divided into short- and long-term measures (Box 12.7). The first involves the ascertainment of single blood glucose concentrations while the second assesses long-term control over the preceding weeks or months.

Capillary blood glucose monitoring
Single blood glucose concentrations are of little use because of the variability in blood glucose throughout the day and from day to day. However, serial blood glucose measurements allow patterns of blood

glucose to be recognized and appropriate adjustment of insulin according to these readings. Modern management of diabetes involves the self-monitoring of capillary blood glucose concentra-

BOX 12.7 **Methods of monitoring glycaemic control**

- Blood glucose
  - intermittent capillary
  - continuous monitoring
- Integrated measures of long-term glycaemic control
  - haemoglobin A_{1c} (HbA$_{1c}$)
  - fructosamine

tions by patients using blood glucose meters that provide the patients with almost instantaneous readings (Fig. 12.11). Patients are usually asked to monitor their blood glucose concentration immediately premeals or approximately 2h after meals.

At present, most blood samples are obtained by finger prick but alternative site testing and noninvasive methods are being developed. Most patients with type 1 diabetes are advised to test their blood glucose concentrations between two and four times a day. However, the principal that any investigation should lead to a change in management should be followed; therefore if patients are unable or unwilling to adjust their insulin then 'testing for testing sake' should be discouraged (Case history 12.5).

CASE HISTORY 12.5

A 47-year-old man, who is treated with soluble insulin three times a day and isophane insulin before bed, presents with the following set of blood results.

	Before breakfast	Before lunch	Before evening meal	Before bed
Insulin dose	10	12	18	30
Home glucose readings	4.0–7.8	2.3–5.2	9.4–13.0	5.0–7.8

What advice would you give?

Answers, see p. 214

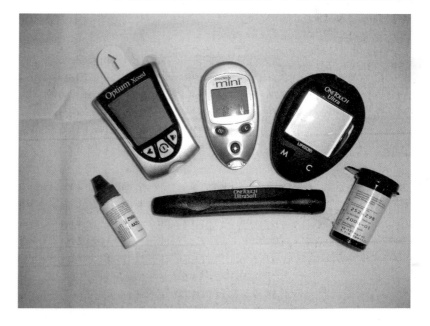

Figure 12.11 Variety of meters used for self-monitoring of capillary blood glucose.

Urinary glucose can be used as a crude index of blood glucose but because of its lack of sensitivity, it should be seen as a last resort only.

Integrated measures of glycaemic control

Glycosylated haemoglobin (HbA_{1c}) is a measure of integrated glycaemic control over the preceding 2 to 3 months. Glucose becomes attached to adult haemoglobin in a nonenzymatic fashion that is dependent on the average concentration of blood glucose. As such, HbA_{1c} correlates well with mean blood glucose concentrations during the previous 2 to 3 months, which reflects the normal lifespan of 117 days for a red blood cell.

The measurement and interpretation of HbA_{1c} has become the currency of most diabetologists' daily work. The HbA_{1c} concentration correlates with the risk of development of microvascular diabetic complications and clinical studies have confirmed the direct benefits of lowering HbA_{1c}. The American Diabetes Association has recommended that the goal of diabetes therapy should be to achieve HbA_{1c} of <7% while the United Kingdom general practitioner contract recommends a target of <7.5%. Nevertheless, it has a number of limitations and so HbA_{1c} should be seen as just one of a number of tools that can used to improve the lives of patients with diabetes (Box 12.8). HbA_{1c} reduction is a means to an end and not an end in itself.

An alternative to HbA_{1c} is fructosamine, which is a measure of glycated serum albumin. It is an index of glycaemic control over the previous 2 to 3 weeks, reflecting the shorter half-life of albumin compared with haemoglobin. As HbA_{1c} assays have improved, fructosamine has been used less frequently.

Diabetic ketoacidosis

Diabetic ketoacidosis is the most severe diabetic emergency and is still associated with a significant mortality (3–5%). It is a state of severe, uncontrolled diabetes caused by insulin deficiency. It is a medical emergency and requires urgent treatment with insulin and fluids to prevent death. Diabetic ketoacidosis occurs more commonly in younger patients but the mortality is higher in older patients.

Many factors can precipitate diabetic ketoacidosis. Infections account for around 30 to 40% of cases, with new cases of diabetes accounting for 10 to 20%. Insulin errors and omissions and noncompliance are also common (15–30%). A common mistake is for patients to stop insulin when they become unwell. Their appetite falls and they reduce the insulin in order to prevent hypoglycaemia. However, the infection often increases insulin requirement. The golden rule is NEVER STOP INSULIN!

Biochemistry of diabetic ketoacidosis

Diabetic ketoacidosis is characterized by hyperglycaemia, metabolic acidosis and hyperketonaemia (Fig. 12.12).

Hyperglycaemia

The absolute insulin deficiency leads to hyperglycaemia secondary to increased hepatic glucose output and diminished peripheral insulin-mediated glucose uptake. This process is accelerated by the presence of catabolic counter-regulatory stress hormones, in particular glucagon and catecholamines,

---

BOX 12.8 Limitations of HbA_{1c}

Analytical variability
- Different methods for HbA_{1c} may give different results but this is largely addressed now by reference method standardization
- Molecular variants of haemoglobin
  - fetal haemoglobin

Biological variability
- Interindividual variability
  - an individual with mean glucose of 10 mmol/L may have an HbA_{1c} value which ranges from 6.0 to 9.0%
  - probably reflects differences in the rates of protein glycation
- Variation in erythrocyte lifespan
  - shortened lifespan can give spuriously low results
    - haemolytic anaemia
    - acute or chronic blood loss
    - pregnancy
    - diabetes may shorten lifespan

Clinical variability
- Predictive link between HbA_{1c} and clinical outcomes is not clear-cut

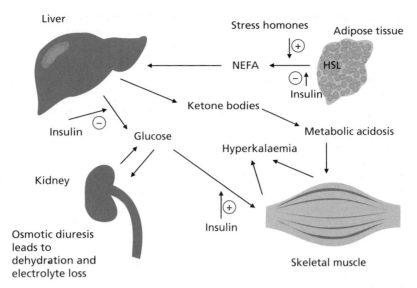

Figure 12.12 Biochemistry of diabetic ketoacidosis. Hormone sensitive lipase (HSL) is sensitive to inhibition by insulin. The insulin deficiency leads to activation of HSL and break down of adipose tissue triglyceride to NEFA, a process which is augmented by stress hormones. The NEFA are transported to the liver where they are converted to acidotic ketone bodies. The acidosis leads to hyperkalaemia, a situation which is worsened because insulin usually leads to transport of potassium into cells with glucose. Hyperglycaemia occurs because of a failure to inhibit hepatic glucose output and a reduction in insulin-mediated glucose uptake. Renal gluconeogenesis is also increased. This leads to an osmotic diuresis and profound electrolyte loss.

but also growth hormone and cortisol that are often elevated in the presence of acute illness. Renal gluconeogenesis is also enhanced in the presence of acidosis. The hyperglycaemia causes an osmotic diuresis and profound dehydration and loss of electrolytes. The loss of electrolytes is worsened because insulin deficiency results in impaired renal sodium reabsorption.

Hyperketonaemia

The lack of insulin leads to an increase in the release of nonesterified fatty acids (NEFA) into the circulation from adipose triglycerides stores. This process is mediated by hormone-sensitive lipase, an enzyme that is inhibited by insulin. Again this process is accelerated by the presence of catabolic counter-regulatory stress hormones. NEFA are transported to the liver where they are partially oxidized to acidic ketones bodies, such as acetoacetic acid and 3-hydroxybutyric acid, and acetone. This occurs because hepatic re-esterification of NEFA to triglyceride is impaired in diabetic ketoacidosis. The ketone bodies are exported from the liver as an alternative fuel supply but build up in the circulation because there is impaired disposal into peripheral tissues, such as muscle and brain, because of the lack of insulin. Plasma ketone body concentrations are commonly elevated 200 to 300 times above normal fasting values. The elevation in NEFA and stress hormones can induce a state of insulin resistance and, as a consequence, hyperglycaemia may take longer to be corrected than in other situations.

Acidosis

Ketones bodies are strong organic acids that associate at physiological pH and generate high concentrations of H^+ ions. These rapidly exceed the buffering capacity of the body and lead to severe metabolic acidosis. In order to compensate for the acidosis, respiratory rate and depth increases (Kussmaul breathing) and ketones bodies may be smelt on the breath, similar to nail varnish remover. Ketone bodies are nauseating and many patients will vomit, which may worsen the dehydration and potassium loss. The metabolic acidosis also has a negative inotropic effect on the heart and exacerbates peripheral vasodilatation. It may also cause respiratory depression and may contribute to insulin resistance.

Metabolic acidosis leads to the exit of intracellular potassium in exchange for hydrogen ions, resulting in hyperkalaemia. One of the actions of insulin is to promote transport of potassium into cells with glucose and therefore lack of insulin further exacerbates hyperkalaemia. Much of this potassium can be subsequently lost in vomit and urine. Thus, although serum potassium may be elevated, there is a severe whole-body deficiency in potassium. The alteration in potassium may lead to cardiac arrhythmias.

Diagnosis of diabetic ketoacidosis

The clinical features of diabetic ketoacidosis are similar to the presenting features of type 1 diabetes, and indeed some patients present with diabetic ketoacidosis. In general, however, they are more severe (Box 12.9).

In order to make the diagnosis the patients must have hyperglycaemia, ketosis and acidosis. Hyperglycaemia should be determined by a blood sample. Ketosis can be detected by measuring urinary ketones and metabolic acidosis should be determined by arterial blood gases. A low venous plasma bicarbonate concentration is further evidence of an acidosis. A common mistake is to describe a hyperglycaemic patient without ketoacidosis as having the diabetic ketoacidosis. These two situations

have different management strategies and therefore it is important to identify patients with diabetic ketoacidosis correctly. It is also important to measure serum electrolytes to look for hyperkalaemia and investigate the cause of the diabetic ketoacidosis.

Management of diabetic ketoacidosis

The treatment of diabetic ketoacidosis is a medical emergency and patients frequently require admission to an intensive care unit or high dependency ward. Treatment of diabetic ketoacidosis involves intravenous rehydration, the administration of insulin and correction of electrolytes, the most important of which is fluid replacement (Table 12.4). Most hospitals have produced guidelines for the management of diabetic ketoacidosis that may differ in detail from Table 12.4. However, the principles underlying the management remain the same.

Patients may have frequently lost up to 10 L, which should be replaced within the first 24 h without overloading the patient. Initially, isotonic saline should be used unless the patient had significant hypernatraemia, in which case hypotonic saline is appropriate. When the blood sugar falls to less than 10 to 15 mmol/L, 5% dextrose can be substituted to prevent hypoglycaemia. Patients are potassium deficient despite initial hyperkalaemia. As insulin is administered, potassium concentrations can fall precipitately and may cause a cardiac arrhythmia if uncorrected. It is therefore important to monitor serum potassium concentrations and replace potassium once the concentration has fallen below 5.0 mmol/L.

Insulin should be administered by continuous intravenous infusion at a rate of around 6 units/h until the blood glucose has fallen to less than 15 mmol/L. Thereafter, the rate can be adjusted to maintain normoglycaemia until the patient is eating again.

These measures will frequently correct the acidosis and sodium bicarbonate should only be used, with the supervision of a senior doctor, if there is persistent acidosis (pH ≤ 7.0) as bicarbonate administration may worsen intracellular acidosis. Sodium bicarbonate may also predispose to cerebral oedema, which is a further cause of death in patients with diabetic ketoacidosis. Repeat arterial blood gases can be used to monitor the resolution of the acidosis but plasma bicarbonate is usually suffi-

---

BOX 12.9 Clinical features of diabetic ketoacidosis

- Polyuria, nocturia
- Thirst
- Nausea and vomiting
- General malaise and weakness
- Cramps
- Kussmaul breathing
- Smells of ketones (pear drops or nail varnish remover)
- Altered conscious level
- Postural hypotension and dehydration

Table 12.4 Management of diabetic ketoacidosis

Fluid
Up to 10 L of fluid may be needed in the first 24 h
  1 L over 15–30 min
  1 L over the next hour
  1 L every 4–8 h depending on fluid deficit
Initially use isotonic (normal) saline unless the patient is significantly hypernatraemic in which case use hypotonic saline
Switch to 5% dextrose once the blood glucose has fallen to <10 mmol/L

Potassium replacement
On average 20 mmol/L KCl should be added to each litre of fluid depending on serum potassium concentration

Plasma potassium	Potassium added
<3.0 mmol/L	40 mmol/L
3–5 mmol/L	20 mmol/L
>5 mmol/L	none

Insulin
Insulin should be given by continuous intravenous infusion and titrated against the plasma glucose. Most hospitals have a
  protocol for the 'sliding scale' but here is a simple one that works:

Blood glucose	Insulin rate
>15 mmol/L	6 units per hour
5–15 mmol/L	3 units per hour
<5 mmol/L	0.5 units per hour
	NB insulin should not be stopped even if glucose is low

Acidosis
50 ml 8.4% bicarbonate should only be given if there is severe acidosis (pH < 7.0) despite adequate fluid replacement

Other measures
Search for the precipitating cause
Insert nasogatric tube in those with impaired conscious level
Consider CVP line especially the elderly or those with cardiac disease
Insert urinary catheter if no urine passed within 4 hours

> **BOX 12.10 Complications of diabetic ketoacidosis**
>
> - Cerebral oedema
> - Adult respiratory distress syndrome
> - Inhalation of vomit
> - Thromboembolism

cient and is less traumatic than repeated arterial punctures.

Cerebral oedema is frequently fatal and the mechanisms responsible for the development of cerebral oedema are unclear (Box 12.10). It is important to ensure that the fluid replacement matches the patient's losses as overaggressive fluid replacement may be one cause of cerebral oedema. If cerebral oedema occurs, intravenous mannitol and mechanical ventilation may be used.

While it is important to monitor fluid balance carefully, there is debate about the need for a urinary catheter. As patients are significantly dehydrated, it is unlikely that they will pass urine for several hours after the initiation of fluid replacement. It therefore seems reasonable to delay the insertion of a urinary catheter for 4 h. A central venous cannula may be required to monitor fluid balance in elderly patients or if cardiac disease is present.

A common cause of death in patients with diabetic ketoacidosis is inhalation of vomit. A nasogastric tube should be inserted if the conscious level is impaired. Adult respiratory distress syndrome occasionally occurs in diabetic ketoacidosis. Features include shortness of breath, central cyanosis and hypoxaemia and a chest radiograph will show bilateral infiltrates that resemble pulmonary oedema. The management involves intermittent positive pressure ventilation and the avoidance of fluid overload.

Thromboembolism is a further potentially fatal complication of diabetic ketoacidosis, which arises from dehydration, increased blood viscosity and coagulability. The place of prophylactic anticoagulation remains controversial and routine anticoagulation is not recommended. It is important to treat the precipitating cause.

Answers to case histories

Case history 12.1

The most likely diagnosis is Addison disease, which is associated with type 1 diabetes. Tiredness, lethargy and postural hypotension are all symptoms of hypoadrenalism. Corticosteroids are insulin antagonists and so the onset of Addison disease is frequently associated with increased hypoglycaemia and a reduction in insulin dose requirement. The increased skin pigmentation results from increased ACTH secretion. A short synacthen test is needed to confirm the diagnosis.

Case history 12.2

The twice-daily regimen is not flexible enough for his lifestyle and so it would be appropriate to discuss whether he would like to go onto a four-times daily insulin regimen. This would give more flexibility for the timing and quantity of food he can eat. A quick-acting analogue may be better for him as this needs to be given only 5 to 10 min before meals.

Case history 12.3

It is almost certain that this man became hypoglycaemic because the dose of insulin was increased inappropriately in hospital. When the patient is sedentary in bed, his insulin requirements will increase and so the dose required to obtain perfect blood control in hospital will almost certainly lead to hypoglycaemia on discharge once the man became more active again. This could have been prevented by reducing the dose back to his preadmission dose on discharge. We know he had good control prior to admission and so this dose was probably right for him.

Case history 12.4

The Diabetes Control and Complications Trial has shown that improved glycaemic control is often achieved at the expense of an increased frequency of severe 'hypos'. In order to regain 'hypo' awareness, it is important that this woman avoids 'hypos' to allow the usual autonomic symptoms to return. From a control perspective this is also important because 'hypos' are frequently followed by episodes of hyperglycaemia as the patient overtreats the 'hypo'. Frequent hypos are often accompanied by large swings in blood sugar. It is also important to inform the woman that she should not drive until her awareness returns. Indeed the licensing authorities may remove her license.

Case history 12.5

It is important to remember that the blood glucose readings have been determined by the previous insulin injection. Therefore as his breakfast readings are satisfactory, this suggests that his night time insulin dose is fine. On a four times a day (basal–bolus) regimen, getting the breakfast glucose right is the key. His readings are too low before lunch and so this implies he is taking too much soluble insulin before breakfast. Unless there are major problems, it is usual to adjust the insulin doses by about 10% and so it would be sensible for him to reduce his breakfast insulin dose to 9 units. His readings before his evening meal are too high suggesting he is taking too little soluble insulin before lunch. A 10% increase to 13–14 units would be appropriate. His prebed readings are fine and so no adjustment is needed to the supper insulin.

CHAPTER 13

13   Type 2 diabetes

LEARNING OBJECTIVES

- To discuss the epidemiology, aetiology and pathogenesis of type 2 diabetes
- To understand the clinical features of type 2 diabetes
- To discuss measures that might prevent, or at least delay, the onset of type 2 diabetes
- To understand the principles of oral hypoglycaemic therapy and their pitfalls

In this chapter we will learn about type 2 diabetes

Introduction

Type 2 diabetes is the commonest type of diabetes, affecting almost 200 million people worldwide. In this chapter we will examine what causes type 2 diabetes and why it is increasing at such an alarming rate. Although insulin can be used to treat type 2 diabetes, most patients are treated with diet alone or diet and oral hypoglycaemic drugs. Some of these have been used for over 50 years but we are currently at a time of much excitement with new drugs just round the corner.

What is type 2 diabetes?

Type 2 diabetes is a heterogeneous disorder that results from an interaction between a genetic predisposition and environmental factors and leads to the combination of insulin deficiency and insulin resistance (Fig. 13.1).

Epidemiology of type 2 diabetes

Type 2 diabetes accounts for around 90% of all cases of diabetes in Western Europe. There are approximately 1.6 million people with diagnosed type 2 diabetes in the UK, with a further 750,000 having undiagnosed type 2 diabetes. The prevalence of diabetes is increasing rapidly. The World Health Organization (WHO) has predicted that, by 2030, the number of adults with diabetes will have more than doubled worldwide, from 177 million in 2000 to 370 million. The incidence of type 2 diabetes increases with age, with most cases being diagnosed after the age of 40 years. This equates to a lifetime risk of developing diabetes of 1 in 10. The demographics of

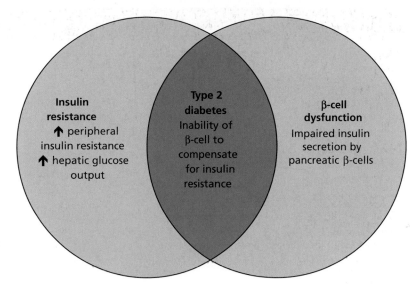

Figure 13.1 What is type 2 diabetes? The two main pathological components of type 2 diabetes are insulin resistance and β-cell dysfunction and failure.

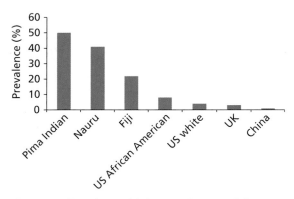

Figure 13.2 Prevalence of diabetes and impaired glucose tolerance in selected populations in the age range of 30–64 years.

Table 13.1 Risk factors for type 2 diabetes

Unmodifiable risk factors	Environmental risk factors
Family history	Obesity
Birth weight	Physical inactivity
Ethnicity	Diet
Age	
Past history of in pregnancy diabetes (gestational diabetes)	
Severe mental illness	

type 2 diabetes are changing, and it is now becoming increasingly common in children and young adults. In certain parts of the United States, the number of new cases of type 2 diabetes among teenagers is the same as for type 1 diabetes.

A marked geographical variation in the prevalence of type 2 diabetes exists (Fig. 13.2). The highest rates of diabetes are found in the Pima Indians of Arizona and in the South Pacific Island of Nauru, where approximately 50% of the adult population has diabetes. In contrast, in the rural communities of China and Chile, the prevalence is less than 1%. In general,

rates of type 2 diabetes are higher in urban populations than rural communities.

Regional and ethnic differences in the prevalence of type 2 diabetes reflect not only differences in environment, but also differences in genetic susceptibility. For example, people from the Indian subcontinent living in Southall have a rate of diabetes which is four times higher than the local Caucasian population.

Aetiology of type 2 diabetes

The risk factors for type 2 diabetes can be divided into those which are unmodifiable and those which are environmental and therefore potentially changeable (Table 13.1).

Genetic predisposition

The heritability of type 2 diabetes is greater than for type 1 diabetes, and is estimated to account for 40 to 80% of total disease susceptibility (Table 13.2). Many patients will have a family history of diabetes, and twin studies show a high concordance rate (60–90%) in monozygotic twins. A maternal history of diabetes confers a higher risk of type 2 diabetes in the offspring than a paternal history of diabetes, possibly through an effect of maternal hyperglycaemia during pregnancy. This may alter the intrauterine environment, which may affect the risk of diabetes. This is discussed further below.

Type 2 diabetes is a polygenic disorder, and it is clear that no single major locus explains its inheritance. There appear to be many candidate genes involved in controlling insulin secretion and action, and these may all play a role in the development of type 2 diabetes.

Approximately 2 to 5% of cases of 'type 2 diabetes' are caused by single gene mutations, such as maturity onset diabetes of the young (MODY). MODY is inherited as an autosomal dominant condition and is caused, in most cases, by a mutation in one of six genes, most commonly HNF1α (Table 13.3 and review Chapter 2).

Environmental factors

The most important environmental risk factors for diabetes are obesity and physical inactivity. The massive explosion in obesity rates worldwide has been largely responsible for the increase in diabetes, and it is estimated that up to 80% of all new cases of diabetes can be attributed to obesity. In the UK, the aver-

Table 13.2 Risk of developing type 2 diabetes for UK relatives of diabetic subjects

Family member	Risk (%)
Monozygotic twin	90
Dizygotic twin	10
Sibling	10
Mother	15–20
Father	15
Both parents	75
General population	3

age body mass index (BMI) of a person with type 2 diabetes is 30.0 kg/m², while in the US, 67% of those with type 2 diabetes have a BMI of more than 27 kg/m², and 46% have a BMI of more than 30 kg/m². The risk of developing type 2 diabetes increases across the normal range of BMI, such that the risk in a middle-aged woman whose BMI is more than 35 kg/m² is 93.2 times greater than in a woman whose BMI is <22.5 kg/m² (Fig. 13.3). In addition to total

Table 13.3 Genetic mutations in MODY

Defective protein	MODY type
Glucokinase	2
Hepatic nuclear factor 1α (also known as transcription factor 1)	3
Hepatic nuclear factor 4α	1
Hepatic nuclear factor 1β (also known as transcription factor 2)	5
Insulin promoter factor-1 (also known as pancreatic duoderum homeobox gene 1)	4
Neurogenic differentiation-1/β2	6

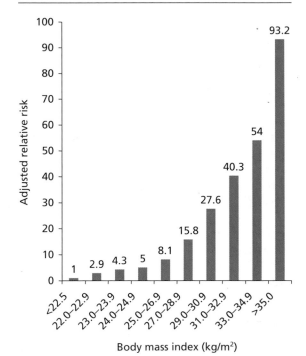

Figure 13.3 Risk of developing diabetes according to body mass index in 114 281 women, US Nurses Health Study. Adapted from Colditz *et al. Ann. Intern. Med.*, 1995, **122**, 481–6.

adiposity, the distribution of fat is also important. For any given level of obesity, the more visceral fat an individual has, the greater their risk of developing diabetes. The importance of obesity is discussed further in Chapter 15.

Physical inactivity is also associated with an increased risk of diabetes. Exercising for around 30 min per day will halve the risk of developing diabetes compared with a sedentary lifestyle. Although some of the difference can be explained by differences in adiposity, around half of this effect can be attributed to exercise patterns.

The intrauterine environment is also considered to be important in the development of type 2 diabetes. Low birth weight and thinness at birth are associated with increasing insulin resistance and diabetes. In contrast to this general observation, it appears that babies born to mothers with diabates are also at increased risk of diabetes, despite the fact that these babies often have a high birth weight. Consequently, the relationship between birth weight and subsequent risk of diabetes is J-shaped.

As diabetes is more common in the elderly, the changing world demographics, with its ageing population, adds a further explanation of the increase in prevalence of diabetes.

Pathogenesis of type 2 diabetes

Under normal physiological conditions, plasma glucose concentrations are maintained within a narrow range, despite wide fluctuations in supply and demand, through a tightly regulated and dynamic interaction between tissue sensitivity to insulin (especially in the liver) and insulin secretion. In type 2 diabetes, these mechanisms break down and, therefore, the two main pathophysiological defects in type 2 diabetes are impaired insulin secretion through a dysfunction of the pancreatic β-cell and impaired insulin action through insulin resistance (Box 13.1).

Insulin resistance

Insulin resistance is defined is an inability of insulin to produce its usual biological effects at physiological concentrations and is a cardinal feature of type 2 diabetes. It is characterized by the impaired ability of insulin to inhibit hepatic glucose output and to stim-

---

BOX 13.1

What is insulin sensitivity?
Insulin sensitivity is the effect of insulin at any given concentration and can be measured in a number of ways to provide a dose–response curve.

What is insulin responsiveness?
Insulin responsiveness refers to the ability of insulin to exert a maximal response. In the situation of reduced insulin responsiveness there is a lower-than-normal maximal response.

What is insulin resistance?
Insulin resistance may be defined as existing when normal insulin concentrations fail to produce a normal biological response. This would lead to a rightward shift of the insulin-response curve.

BOX 13.2 Consequences of insulin resistance

- Skeletal muscle
  — reduced glucose uptake into skeletal muscle
- Adipose tissue
  — failure to suppress lipolysis in adipose tissue leading to increased circulation of nonesterified fatty acids (NEFA)
- Liver
  — reduced ability to inhibit hepatic glucose output
  — increased NEFA stimulates gluconeogenesis and glucose production, and triglyceride synthesis
- Vasculature
  — impaired endothelial function
  — increased stiffness of arteries
  — procoagulation
- Increased sympathetic tone
  — through an action of insulin on the hypothalamus
- Hyperuricaemia
  — insulin reduces renal uric acid clearance and this action is preserved

---

ulate glucose uptake into skeletal muscle. Insulin also fails to suppress lipolysis in adipose tissue (Box 13.2).

The mechanisms leading to the development of

insulin resistance are not fully understood but may occur at many levels of insulin signalling (Box 13.3). It would appear that in type 2 diabetes, most insulin resistance is caused by defects in postreceptor signalling (review Fig. 3.6).

β-cell dysfunction

Insulin resistance does not explain the whole story because patients with type 2 diabetes are no more insulin resistant than the most insulin resistant quartile of the general population. Indeed, only around 20% of those with this degree of insulin resistance develop diabetes. Abnormalities in β-cell function are found early in the natural history of type 2 diabetes and in first-degree relatives of subjects with type 2 diabetes, suggesting that they are an integral component of the pathogenesis of type 2 diabetes.

Insulin is secreted in a characteristic biphasic pattern in response to glucose: an acute first phase lasting a few minutes followed by a sustained second phase. The major β-cell abnormalities in type 2 diabetes are a marked reduction in first-phase insulin secretion and, in established diabetes, an attenuated second phase (Fig. 13.4).

BOX 13.3 Potential mechanisms of insulin resistance

- Absent or reduced number of insulin receptors
  - high circulating insulin concentrations suppress the number of hormone receptors present on cell surface, so called 'down regulation'
- Abnormal insulin receptor
  - failure of insulin to bind to insulin receptor
  - failure of insulin binding to activate insulin receptor—no autophosphorylation, no activation of tyrosine kinase
- Postreceptor signalling
  - down-regulation, deficiencies or genetic polymorphisms of postreceptor signalling molecules such as tyrosine phosphorylation of the insulin receptor, IRS proteins or PI-3 kinase
- Abnormalities of GLUT 4 translocation and function
- Accumulation of skeletal muscle triglyceride—so called 'lipotoxicity'

IRS, insulin receptor substrate; PI-3, phosphatidylinositol-3.

By the time of diagnosis, mean β-cell function is already less than 50%, and a further deterioration of β-cell function of around 4% per year is seen after the diagnosis. Extrapolation of the observed rate of β-cell decline suggests that the loss of β-cell function begins at least a decade prior to the diagnosis. This progressive loss of β-cell function explains why patients require escalations in the number and doses of oral hypoglycaemic agents with time, and why eventually they become refractory to the oral treatments and require insulin.

The mechanisms underlying the β-cell dysfunction remain unclear and are likely to be multifactorial (Table 13.4). As well as genetic factors, a number of environmental factors, including early-life malnutrition, obesity, and hyperglycaemia and hyperlipidaemia, may all accelerate the decline in β-cell function.

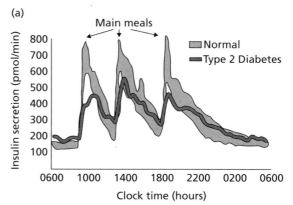

(a)

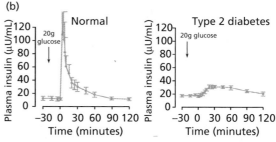

(b)

Figure 13.4 (a) Insulin secretion of people with type 2 diabetes throughout a 24-hour period compared with normal insulin secretion. Redrawn from O'Meara et al. Am. J. Med. 1990, **89**, 11S–16S. (b) Loss of early-phase insulin release in type 2 diabetes. The first abnormality in insulin secretion seen in type 2 diabetes is a loss of early-phase insulin release. This is compensated by an exaggerated second-phase response which can cause hypoglycaemia 3 to 4 hours after a meal. With time, second-phase insulin secretion is lost too. Redrawn from Ward WK et al. Diabetes Care 1984, **7**, 491–502.

Table 13.4 Possible mechanisms of β-cell dysfunction

Innate	Acquired
Genetics	Glucose toxicity
In utero malnutrition	Lipotoxicity
	Obesity
	Hormonal
	Inadequate incretin stimulation
	Increased glucagon secretion

Incretins are hormones released by the gut in response to food ingestion that augment insulin release and include GLP-1 and GIP. New drugs for the treatment of type 2 diabetes that mimic these hormones have recently been licensed for treatment of type 2 diabetes.

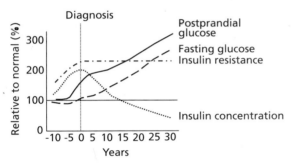

Figure 13.5 Natural history of insulin resistance and insulin secretion in type 2 diabetes. As insulin sensitivity falls, the β-cell responds by increasing insulin secretion to compensate and to maintain glucose concentrations within the normal range. The maximal insulin secretory capacity is eventually reached and, beyond that point, insulin secretion declines. The blood glucose concentrations rise, initially in the postprandial period, as the individual develops impaired glucose tolerance before the onset of frank diabetes.

There has been much discussion about the relative roles of insulin resistance and β-cell function in the natural history of diabetes, since both components occur early in the disease process. One model for the development of diabetes is as follows (Fig. 13.5). As insulin sensitivity falls, the β-cell responds by increasing insulin secretion to compensate and to maintain glucose concentrations within the normal range. The maximal insulin secretory capacity is eventually reached and, beyond that point, insulin secretion declines. The blood glucose concentrations rise, initially in the postprandial period, as the individual develops impaired glucose tolerance before the onset of frank diabetes.

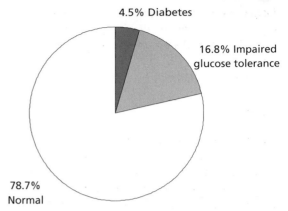

Figure 13.6 Prevalence of undiagnosed glucose intolerance from the Isle of Ely Diabetes Project. In the Isle of Ely project, 1122 people aged 40–65 years without known diabetes, from one general practice, underwent a standard 75 g oral glucose tolerance test and were classified according to WHO criteria. Williams *et al. Diabet. Med.*, 1995, **12**, 30–5.

This process may, however, be reversible. Although around 2 to 5% of individuals with impaired glucose tolerance will progress to diabetes each year, many revert to normal. Intensive lifestyle intervention at this stage can reduce incident diabetes and so people falling into these categories should be managed actively with advice about their diet and exercise.

Prognosis

Type 2 diabetes is also associated with premature mortality, predominantly through cardiovascular disease. Approximately one in 17 of the general population will die as a result of type 2 diabetes. Cardiovascular complications are discussed in Chapter 15.

Clinical features of type 2 diabetes

Type 2 diabetes has a gradual and insidious onset, with nearly one-third of cases being identified as an incidental finding or on the coronary care unit, when an asymptomatic individual suffers a myocardial infarction. The diagnosis is often delayed, and some degree of hyperglycaemia may have been present for more than 20 years before the diagnosis is confirmed. This accounts for the 750,000 people with undiagnosed diabetes in the UK (Fig. 13.6).

Around 50% of patients with type 2 diabetes are diagnosed as a result of the typical diabetic symptoms of polyuria, nocturia, thirst, tiredness and blurred vision; a further 16% of patients are diagnosed after presenting with an infection.

Hyperosmolar nonketotic coma

Hyperosmolar nonketotic coma (HONK) is a medical emergency and is characterized by the hyperglycaemia, dehydration and uraemia without significant ketosis or acidosis. It occurs in middle-aged or elderly patients with type 2 diabetes and may be the presenting feature in around 25% of individuals. Afro-Caribbean individuals appear to be at a higher risk of developing HONK (Box 13.4).

HONK may be complicated by thromboembolism or rhabdomyolysis and carries a mortality rate of approximately 15%. The management is similar to the treatment of diabetic ketoacidosis, with fluid and electrolyte replacement and intravenous insulin (Table 12.4). Following correction of the HONK, patients may only require treatment with lifestyle modification.

Prevention of diabetes

One of the most exciting areas in diabetes at present is the possibility that type 2 diabetes can be prevented or at least delayed by both lifestyle and pharmacological interventions (Case history 13.1).

Lifestyle intervention aimed at reducing weight, the amount of fat, in particular saturated fat, in the diet while increasing the amount of dietary fibre and exercise have been shown to reduce diabetes by a half over a 3-year period. Public health policies are therefore urgently required that will encourage people to follow a healthy lifestyle and prevent the development of impaired glucose tolerance and diabetes. Primary prevention strategies should target individuals at especially high risk of developing type 2 diabetes, including those with prediabetes, first-degree relatives of people with type 2 diabetes, women with a history of gestational diabetes, individuals with

---

BOX 13.4 Precipitating causes of hyperosmolar nonketotic coma

- Infection
- Myocardial infarction
- Drugs
  - Diuretics
  - Steroids
  - Omission of oral hypoglycaemic drugs

BOX 13.5 Measures to reduce the incidence of diabetes

- Lifestyle
  - ↓ weight by 5% (ideally to BMI <25)
  - ↓ fat intake to <30% of energy intake
  - ↓ saturated fat to <10% of energy intake
  - ↑ fibre to >15 g/1000 g
  - take at least 30 min/day of aerobic and muscle strengthening exercise
- Pharmacological
  - merformin
  - orlistat (intestinal lipase inhibitor)
  - acarbose (α-glucosidase inhibitor)
  - troglitazone (thiazolidinedione)
  - ?blockade of the renin–angiotensin system— ACE inhibitors, angiotensin receptor blockers

These drugs will be considered in greater detail below. Randomized clinical trials have shown that the first four drugs can reduce diabetes but with a lesser effect than lifestyle intervention. Post-hoc analysis suggested that blockade of the renin–angiotensin system may reduce diabetes. Troglitazone has been withdrawn from the market but trials of other thiazolidinediones are currently underways.

CASE HISTORY 13.1

A 35-year-old woman developed gestational diabetes which required treatment with insulin during her third pregnancy. She has a strong family history of diabetes and was significantly overweight (BMI 28.2 kg/m²) prior to her pregnancy.

What advice and treatment will you offer her?

Answers, see p. 233

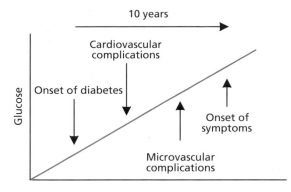

Figure 13.7 The imperative for screening. It is estimated that many patients have diabetes for up to a decade before the onset of overt symptoms. However, diabetic complications can progress in asymptomatic individuals. For example, approximately 20% of people with newly diagnosed diabetes have retinopathy at presentation and diabetes is frequently diagnosed following a myocardial infarction.

other features of the metabolic syndrome (Box 14.12) and those with severe mental illnesses.

In addition to lifestyle intervention, several drugs have been shown to reduce diabetes (Box 13.5).

Screening for diabetes

The high prevalence of undiagnosed diabetes and the proportion of patients with evidence of complications at diagnosis create a strong imperative for screening (Fig. 13.7). Many possible screening methods have been shown to be feasible, acceptable and accurate, but there is still debate about *whom* to screen.

Universal screening for diabetes is currently impractical because of the burden that would be placed upon general practice but there is justification for screening of high-risk groups in whom undiagnosed diabetes is prevalent (Box 13.6).

Although the oral glucose tolerance test is relatively simple and inexpensive, and is the gold standard test for diabetes, it is not suitable for routine screening. A fasting plasma glucose has been endorsed by the WHO, American Diabetes Association and Diabetes UK as a suitable test for screening. This test is more convenient than the oral glucose tolerance test but lacks sensitivity and may miss a large number of individuals with diabetes (Table 13.5).

BOX 13.6   Groups who should be screened for diabetes within targeted populations

(a) White people aged over 40 years and people from Black, Asian and minority ethnic groups aged over 25 with one or more of the risk factors below:
  — a first degree family history of diabetes and/or
  — who are overweight/obese/morbidly obese with a BMI of 25–30 kg/m^2 and above, and who have a sedentary lifestyle* and/or
  — waist measurement of over ≥ 94 cm for White and Black men and ≥ 80 cm for White, Black and Asian women, and ≥ 90 cm for Asian men
(b) People who have ischaemic heart disease, cerebrovascular disease, peripheral vascular disease or treated hypertension
(c) Women with a past history of gestational diabetes
(d) Women with polycystic ovary syndrome who have a BMI ≥ 30 kg/m^2
(e) People who are known to have impaired glucose tolerance or impaired fasting glycaemia
(f) People who have severe mental health problems
(g) People who have hypertriglyceridemia not due to alcohol excess or renal disease

The more risk factors that a person has the more likelihood of being at risk of diabetes, however just being over 40 years if White or 25 years if Black, Asian or of ethnic origin is not necessarily a risk factor in itself.

Reference: Diabetes UK 2006

*Though more accurate than body weight alone, BMI may overestimate body fat in people who are very muscular or understimate fat mass in those who have lost muscle mass

---

Table 13.5 Comparison of screening tests for diabetes

Test	Specificity (%)	Sensitivity (%)
Fasting plasma glucose	84–99	40–95
Random plasma glucose	92–98	50–69
HbA$_{1c}$	79–100	35–98

Specificity: the probability that the screening test is negative if the person does not have diabetes. This is also known as true negative rate.
Sensitivity: the probability that the screening test is positive if the person has diabetes. This is also known as the true positive rate.

Although a random plasma glucose measurement may be unreliable, it does have certain merits. It is easy to perform and has reasonable sensitivity and specificity. The value of a glycosylated haemoglobin as a screening test is unproven and therefore not recommended. However, when combined with a fasting or random glucose, it may improve the sensitivity and specificity of the test.

It is important that structured screening programmes, especially in high-risk groups, are established to ensure that the burden of undiagnosed diabetes is reduced. As the management of diabetes is increasingly becoming part of primary care, screening for diabetes should be undertaken within community practice, where possible. Many primary healthcare services are overstretched and other settings may be required; for example, an increasing number of pharmacists are also offering local screening services is based upon a random blood test.

Management of type 2 diabetes

The aims of management of type 2 diabetes are identical to those of type 1 diabetes.
- Save life
- Alleviate symptoms
- Achieve good control to minimize long-term complications
- Avoid iatrogenic side-effects such as hypoglycaemia

There are additional challenges for patients with type 2 diabetes. Many are asymptomatic and may be reluctant to start lifestyle change and drug therapy without obvious immediate benefit. Nevertheless, improvements in glycaemic control are associated with a reduction in microvascular complications and therefore a major challenge for health-care professionals is to educate patients about the long-term morbidity and mortality associated with type 2 diabetes, with the aim of motivating patients to make the appropriate management steps.

Type 2 diabetes is treated in a step-wise approach, starting with lifestyle modification by dietary manipulation and increasing daily physical activity, which is the cornerstone of management. If adequate control is not obtained, then oral hypoglycaemic agents are required, initially alone but subsequently in combination. Finally, insulin therapy with or without oral therapy is needed (Fig. 13.16).

Diet

The principles of the dietary changes that need to be adopted by a patient with type 2 diabetes are identical to those with type 1 diabetes and have been outlined in Chapter 12. In brief, patients should reduce the amount of refined sugar and fat while increasing the proportion of complex carbohydrate and fibre. Many patients with type 2 diabetes are also overweight or obese and therefore the diet should have a moderate calorie deficit to allow the patient to lose weight (Case history 13.2). The management of obesity is covered in greater detail in Chapter 15.

Exercise

Patients should be encouraged to exercise for at least

> **BOX 13.7 Benefits of exercise**
> - Improved insulin sensitivity with or without weight loss
> - Reduced blood glucose
> - Reduced blood pressure
> - Improved lipid profile
> - Increased longevity

CASE HISTORY 13.2

A 56-year-old office manager presented with thirst, polyuria and tiredness. He admits to consuming large quantities of carbonated cola drink. He weighs 90 kg. His fasting blood glucose is 10.0 mmol/L and postprandial glucose is 25.6 mmol/L.

How would you manage him?
Would you consider drug therapy at this time?

Answers, see p. 233

30 min a day to improve their glycaemic control and reduce their cardiovascular risk (Box 13.7). Both aerobic and strength training are beneficial and the best exercise for the patient is the one that they will still be undertaking many years from the diagnosis. Exercise is not equivalent to sport and practical advice, such as suggesting patients walk more by alighting the bus one stop early on journeys to and from work or use stairs rather than lifts, are helpful.

Care should be used when advising patients with peripheral neuropathy. It is important to ensure that they wear natural fibres and well fitting sports shoes to reduce the risk of foot ulceration.

Oral hypoglycaemic agents

When diet and exercise fail to maintain normoglycaemia, oral hypoglycaemic agents are required in addition to, not instead of, lifestyle management. The oral hypoglycaemic agents require some residual insulin secretory capacity to be effective and therefore are ineffective alone in patients with type 1 diabetes. There are three categories of oral agents (Fig. 13.8):

- Insulin secretagogues
- Insulin sensitizers
- Inhibitors of glucose absorption from the gastrointestinal tract

Drugs from different categories can be combined as the blood glucose concentrations increase with the progressive loss of β-cell function.

Insulin secretagogues

Insulin secretagogues, such as sulphonylureas and meglitinides, stimulate insulin release from the pancreas. The properties of ideal insulin secretagogues are as follows:

- Rapid restoration of early-phase insulin release to reduce postprandial glucose excursions
- Plasma insulin should be returned to preprandial levels as soon as possible to prevent between-meal hypoglycaemia

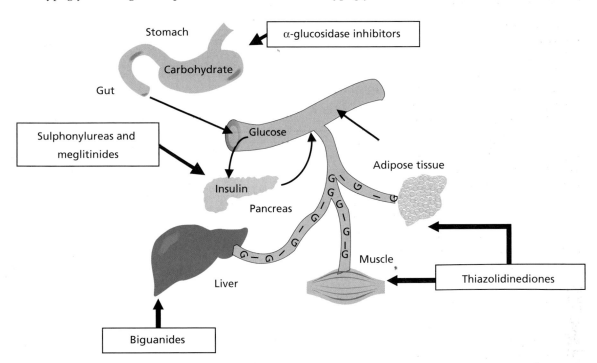

Figure 13.8 Primary sites of action of oral antidiabetic agents. Different antidiabetic agents target distinct sites as part of their primary mechanism of action in reducing hyperglycaemia. Sulphonylureas and meglitinides stimulate insulin release from the pancreas. Biguanides, such as metformin, primarily suppress hepatic glucose output. α-glucosidase inhibitors (acarbose) delay digestion and absorption of carbohydrates in the gastrointestinal tract. Thiazolidinediones decrease insulin resistance in adipose tissue, skeletal muscle and liver.

- Suitable for use in combination with a treatment for insulin resistance

Sulphonylureas

The hypoglycaemic effects of sulphonamide antibiotics were first recognized during a typhoid epidemic at the beginning of the 20th century. Following this observation, sulphonylureas were developed to treat diabetes (Table 13.6).

Mechanism of action. Sulphonylureas act mainly by increasing the release of insulin from the pancreatic β-cells in response to stimulation by glucose (Fig. 11.8). Following binding to the sulphonylurea receptor, there is a closure of the K^+ ATP channel in the cell membrane which leads to a rise in intracellular calcium and insulin release. The *in vivo* potency of sulphonylureas approximates to their potency to inhibit the K^+ ATP channel *in vitro*. Although there is individual variability, sulphonylureas will lead to a reduction in HbA_{1c} of approximately 1.5 to 2.0%.

Side-effects. The commonest side-effect of sulphonylureas is weight gain (Box 13.8). When a patient has poorly controlled diabetes, energy expenditure increases through glycosuria and an increase in basal metabolic rate. As glycaemic control improves, energy expenditure decreases with the reduction in glycosuria and basal metabolic rate. Unless the patient increases voluntary energy expenditure or reduces caloric intake, weight gain is inevitable. This weight gain may occur with any hypoglycaemic agent but appears to be particularly marked with sulphonylureas, thiazolidinediones and insulin. The weight gain with sulphonylureas and insulin may result from hyperinsulinaemia between meals. Patients may increase their food intake to prevent hypoglycaemia at this time.

The second major side-effect of sulphonylureas is hypoglycaemia, which occurs at a rate of 0.2 episodes per 1000 patients per year. The action of the drugs prevents the normal physiological reduction in insulin secretion when blood glucose concentrations

---

BOX 13.8 Side-effects of oral hypoglycaemic agents

- Sulphonylurea
  - weight gain
  - hypoglycaemia
  - hyponatraemia
  - alcohol flushing (chlorpropamide)
  - ?worsening of myocardial ischaemia
  - ?acceleration of β-cell loss
- Metiglinides
  - weight gain
  - hypoglycaemia
- Metformin
  - gastrointestinal upset
  - lactic acidosis
- Thiazolidinedione
  - weight gain
  - oedema
  - cardiac failure
  - hepatotoxicity (troglitazone)
- Acarbose
  - gastrointestinal upset

Table 13.6 Properties of different sulphonylureas

Drug	Half-life	Duration of action	Route of elimination	Active metabolite
1st generation				
Acetohexamide	Medium	Medium	Hepatic	+
Chlorpropamide	Very long	Very long	Hepatic and Renal	+
Tolazide	Short	Medium	Hepatic	+
2nd generation				
Tolbutamide	Short	Short/medium	Hepatic	
Glibenclamide	Very short	Long	Hepatic	?
Gliclazide	Medium	Medium	Hepatic	
Glipizide	Very short	Short/medium	Hepatic	
Gliquidone	Long	Long	Hepatic	+
Glimepiride	Short	Medium/long	Hepatic	

fall. Patients with severe hypoglycaemia on sulphonylureas need admission to hospital for observation
and glucose support for up to 48h until the drug has
cleared from the circulation. Hypoglycaemia is a particular worry in the elderly when the clearance of the
drugs is reduced and in whom the signs of hypoglycaemia may be masked. It may also occur in renal failure or during intercurrent infection.

Some of the older sulphonylureas, such as chlorpropamide, are associated with hyponatraemia because they increase the sensitivity of the distal tubule
to antidiuretic hormone.

There is concern that the sulphonylureas may
worsen cardiovascular events in patients with type 2
diabetes. Potassium channels exist within cardiac
myocytes and are the target of the antianginal drug
nicorandil. Some of the more modern sulphonylureas have lower affinity for the cardiac potassium
channels and therefore may be less of a worry.

There is also concern that the sulphonylureas may
hasten β-cell loss by increasing the work rate in an already 'exhausted cell' thereby achieving short-term
control at the expense of worsening long-term control.

Meglitinides or postprandial regulators
There are two drugs in the postprandial regulator
class: nateglinide and repaglinide (Fig. 13.9).
Repaglinide is the nonsulphonylurea component of
glibenclamide while nateglinide is derived from
D-phenylalanine.

Mechanism of action. They also stimulate insulin release by closing the K⁺ ATP channel, but they bind to
a different, but closely related, site on the β-cell from
sulphonylureas. They are designed to restore the
early phase postprandial insulin response to glucose
without prolonged stimulation during subsequent
periods of fasting. The glycaemic control achieved
with the meglitinides is generally less than that with
other oral hypoglycaemic drugs and so the place of
meglitinides in therapy compared to sulphonylureas
is not yet established.

Side-effects. Hypoglycaemia may occur but less than
with sulphonylureas because of the short duration of
action. There is less weight gain because of the reduced need to snack between meals.

Insulin sensitizers
These drugs have no effect on insulin secretion but

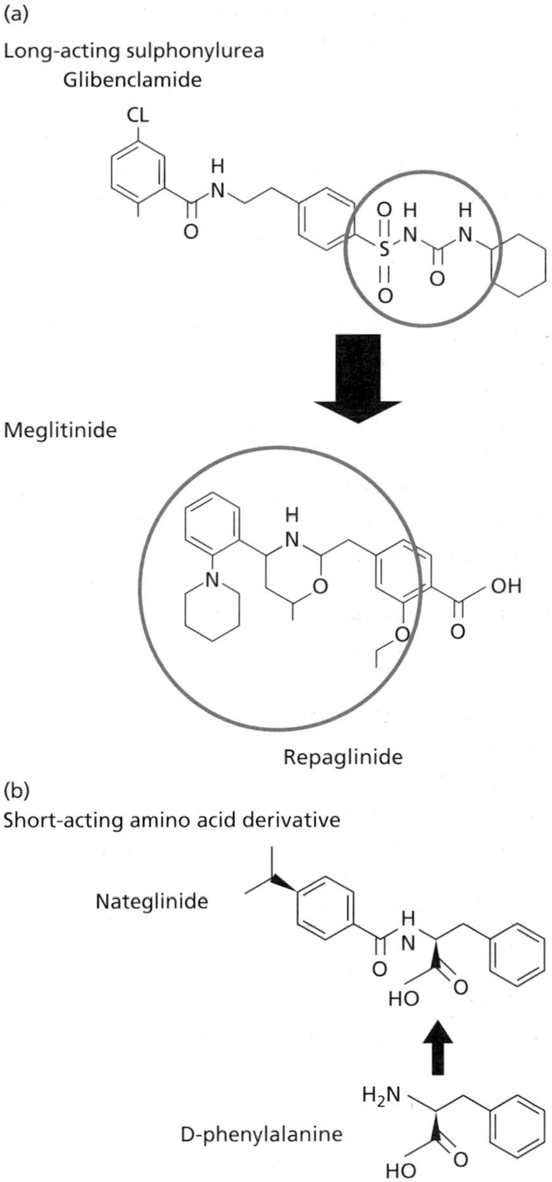

Figure 13.9 The development of the postprandial
regulators. (a) Repaglinide. (b) Nateglinide. Repaglinide is
derived from longer acting sulphonylureas while
nateglinide is derived from the amino acid D-phenylalanine.

improve the effectiveness of the insulin that is present within the circulation.

Biguanides
The biguanide are derived from guanidine and
the only one currently available is metformin (Fig.
13.10). Although this drug has been available for

many years its mode of action is still not fully understood. Its major actions are:

- To increase glucose uptake in skeletal muscle and adipocytes
- To suppress hepatic gluconeogenesis
- To reduce glucose absorption from the small intestine at high concentrations of metformin

Recent work suggests that metformin acts through the stimulation of AMP kinase, which is an intracellular energy sensor that is usually stimulated during exercise or hypoxia. Stimulation of AMP kinase leads to activation of glucose transporters and facilitates substrate uptake into the cell. Metformin may also suppress appetite and help achieve weight loss, which is useful in patients who are overweight.

Metformin may be used in combination with either sulphonylureas or insulin and is associated with a reduction in HbA1c of around 1.5 to 2%. As well as its effect on glycaemic control, unlike sulphonylureas and insulin, metformin appears to have a cardioprotective effect. The UK Prospective Diabetes Study has shown that metformin is associated with reduced cardiovascular mortality and morbidity.

Side-effects. The use of metformin is limited by the high prevalence of gastrointestinal side-effects including anorexia, nausea, abdominal discomfort and diarrhoea. The side-effects can be reduced by starting the metformin at a low dose and gradually increasing the dose until a therapeutic effect as achieved. A slow release preparation of metformin has recently been released and this appears to be better tolerated.

The most worrying side-effect of metformin is potentially fatal lactic acidosis. The use of metformin is associated with an increase in lactate production because of inhibition of pyruvate metabolism. In situations where there is impaired clearance of lactate or an increase in anaerobic metabolism, such as shock, lactic acidosis can result. The use of metformin is therefore contraindicated in renal impairment, cardiac failure and hepatic failure.

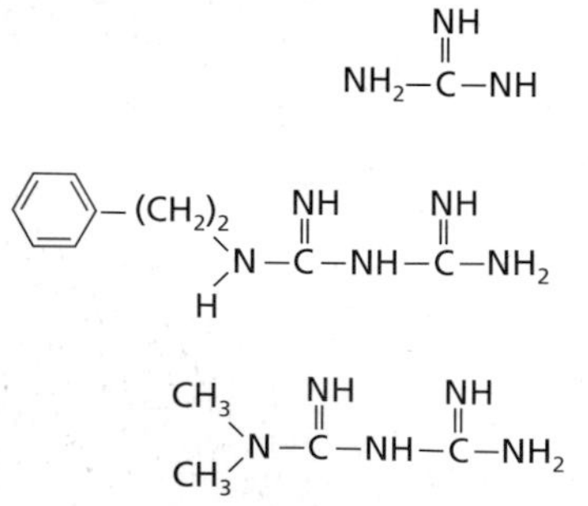

Thiazolidinediones or 'glitazones'

Thiazolidinediones have only recently been available for clinical use and include pioglitazone and rosiglitazone (Fig. 13.11).

Mechanism of action. Thiazolidinediones bind to the nuclear hormone receptor peroxisome proliferator-activated receptor-gamma (PPARγ) in the cell nucleus (Fig. 13.12). This receptor is part of a larger family of nuclear hormone receptors and, at present, its natural ligand is unknown, although fatty acids will bind PPARγ with a low affinity. After binding to the thiazolidinedione, PPARγ then associates as a heterodimer with the retinoid X receptor (RXR) in the cell nucleus, similar to the thyroid hormone receptor, (Fig. 3.20) and binds to PPARγ response elements in the promoter domains of insulin target genes (Fig. 13.13).

PPARγ receptors are particularly abundant in adipose tissue and it is thought that adipose tissue is the major site of action of these drugs. Thiazolidinediones enhance glucose and fatty acid uptake and utilization in adipocytes. They also induce differentiation of preadipocytes and reduce the secretion of a number of cytokines by fat that inhibit insulin action. Reduced availability of fatty acids to muscle improves insulin sensitivity in muscle cells through the Randle cycle (Box 13.9). The thiazolidinediones finally reduce hepatic glucose output (Fig. 13.14).

As the effect on blood glucose is indirect, it may take up to 3 months to reach a maximal effect. The magnitude of the effect on blood glucose is similar to that seen with metformin and sulphonylureas. In addition to reducing the plasma glucose concentration, thiazolidinediones also improve diabetic dyslipidaemia. Pioglitazone, in particular, decreases plasma triglyceride and increases plasma HDL cholesterol concentrations through increased lipolysis of triglycerides in VLDL. The plasma LDL fraction may also become larger and less dense and therefore less atherogenic. This action may be important in

Figure 13.10 Structure of guanidine, phenformin (phenethylbiguanide), and metformin (dimethylbiguanide).

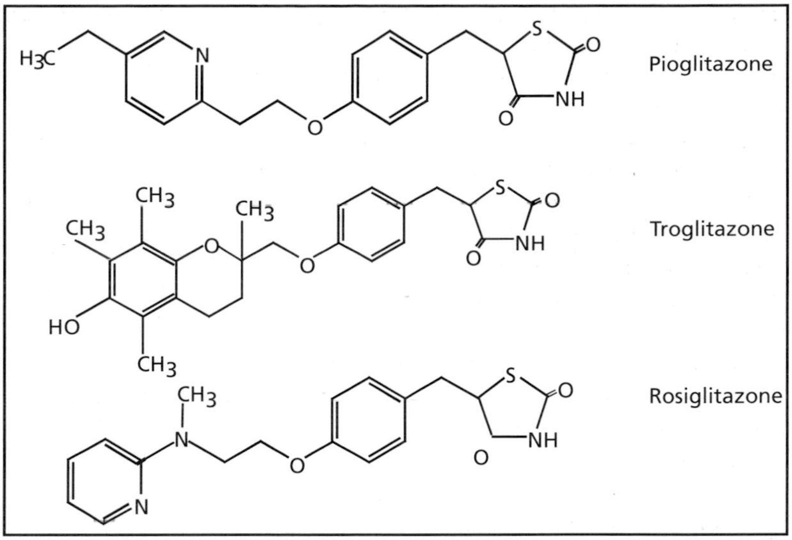

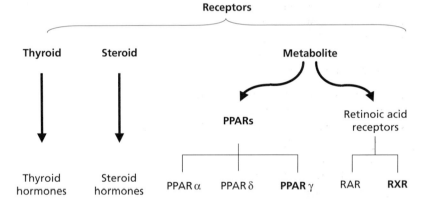

Figure 13.11 Structure of thiazolidinediones. Troglitazone was withdrawn from the market because of hepatotoxicity.

Figure 13.12 Ligand-activated nuclear hormone receptors—an expanding family. Thiazolidinediones bind to PPARγ receptors. These are metabolite nuclear hormone receptors for which the natural ligand is unclear. They fall into the same category of hormone receptors as thyroid and steroid hormone receptors. PPARγ, peroxisome proliferator-activated receptor; RXR, retinoid X receptor; RAR, retinoid acid receptor α.

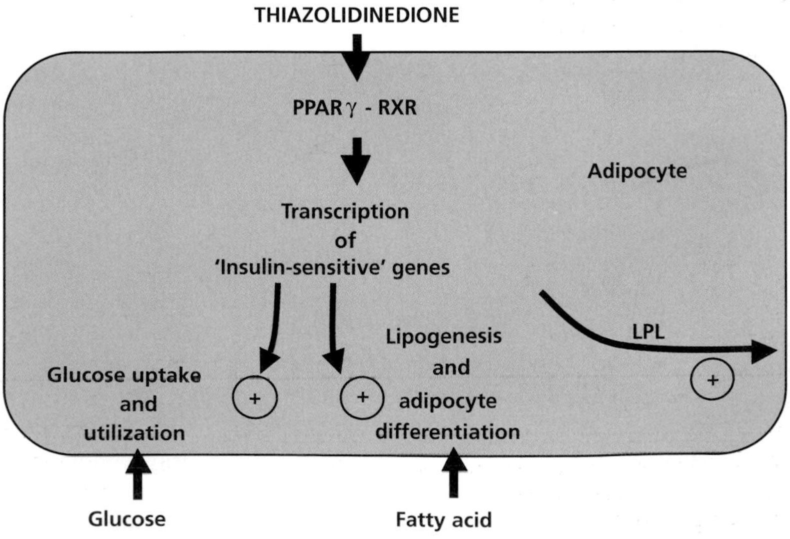

Figure 13.13 Thiazolidinediones: mode of action. After the thiazolidinedione binds to the PPARγ receptor, it associates as a heterodimer with the retinoid X receptor (RXR) in the cell nucleus, and binds to PPARγ response elements in the promoter regions of insulin target genes.

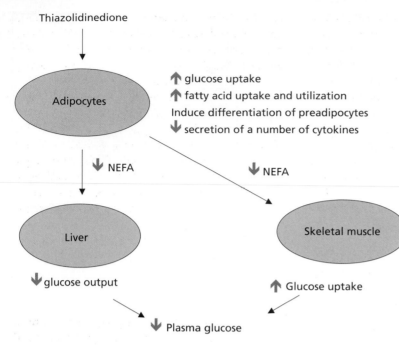

Figure 13.14 How thiazolidinediones enhance insulin action and normalize blood glucose. Thiazolidinediones enhance glucose and fatty acid uptake and utilization in adipocytes. They also induce differentiation of preadipocytes and reduce the secretion by fat of a number of cytokines that inhibit insulin action. Reduced availability of fatty acids to muscle increases glucose uptake and utilization in muscle cells through the Randle cycle. The thiazolidinediones also reduce hepatic glucose output.

BOX 13.9 What is the Randle cycle?

- Cells are able to utilize either fatty acids or glucose as fuels and are able to switch from one substrate to another depending on the supply
- When fatty acid concentrations fall, the uptake and utilization of glucose increases
- When glucose concentrations fall, the uptake and utilization of fatty acids increases

---

reducing the burden of cardiovascular disease and is discussed in more detail in Chapter 14.

There is some preliminary evidence to suggest that thiazolidinediones may affect disease progression and there are ongoing trials to assess whether these drugs can be used to prevent diabetes or reverse the pathological processes.

Side-effects. The commonest side-effect associated with thiazolidinediones is weight gain. Patients gain a significant amount of fat which appears paradoxical, given that obesity is associated with increasing insulin resistance. The answer to this is the distribution of weight gain. Fat is particularly deposited around the hips and thighs and, if anything, the metabolically more important intra-abdominal fat is reduced.

The thiazolidinediones are associated with significant fluid retention and may precipitate overt cardiac failure in those at risk. The fluid retention may also be responsible for some of the weight gain and a dilutional anaemia. Severe liver toxicity was observed with troglitazone and led to its withdrawal from the market but this does not appear to result from treatment with pioglitazone or rosiglitazone. Indeed investigators are now considering the use of these drugs, as well as metformin, to treat nonalcoholic steatohepatitis.

Inhibitors of glucose absorption from the gastrointestinal tract

Guar gum has been used as an additional source of soluble fibre to reduce carbohydrate absorption from a meal. Large quantities are required and the lack of clinical benefit has limited its use.

Acarbose

Acarbose was designed specifically to inhibit α-glucosidase inhibit α-glucosidase in the brush border of the small intestine and reduce glucose uptake from the gut (Fig. 13.15). Carbohydrate digestion involves several enzymes that sequentially degrade complex polysaccharides such as starch into monosaccharides such as glucose. Digestion of carbohydrates is begun by amylases from the saliva and pancreas and is followed by the digestion of oligosac-charides by β-galactosidases, such lactase, and various α-glucosidase enzymes which hydrolyse disaccharides in the small intestinal brush border.

Acarbose binds with a higher affinity to α-glucosidase enzymes and thereby inhibits break-down of dietary carbohydrate. Digestion and absorption of glucose after a meal is slowed and, as a result, the postprandial peak of blood glucose is reduced and blood glucose concentrations are more stable through the day. Its clinical effectiveness is limited by its lack of efficacy and side-effects. The maximum reduction in HbA_{1c} is approximately half of that of metformin or sulphonylureas.

Side-effects. The major side-effects associated with a acarbose are gastrointestinal and include flatulence, abdominal distension and diarrhoea as unabsorbed carbohydrate is fermented in the bowel.

Which drug and when?

For many years sulphonylureas were the first-line agent for patients with diabetes. Recently it has been shown that metformin is the only drug to improve longevity and reduce cardiovascular mortality and so the preferred first-line agent for all patients who are not underweight is now metformin (Fig. 13.16). When metformin can no longer achieve adequate glycaemic control, sulphonylureas are commonly the next step (Case history 13.3). Thiazolidinediones may be used in combination with either metformin or sulphonylureas for those that are unable to tolerate the other hyperglycaemic drugs. The additional, po-

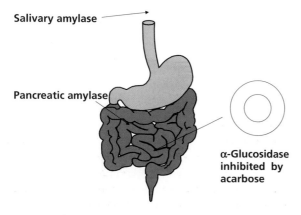

Figure 13.15 Gastrointestinal carbohydrate digestion and the site of action of acarbose. Circles are a section through gut.

tentially beneficial cardiovascular and disease modi-fying effects of thiazolidinediones has led to calls for these drug to be used earlier in the natural history of diabetes. Ongoing trials of thiazolidine-diones may well lead to changes in the current guidelines.

At present there is limited evidence about the use of triple therapy of metformin, sulphonylureas and thia-zolidinediones. However, many clinicians are using this combination to delay a move to insulin. This is particularly important for individuals, for example professional drivers, whose livelihood would be af-fected by this therapeutic change (see Chapter 14).

For thin individuals, where the predominant de-fect is β-cell failure, sulphonylureas are the first-line agent. If these measures fail, patients should move to insulin therapy earlier rather than later.

Insulin

If it is impossible to maintain good glycaemic control with oral hypoglycaemic agents, patients will need to be treated with insulin. Patients are usually treated with once-daily, long-acting insulin at night, twice-daily mixed insulin or with a basal–bolus regimen. There are advantages and disadvantages with each of these approaches and therefore the insulin regi-men must be discussed with the patient. Previously, when patients were changed to insulin, the oral hypoglycaemic agents would be stopped. Recently, there has been an increasing usage of oral hypogly-caemic agents with insulin with the commonest combination being insulin and metformin. The metformin acts as an insulin sensitizing agent and can reduce the number of hypoglycaemic episodes and weight gain associated with insulin therapy. When once daily long-acting insulin is used, this con-trols the glucose concentrations overnight and com-binations of oral hypoglycaemic agents are used to control the daytime glucose levels. The thiazoline-diones are not licensed to be combined with insulin in Europe and Japan because of the risk of cardiac failure but this combination has been used success-fully in the USA.

Emerging Therapies for type 2 diabetes

Therapies based on glucagon-like peptide 1

Certain cells within the gastrointestinal tract secrete

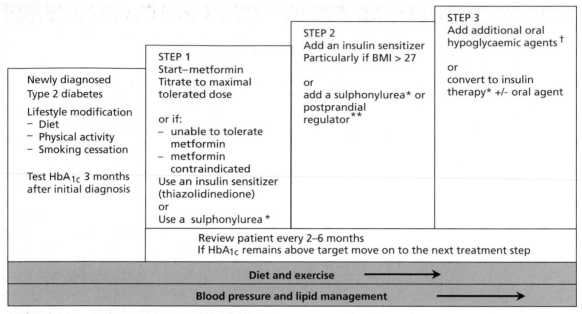

*Clinicians should be alert to the risk of hypoglycaemia with insulin, sulphonylurea and postprandial glucose regulators

**Postprandial glucose regulators may be of particular use in patients with nonroutine daily patterns

†Acarbose may be considered as an alternative agent in patients unable to use other oral therapies. Insulin sensitizers are not licensed in combination with insulin

Figure 13.16 The stepwise management of type 2 diabetes.

CASE HISTORY 13.3

A 45-year-old woman has had diabetes for 10 years. She has a BMI of 28 kg/m^2. She has been treated with glibenclamide 15 mg daily and has poor diabetic control (HbA$_{1c}$ 11.0%). She has background retinopathy and mild renal impairment (Creatinine 157 µmol/L).

What would you do next?

Answers, see p. 233

---

several hormones, collectively known as incretins, that stimulate insulin secretion. These hormones include glucagon-like peptide 1 (GLP-1) and gastric inhibitory peptide (GIP). The incretin effect is markedly impaired or absent in patients with type 2 diabetes because of decreased secretion of GLP-1 and a loss of the insulinotropic effects of GIP and so several years ago it was reasoned that replacement of these hormones may lead to improved metabolic control. Although GIP replacement has little effect on insulin secretion, glycaemic control was greatly improved by administration of exogenous GLP-1. However, the native peptide is of limited clinical use

because it is almost immediately degraded by the enzyme dipeptidyl peptidase IV (DPP-IV).

The discovery of DPP-IV-resistant GLP-1 analogues (incretin mimetics) was pursued in parallel with the development of inhibitors of DPP-IV. The first incretin mimetic, exenatide, has now been introduced into clinical practice in the USA and was originally isolated from the saliva of the Gila monster, a poisonous lizard from the deserts of Arizona. It is administered by twice daily subcutaneous injection and in clinical trials resulted in a lasting reduction of HbA$_{1c}$ of ~0.8%. Adverse effects were mild and generally gastrointestinal. A further welcome side-effect was steady weight loss over 2 years, predominantly through diminution of appetite. It has been argued that these drugs may be able to slow or prevent the apparently inevitable progression of type 2 diabetes because GLP-1 has trophic effects on the β-cell but this issue is unresolved. Other DPP-IV-resistant GLP-1 analogues are also in development.

The DPP-IV inhibitors currently in phase III trials also appear to provide some lasting improvement in HbA_{1c}. While they have the advantage of being administered orally, unlike the incretin analogues, DPP-IV inhibitors have no effect on weight and are perhaps not such potent insulin secretagogues.

Therapies based on amylin

Amylin is a peptide hormone that is co-secreted with insulin from the pancreatic β-cell and is deficient in individuals with diabetes. It inhibits glucagon secretion, delays gastric emptying, and acts to enhance satiety.

Pramlintide is an amylin analogue, which is administered by subcutaneous injection prior to meals, in order to reduce postprandial glucose levels. It leads to a reduction in HbA_{1c} of ~0.6% and is associated with modest weight loss.

Answers to case histories

Case history 13.1

This woman is at considerable risk of diabetes in the future. Around 50% of woman with gestational diabetes develop diabetes within 10 years of the index pregnancy. She needs support to help her change her lifestyle to reduce her risk. She needs dietary advice to help her lose weight and she should increase the amount of exercise she takes as this will reduce her risk over and above any effect on weight. It is debatable at this stage whether she should have drug therapy. Although both metformin and orlistat have been shown to reduce the risk of diabetes, the size of the effect is smaller than lifestyle modification and so the emphasis should be placed on the latter. As diabetes is frequently asymptomatic in its earliest stages, it is important to screen this woman for diabetes every 1 to 3 years.

Case history 13.2

This man presents with classical diabetic symptoms and has a diagnostic blood test. Given his age and size it is most likely he has type 2 diabetes but it is important to be aware that type 1 diabetes can occur in this age group. Lifestyle modification—particularly avoidance of sugary drinks—is the most important aspect of this man's treatment, although there may be an indication to use a sulphonylurea in the short term (<6 weeks) to improve his symptoms while he is adjusting to his new lifestyle. The diet and exercise should also help him to lose weight.

Case history 13.3

This woman has poor glycaemic control and it is likely that improving her control will make her feel better. She is overweight and it is always worth re-emphasizing lifestyle change. She is already on a maximal dose of glibenclamide and so a second agent is needed. As she has renal impairment, metformin is contraindicated and so a thiazolidinedione would be the treatment of choice. This will take several months to reach maximal efficacy. She may ultimately require insulin.

14 Complications of diabetes

LEARNING OBJECTIVES

- To discuss the cause of microvascular and macrovascular complications
- To understand the importance of screening for complications

- To understand the strategies to prevent and treat complications
- To discuss diabetes in pregnancy
- To understand the psychosocial aspects of diabetes

In this chapter we will learn about the complications of diabetes

Introduction

Since the introduction of effective treatment that allows patients with diabetes to live through the acute metabolic consequences of diabetes, it has become apparent that diabetes is associated with a number of chronic microvascular complications that affect the eyes, kidneys and nerves. Furthermore, patients with diabetes have a higher incidence of macrovascular complications such as myocardial infarction, stroke and peripheral vascular disease (Fig. 14.1). Pregnancy outcomes for women with diabetes are also worse than in the general population. Finally, diabetes is associated with a number of psychosocial sequelae. These complications of diabetes adversely affect the quality of life of people with diabetes and will be considered in turn, together with the underlying causes and treatment.

Microvascular complications

Microvascular complications affect over 80% of individuals with diabetes and are present in approximately 20–50% of patients with newly diagnosed type 2 diabetes (Fig. 14.2). The prevalence of microvascular complications increases with increasing duration of diabetes.

Pathogenesis of microvascular complications

The pathogenesis of diabetic microvascular complications is not fully understood and is likely to be multifactorial (Box 14.1).

Hyperglycaemia
Chronic hyperglycaemia undoubtedly predisposes to the generation of microvascular complications

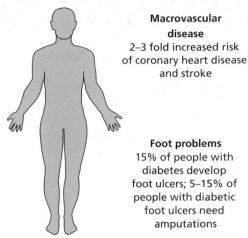

Retinopathy
Most common cause of blindness in people of working age

Nephropathy
16% of all new patients needing renal replacement therapy have diabetes

Erectile dysfunction
May affect up to 50% of men with long-standing diabetes

Macrovascular disease
2–3 fold increased risk of coronary heart disease and stroke

Foot problems
15% of people with diabetes develop foot ulcers; 5–15% of people with diabetic foot ulcers need amputations

Figure 14.1 The chronic complications of diabetes.

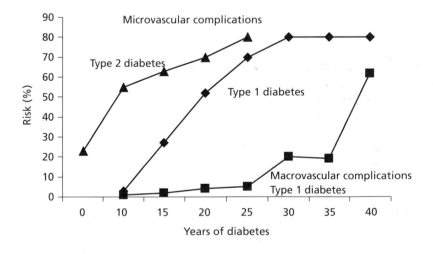

Figure 14.2 Cumulative prevalence of diabetic complications in patients with diabetes. Note that at least 20% of patients with newly diagnosed type 2 diabetes already have microvascular complications. This reflects the long duration of asymptomatic disease before diagnosis.

BOX 14.1 Why do microvascular complications occur?

- Hyperglycaemia
  - development of advanced glycation end-products (AGE)
  - activation of the sorbitol pathway
  - activation of several intracellular kinases—protein kinase Cβ
  - activation of cytokines—transforming growth factorβ (TGFβ) and vascular endothelial growth factor (VEGF)

- Abnormalities in the growth hormone–insulin like growth factor axis
- Hypertension
  - swamping of normal capillary autoregulation
  - activation of the renin–angiotensin system

Genetic polymorphisms in proteins of these systems may explain some of the genetic differences in the predisposition to complications.

and, indeed, the diagnosis of diabetes is based on the concentration of glucose that is associated with the development of microvascular complications, and retinopathy in particular. Studies of patients with either type 1 or type 2 diabetes have shown that improved glycaemic control will reduce the incidence of microvascular complications.

The underlying mechanism linking hyperglycaemia with the development of microvascular complications is not fully understood and is likely to be multifactorial. There are several candidate intracellular mechanisms, including the development of advanced glycation end-products, activation of the sorbitol pathway and activation of several intracellular kinases, as well as damage to the microcirculation (Fig. 14.3).

Advanced glycation end-products (AGE)

If proteins are exposed to glucose over a prolonged period, glucose becomes attached to the protein through a mechanism which is independent of enzymatic action. Early glycation products are reversible (Box 14.2) but eventually the proteins undergo irreversible changes through cross linking to form advanced glycation end-products (AGE).

AGE proteins accumulate in proportion to hyperglycaemia and time and do not function normally. They promote extracellular matrix accumulation and generation of reactive oxygen species, both of which damage cellular function.

Inhibitors of the AGE reaction or antioxidants have been tried to reduce the rate of microvascular complications but have been largely unsuccessful. The reason for this may be the high quantity of

---

BOX 14.2 Glycosylated haemoglobin

- We utilize the first part of the AGE reaction when we assess glycaemic control
- Glycosylated haemoglobin is an early glycation product formed by the nonenzymatic attachment of glucose to the N terminal of the β chain of haemoglobin

---

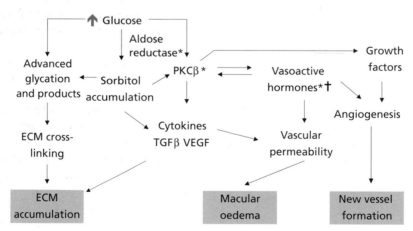

Figure 14.3 Molecular mechanisms that may be important in the generation of microvascular complications. There is no one mechanism that explains the development of microvascular diabetic complications. Hyperglycaemia affects a number of biochemical pathways leading to the accumulation of advanced glycation end-products (AGEs) and sorbitol through the polyol pathway. Hyperglycaemia also activates PKCβ. AGE accumulation leads to deposition of material in the extra cellular matrix (ECM). This impairs the function of the tissue, e.g. kidney. Sorbitol and PKCβ activation, in turn, lead to the secretion of a number of cytokines and growth factors that affect vascular permeability and angiogenesis. *Genetic factors are also important in the development of microvascular complications. Polymorphisms in the aldose reductase enzyme, PKCβ and vasoactive hormones may account for some of the genetic difference. † Hypertension is a strong risk factor for the development of complications. Increased tissue blood flow may affect the function of the vasoactive hormones.

dietary AGE products that result from many cooking processes. The ingestion of AGE products may then swamp any effect of the drug to reduce cellular formation of AGE proteins.

Sorbitol pathway

In situations where there is excess glucose, glucose can be metabolized to sorbitol via the polyol pathway under the action of the aldose reductase enzyme. This pathway utilizes NADPH and NAD^+. The depletion of NADPH leads to decreased reduced glutathione. The latter is an important scavenger of reactive oxygen species and therefore depletion of reduced glutathione leads to excess reactive oxygen species, which are damaging to the cell.

The formation of sorbitol can be inhibited by blocking the aldose reductase enzyme. Clinical trials of aldose reductase inhibitors, however, have been largely disappointing and have not led to reductions in the prevalence of microvascular complications. The reason for the lack of efficacy is not clear but may reflect the multiple intracellular pathways involved and so blockade of one pathway may be insufficient to prevent damage.

Activation of protein kinase Cβ

The β-isoform of protein kinase C (PKCβ) is an intracellular kinase belonging to a family of protein serine–threonine kinases (Fig. 3.16). When glucose is metabolized to diacylglycerol, the expression of PKCβ is increased. PKCβ increases the expression of a number of mitogenic cytokines, such as transforming growth factor β (TGFβ) and vascular endothelial growth factor (VEGF). Animal experiments using PKC inhibitors have shown that macular oedema can be reduced in an experimental model of retinopathy and clinical trials in humans are on-going.

Cytokines

TGFβ and VEGF expression are increased by AGE products and hypoxia as well as PKCβ. Both cytokines increase vascular permeability and angiogenesis, which may be responsible for the macular oedema and new vessel formation seen in diabetic retinopathy. Polymorphisms in the genes of these cytokines have been associated with an increased risk of retinopathy and may explain some of the genetic

difference in the risk of developing microvascular complications.

Haemodynamic theory of diabetic complications

It is clear that chronic hyperglycaemia is not the whole explanation as it is well recognized that the appearance of new microvascular complications in patients who have remained complication free for 20 years is unusual, suggesting that some, as yet unknown, mechanism may protect against the development of complications. This is supported by twin studies showing that complications are more likely to occur in both identical twins than nonidentical twins, indicating that certain genotypes may predispose or protect against the generation of microvascular complications.

Hypertension is also important in the pathogenesis of microvascular complications and may be more important than hyperglycaemia in the progression of microvascular complications once complications are present.

The *haemodynamic* theory proposes that:

- Microvascular complications result from chronic abnormalities in the blood flow through capillary beds. Hyperglycaemia by an osmotic effect initiates the process by swamping the normal autoregulatory mechanisms that limit blood flow through a tissue.
- After this initial damage, high flow rates that are increased in patients with hypertension lead to tissue damage.

This hypothesis is supported by the observation that retinopathy is often much better in the ipsilateral eye when a patient has a carotid artery stenosis. This hypothesis also explains why microvascular complications occur in tissues where there is a high capillary blood flow. Aggressive treatment of blood pressure to values less than 130 to 140/80 mmHg has been shown to slow the progression of microvascular complications.

The renin–angiotensin system

There is evidence to suggest that blockade of the renin–angiotensin system can slow the progression of microvascular complications to a greater extent than other blood pressure lowering agents, suggesting the renin–angiotensin system may have a role in the generation of microvascular complications. The evidence is best in the treatment of nephropathy where both ACE inhibitors and angiotensin receptor blockers have been shown to be effective, but there is tantalizing preliminary data that may suggest the ACE inhibitors also slow the progression of retinopathy.

The growth hormone–insulin-like growth factor axis

The growth hormone–insulin-like growth factor axis has also been implicated in the generation of microvascular complications for a number of reasons:

- In 1953, Poulsen presented the case of a woman with type 1 diabetes and background diabetic retinopathy, which regressed after she developed panhypopituitarism after postpartum pituitary necrosis.
- In the 1960s, pituitary ablation was shown to result in a regression of diabetic retinopathy, which could be related to the degree of GH deficiency.
- Patients with type 1 diabetes and GH deficiency have decreased rates of retinopathy.

This area remains controversial because there is no evidence that GH replacement therapy causes an increased incidence of retinopathy in GH-deficient patients with or without diabetes. In patients with diabetes, the GH–IGF axis does not function normally; the reduced portal concentrations of insulin that inevitably accompany subcutaneous administration of insulin result in reduced hepatic production of IGF1. This leads to reduced feedback to the pituitary gland and GH hypersecretion. Growth hormone concentrations are typically up to two to three times higher in individuals with diabetes compared with healthy subjects. It is possible that correction of the GH hypersecretion by administration of IGF1 may reduce the risk of developing microvascular complications. Although effective, pituitary ablation was associated with significant morbidity and mortality and has been superseded by retinal photocoagulation. Somatostatin and GH receptor antagonists have been shown to have some benefit in clinical trials to reduce microvascular complications.

Clinical features of microvascular complications

Retinopathy

Aetiology
The most important way that diabetes can affect the

eye is the development of retinopathy, which is the commonest cause of blindness in the UK in people under the age of 60 years (Box 14.3). Retinopathy is also important because it develops in an insidious way and is almost invariably asymptomatic until a patient has a catastrophic intraocular sight-threatening haemorrhage. This is a tragic situation because retinopathy is treatable and so with adequate screening most cases of blindness are preventable.

Natural history of diabetic retinopathy
Retinopathy proceeds through a natural history that begins with background retinopathy, before moving to preproliferative retinopathy and finally to proliferative retinopathy (Box 14.4; Plates 14.1–14.8, facing p. 246).

Screening and diagnosis of retinopathy
As retinopathy is asymptomatic, screening for retinopathy is essential in order to prevent blindness. It is recommended that every patient receives an annual eye test, which involves a check of visual acuity and fundoscopic examination. Visual acuity should be also checked through a pin hole to assess macula vision. Traditionally, the examination of the fundus has been performed by a trained physician using an ophthalmoscope having dilated the patient's pupils. More recently, however, it has been shown that reti-

---

BOX 14.3 Ways in which diabetes can affect the eye

- Retinopathy
- Cataract
  - diabetes increases the rate of age-related cataract formation
  - there is a diabetes-specific cataract that generally affects young patients with type 1 diabetes and may progress rapidly
- Refractory defects
  - hyperglycaemia may alter the osmotic pressure within the lens leading to temporary refractive defects
- Glaucoma
  - prevalence is increased in patients with diabetes
- Infection

BOX 14.4 Features of different stages of diabetic retinopathy

- Background retinopathy
  - dots (microaneurysms)
  - blots (small intraretinal haemorrhages)
  - hard exudates—lipid exudates that often form in a circle around a leaking blood vessel
- Maculopathy
  - background retinopathy occurring around the macula
  - may cause reduction in visual acuity
  - may be associated with macula oedema
  - more common in type 2 diabetes
- Preproliferative retinopathy
  - cotton wool spots that result from retinal ischaemia
  - intraretinal microvascular abnormalities (IRMA)—clusters of irregular branched vessels in the retina and may represent early new vessel formation
  - venous changes—beading, which appears as segmental dilatations, loops, reduplication
- Proliferative retinopathy—new vessels formation
  - caused by growth factors that are secreted in response to the retinal ischaemia
  - these are friable and have a high tendency to bleed
  - the haemorrhage can lead to temporary or permanent blindness
  - categorized according to whether they occur at the disc (NVD) or elsewhere (NVE)

BOX 14.5 Indications and urgency for referral to an ophthalmologist

- Maculopathy — 1 month
- Preproliferative — 1 month
- Proliferative — 1 week
- Sudden loss of vision — Same day
- Retinal detachment — Same day
- Cataract — Nonurgent

nal photography is able to identify retinopathy more reliably than traditional methods. Furthermore, retinal photography provides a permanent record for comparison and for these reasons the preferred method of screening is photography.

Management of retinopathy

The optimal management of diabetic retinopathy involves the close liaison between ophthalmology and diabetic services (Box 14.5).

There is good evidence that retinopathy can be prevented by good glycaemic control. The Diabetes and Complication and Control Trial has shown that by lowering glycosylated haemoglobin by 2% in patients with type 1 diabetes, the incidence and progression of retinopathy was more than halved.

Similarly, in patients with type 2 diabetes, a reduction in glycosylated haemoglobin by 1% resulted in a 21% reduction in retinopathy. Tight blood pressure control has also been shown to reduce retinopathy and the best results are obtained in patients who have both good glycaemic and blood pressure control. At present no other medical therapies are licensed to prevent or treat retinopathy.

Once a patient has developed preproliferative or proliferative retinopathy or maculopathy, further treatment by laser photocoagulation is needed (Plate 14.4–14.8, facing p. 246). The principle of laser treatment is that by destroying peripheral parts of the retina, the ischaemic stimulus for new vessel formation is reduced. In essence, peripheral vision is sacrificed for central vision but laser treatment is effective in reducing for the loss of vision.

Patients may need vitrectomy (removal of the vitreous) if an intravitreal haemorrhage fails to clear. After the onset of blindness, patients should be advised to register blind and may require additional aids to help them monitor their diabetes.

Nephropathy

Aetiology

Diabetic nephropathy is a common cause of established renal failure, accounting for around 16% of new patients requiring renal replacement therapy. The risk of developing nephropathy is lower in patients with type 2 diabetes than in type 1 diabetes because of the generally later onset of type 2 diabetes. Despite this, patients with type 2 diabetes requiring renal replacement therapy outnumber patients with type 1 diabetes because of the much greater prevalence of type 2 diabetes.

The development of nephropathy is also associated with premature cardiovascular mortality. The risk of developing cardiovascular disease is increased by two- to threefold in those with microalbuminuria, the earliest sign of nephropathy, and 10-fold with frank proteinuria. Around one-third of proteinuric diabetic patients die from cardiovascular disease before they develop established renal failure.

Natural history of diabetic nephropathy
The earliest effect of diabetes on the kidney is an increase in glomerular filtration rate. The kidney enlarges through expansion of tubular tissue but there is no change in serum creatinine or blood pressure. As diabetic nephropathy progresses, there is a progressive increase in urinary albumin excretion and diminished renal function, which results from pathological basement membrane thickening, atrophy and interstitial fibrosis (Table 14.1).

The initial stage of diabetic nephropathy is microalbuminuria, which is defined as a higher than normal albumin excretion that cannot be detected by standard urine albustix test, and affects around 50% of patients with diabetes. Protein excretion returns to normal in around 30% of people with microalbuminuria while only 20% of patients will have progressive renal disease. These patients will develop intermittent overt proteinuria before developing persistent overt proteinuria. Occasionally, protein excretion can reach a level that causes the nephrotic syndrome. Glomerular filtration rate and serum creatinine only become abnormal after the development of frank proteinuria. Hypertension affects virtually all patients with persistent proteinuria and some patients will also develop peripheral oedema.

Screening and diagnosis of diabetic nephropathy
Around two-thirds of patients with overt proteinurla will ultimately develop established renal failure. In contrast, if interventions are put in place when the patient has microalbuminuria, this progression can be halted at best and delayed at worst. As microalbuminuria is asymptomatic, it is important to screen for this on an annual basis using either a urinary albumin to creatinine ratio or more sensitive dipsticks. Before microalbuminuria can be confirmed, three tests should be positive and other causes of proteinuria excluded. Although not very sensitive, it is recommended that serum creatinine is measured on an annual basis. The estimated glomerular filtration rate can be calculated from this (Box 14.6).

BOX 14.6 Estimated glomerular filtration rate (GFR)

$$GFR = 186 \times \{[(\text{serum creatinine})/88.4]^{-1.154}\} \times \text{age (years)}^{-0.203}$$

GFR: $mL/min/1.73\,m^2$
Creatinine: $\mu mol/L$

If the patient is female the result of the formula is multiplied by 0.742
If the patient is of Black ethnicity the result of the formula is multiplied by 1.21

Table 14.1 Five stages of diabetic nephropathy

Test	Normal	Microalbuminuria	Persistent proteinuria	Renal impairment	Established renal failure
Albuminuria (mg/day)	<20	20–300	>300 Up to 15 g/day	>300 Up to 15 g/day	>300 Can fall
GFR (ml/min)	High/normal	High/ normal	Normal/Decreased	Decreased	Decreased ++
Serum creatinine (umol/L)	Normal 60–150	Normal 60–150	High Normal 80–120	High 120–400	Very high >400
BP	Normal	Small increase	Increased	Increased	Increased
Signs	None	None	+/−Oedema	+/−Oedema	Uraemic symptoms

Management of diabetic nephropathy

It is important that there is a locally defined protocol for the referral of patients with diabetes mellitus and microalbuminuria to a specialist diabetes team. The management of these patients consists of normalization of blood pressure and correction of cardiovascular risk factors. There is also good evidence that treatment with ACE inhibitors or angiotensin receptor blockers will slow the progression of the nephropathy. Glycaemic control should be optimized.

Referral to a nephrology unit is generally recommended when the serum creatinine approaches 200 to 250 μmol/L or GFR falls below 60 mL/min/1.73 m². Referral to a nephrologist should also be considered if there is increasing proteinuria without diabetic retinopathy because this is a sign of nondiabetic renal damage.

Renal replacement therapy can be provided by haemodialysis, continuous ambulatory peritoneal dialysis or renal transplantation. Renal transplantation is considered the treatment of choice for patients under the age of 60 years and the 5-year survival following transplantation is now as good as that in a nondiabetic population.

Neuropathy

Aetiology

Neuropathy affects 20 to 50% of patients with type 2 diabetes, and its sequelae, such as foot ulceration and amputation, cause considerable morbidity and mortality (Box 14.7). Diabetic neuropathy can be divided into acute reversible neuropathy and other persistent neuropathies, such as distal symmetrical and focal and multifocal neuropathies.

Hyperglycaemic neuropathy. Hyperglycaemia slows nerve conduction and causes uncomfortable sensory symptoms in those with poor glycaemic control.

Distal symmetrical neuropathy. The most common neuropathy is distal symmetrical neuropathy which is frequently called 'peripheral neuropathy'. It results from damage to the axon tips that begins in the longest nerves. This explains why symptoms occur in a 'glove and stocking' distribution. Sensory loss is the most obvious component leading to numbness but patients might also complain pain or altered sen-

---

BOX 14.7 Classification of diabetic neuropathy

Acute reversible
- Hyperglycaemic neuropathy

Persistent
- Symmetrical
  - distal symmetrical neuropathy (peripheral neuropathy)
  - acute painful neuropathy
- Focal and multifocal
  - pressure palsies—carpal tunnel syndrome (median nerve), ulnar nerve compression at the elbow
  - mononeuropathies—diabetic amyotrophy (femoral nerve), III and VI cranial nerves, truncal
- Autonomic

---

sation. The pain is often described as burning or like an electrical shock and may be accompanied by paraesthesiae.

Pressure palsies. Diabetic nerves are more susceptible to mechanical injury at sites of compression or entrapment. The most common is the carpal tunnel syndrome which is caused by compression of the median nerve leading to paraesthesiae and numbness in the lateral three and a half fingers. Most patients respond to surgical decompression.

Mononeuropathies and radiculopathies. Patients with diabetes are more prone to develop mononeuropathies of the third or sixth cranial nerves or trunk. Damage to nerve roots is also more common in those with diabetes. The aetiology of the mononeuropathies and radiculopathies is unclear but the rapid onset suggests a vasculitic or inflammatory process. The commonest radiculopathy is femoral amyotrophy in which there is involvement of the lumboscral nerve roots, plexus and femoral nerve. The patients present with continuous thigh pain, wasting and weakness of the quadriceps and sometimes weight loss. The knee-jerk reflex is also lost.

Recovery of the mononeuropathies or radiculopathies is usually spontaneous but may take many months.

Management of painful diabetic neuropathy

The management of diabetic neuropathy is often difficult (Fig.14.4). It is important to exclude other causes of neuropathy such as vitamin B_{12} deficiency, alcohol excess and renal dysfunction. Some patients will respond to a bed cradle or protective film that prevents the affected limb from being touched or rubbed. Simple analgesics such as paracetamol, aspirin, and codeine phosphate are usually ineffective in the treatment of neuropathy but may provide some relief. Burning pain can be controlled by tricyclic antidepressants such as amitriptyline and imipramine. Anticonvulsants, such as carbamazepine and gabapentin, may also be of benefit. Where the pain is localized, capsaicin may be useful when applied as a cream to the skin.

Autonomic neuropathy

In patients with longstanding diabetes, autonomic neuropathy may develop (Box 14.8). Symptoms are unusual but may be distressing.

The diabetic foot

Foot problems are a major cause of morbidity in patients with diabetes (Case history 14.1). Fifteen per cent of people with diabetes develop foot ulcers, and 5 to 15% of these people require foot amputations (Plate 14.9, facing p. 246). Foot ulceration is the commonest reason for hospitalization and the most expensive complication of diabetes.

Diabetic foot ulcers are caused by a combination of neuropathy and ischaemia and are frequently complicated by infection (Box 14.9). Infected diabetic foot

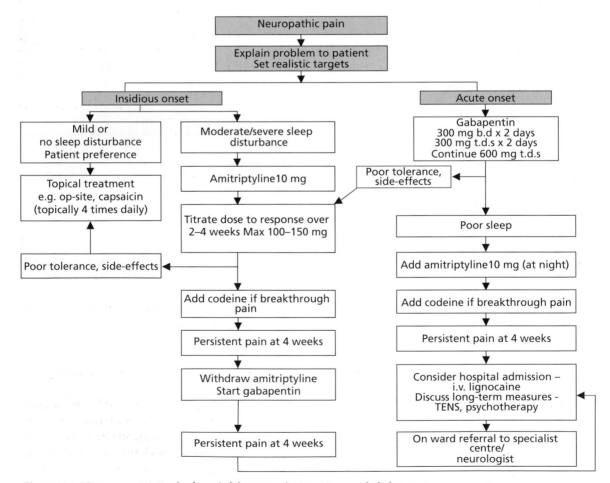

Figure 14.4 Management strategies for painful neuropathy in patients with diabetes.

BOX 14.8 Symptoms and signs of autonomic neuropathy

- Gastrointestinal
  - gustatory sweating
  - oesophageal dysmotility
  - gastroparesis
  - diabetic diarrhoea
- Cardiovascular
  - postural hypotension
  - abnormal cardiovascular reflexes
  - cardiorespiratory arrest
  - neuropathic oedema
  - increased peripheral blood flow
- Genitourinary
  - neuropathic bladder
  - erectile dysfunction in men, sexual dysfunction in women
- Musculoskeletal
  - Charcot arthropathy
- Metabolic
  - blunted counter regulation responses to hypoglycaemia
- Eyes
  - abnormal papillary reflexes

BOX 14.9 Cause of diabetic foot ulcers

Neuropathy
- Peripheral neuropathy results in a loss of pain sensation
  - patients are unaware of injury to their feet
- Motor neuropathy leads to a characteristic posture of a raised arch and clawed toes
  - concentrates pressure on to the metatarsal heads and heel
  - callus production is stimulated at these pressure points
  - haemorrhage or necrosis, which commonly occurs within the callus, can break through to form an ulcer
- Autonomic neuropathy
  - reduced sweating leads to dry and cracked skin; this can perform a portal of entry for infection
- Charcot arthropathy

Peripheral vascular disease
- The reduced blood supply to the feet may compromise both nutrition and oxygen

Infection

CASE HISTORY 14.1

A 56-year-old woman develops an infected foot ulcer after a night out at a club. She has had diabetes for 7 years and is treated with metformin 500 mg three times daily and gliclazide 80 mg twice daily. Her HbA_{1c} is 9.0%.

What is your immediate management?
What are your long-term plans?

Answers, see p. 251

ulcers should be considered as medical emergencies as early inattention can result in massive tissue loss and the need for amputation. Foot ulcers require radical debridement and relief of pressure by bed rest or the use of contact casting. Infection should be treated with appropriate antibiotics and it may be necessary to perform revascularization of ischaemic limbs (Plates 14.10–14.12, facing p. 246).

Charcot arthropathy
Charcot arthropathy is a rare complication of severe neuropathy, both peripheral and autonomic, and longstanding diabetes. Charcot arthropathy can be divided into three phases:
- Acute onset
- Bony destruction
- Radiological consolidation and stabilization.

Acute onset. Patients present with an acutely swollen, hot foot and about a third have pain (Plate 14.13, facing p. 246). The initiating event may be an injury, which is often trivial, that causes bone fracture. A radiograph at this time may be normal but a technetium bone scan will detect bony destruction.

Charcot arthropathy	Cellulitis
Oedema may resolve with elevation	Typical signs of infection are usually present
	Generalized signs may be present
	More likely if ulcer is present
	Particularly if discharge present

Table 14.2 Features to differentiate acute Charcot from cellulitis

Table 14.3 Dos and don'ts of foot care

Do	Don't
Wash feet daily	Use corn cures
Check feet daily	Use hot water bottle
Seek urgent treatment of problems	Walk barefoot
See a chiropodist regularly	Cut corns / callosities
Wear sensible shoes	Treat foot problems yourself

> **BOX 14.10 Sites to be tested with monofilament**
>
> - Plantar aspect of first toe
> - 1st, 3rd and 5th metatarsal heads
> - Plantar surface of heel
> - Dorsum of foot

It is important to differentiate between Charcot arthropathy and cellulitis (Table 14.2). This can be difficult and so, if in doubt, both conditions should be treated. Acute gout and deep vein thrombosis may also masquerade as Charcot arthropathy.

The aim of treatment of Charcot arthropathy is to prevent or minimize bony destruction. The foot is immobilized in a nonweight-bearing cast, which should be checked and replaced regularly. The casting should be continued until the swelling and temperature in the foot has resolved.

Bony destruction. If treatment of the acute stage is delayed, the foot can become deformed as bone is destroyed. These changes often develop very rapidly, over a few weeks. The deformity can predispose the foot to ulceration, particularly on the plantar surface of a 'rockerbottom' deformity (Plate 14.14, facing p. 246). Treatment of this stage is also by immobilization.

Radiological consolidation. Ultimately, the destructive process stabilizes after 6 to 12 months. Rehabilitatione is always necessary after a long period in a cast.

Screening for peripheral neuropathy
As the treatment of diabetic foot ulcers is difficult, prevention is vital. It is important to examine the patient's feet regularly and to educate our patients about the risks to their feet (Table 14.3).

Foot screening consists of four parts:
- Enquiry for past or present ulceration
- Inspection for abnormalities
- Testing for neuropathy
- Palpation of foot pulses to detect ischaemia

There has been considerable discussion about the optimal means of testing for neuropathy. Examination of the feet may reveal distal loss of sensory modalities, such as vibration sense, touch, pinprick, joint position sense and temperature. Formal measurements of vibration sense with a biothesiometer and nerve conduction studies have not been used routinely in clinical practice. This has meant that there has been a lack of standardization of assessments of neuropathy in clinical practice. More recently, the introduction of a 10-g monofilament has allowed reproducible assessments of neuropathy. The monofilament is applied perpendicular to the foot and buckles at a force of 10 g (Box 14.10). Ability to feel that level of pressure provides protective sensation against foot ulceration. The test is repeated at various sites to detect any area where protective pain sensation is lost.

Sexual problems of diabetes
Erectile dysfunction
Erectile dysfunction is a major sexual problem among men with diabetes (Case history 14.2). Its prevalence increases with age, such that around

---

CASE HISTORY 14.2

A 55-year-old man with a 10-year history of diabetes complains of impotence. He has no early morning erections. He shaves normally and has a good relationship with his wife. He drinks half a bottle of wine daily. In addition to diabetes, he has hypertension, for which he takes atenolol and nifedipine, and hypercholesterolaemia for which he takes simvastatin.

What are the possible causes for his erectile dysfunction?
What treatment would you suggest?

Answers, see p. 251

60% of men with diabetes over the age of 60 years are affected. The overall prevalence is around 35 to 40%.

Penile erection occurs following the flow of blood into the erectile tissue. Nitric oxide-mediated vascular smooth muscle relaxation of the corpus cavernosum produces expansion of the cavernosal space and compression of the outflow venules. This allows blood to flow into, but not out of, the penis. Erectile dysfunction in diabetes mainly results from autonomic neuropathy and endothelial dysfunction. However, there are other factors that contribute to erectile dysfunction, including drugs, psychological, neurological, endocrine and metabolic disorders.

When a man complains of erectile dysfunction, it is important to take a detailed history to assess whether there are reversible causes. General treatment measures include improving glycaemic control, reducing alcohol intake and withdrawing drugs that may impair erection.

First-line pharmacotherapy is with phosphodiesterase type 5 inhibitors, such as sildenafil, vardenafil and tadalafil. These agents act by inhibiting the breakdown of cyclic GMP, which is a second messenger of nitric oxide. They enhance erections under conditions of sexual stimulation and so the drugs are taken before intended sexual activity. They are effective in around 50 to 60% of diabetic man. Phosphodiesterase type 5 inhibitors may cause severe acute hypotension when used concomitantly with nitrates.

Other treatment options include the use of prostaglandin E, which can be administered by injection into the corpus cavernosum or transurethrally. Apomorphine, a dopamine agonist, has recently been introduced. Vacuum devices allow blood to be drawn into the penis while a constriction band around the base of the penis prevents blood leaving the penis and thereby maintains the erection. There is also a limited role for surgical insertion of penile prostheses.

Sexual dysfunction in women

Although less common than in men, women with diabetes may also have sexual problems. There is an increased risk of vaginal dryness and impaired sexual arousal. Genitourinary infections, in particular candidiasis, are common in diabetic women. Urinary tract infections are frequent in women with poorly controlled diabetes, particularly if there is autonomic neuropathy and bladder distension.

Macrovascular disease

Aetiology

Diabetes confers a two- to fourfold increased risk of myocardial infarction and stroke in men, and up to a 10-fold increased risk in premenopausal women, who lose their normal premenopausal protection against cardiovascular disease. Mortality following a myocardial infarction is far greater in people with diabetes, with 60 to 75% of diabetics dying from cardiovascular disease. These statistics, coupled with the observation that people with diabetes who have not had a previous myocardial infarction share the same risk of having a myocardial infarction as nondiabetic patients who have had a myocardial infarction, has begun to shift the focus of management of diabetes from purely glucose control to a greater emphasis on arterial risk-factor management.

Pathogenesis

The pathogenesis of atheroma in diabetes is identical to that in nondiabetic people but it develops earlier and faster and is more extensive and widespread (Box 14.11). There are also major functional abnormalities in the endothelium, which include increased endothelial adhesiveness, impaired vasodilatation, enhanced haemostasis and increased permeability.

Hyperglycaemia

There are several mechanisms by which hyperglycaemia and advanced glycation end-products (AGEs) might contribute to macrovascular disease. AGEs cross-link vessel wall proteins that cause thickening and dysfunction of the subintimal layer. AGEs also generate toxic, reactive oxygen species that quench the vasodilator nitric oxide and so favour vasoconstriction. The AGEs also interact with specific receptors on the endothelium, smooth muscle cells, monocytes and macrophages and lead to up regulation of procoagulant and adhesion proteins.

Nevertheless, the relationship between glycaemic control and macrovascular disease is relatively weak and hyperglycaemia *per se* is insufficient to explain the increased prevalence of cardiovascular disease in diabetes. Furthermore, in the UK Prospective Diabetes Study (UKPDS) in patients with type 2 diabetes, improved glycaemic control had no significant effect on cardiovascular mortality and a borderline effect on myocardial infarction. The exception to this was the group of patients treated with metformin who had a significant reduction in cardiovascular death and events. There is some preliminary evidence to suggest that treatment with thiazolidinediones may reduce cardiovascular events but this may not be through their hypoglycaemic effect as these drugs have direct vascular effects.

Traditional cardiovascular risk factors

The traditional cardiovascular risk factors in nondiabetic population, such as smoking, hypertension and hyperlipidaemia, also operate in patients with diabetes. It has been known for over a century that cardiovascular risk factors tend to cluster within the same individuals and so patients with diabetes have higher prevalence rates of cardiovascular risk factors than the general population. In the Munster Heart Study, for example, 49% of individuals with diabetes had hypertension, 24% had a low HDL-cholesterol, and 37% had hypertriglyceridaemia compared with 31%, 16% and 21%, respectively, in nondiabetic subjects.

Diabetes is associated with a dyslipidaemia that is characterized by elevated serum triglyceride concentrations, low high-density lipoprotein (HDL) concentrations and small dense low-density lipoproteins. These abnormalities of dyslipidaemia are not reversed completely by tight glycaemic control. Hypertension is twice as common in patients with diabetes is in the general population, particularly in those who have microalbuminuria.

This concept of cardiovascular risk clustering was taken a step further by Gerald Reaven when he proposed that insulin resistance and its compensatory hyperinsulinaemia predisposed individuals to hypertension, dyslipidaemia and diabetes. The clustering has been termed the 'metabolic syndrome' (Box 14.12). The increased prevalence of metabolic syndrome features in people with diabetes largely explains the excess CVD in these patients.

Management of cardiovascular disease

Management of cardiovascular complications involves the aggressive management of each of the risk factors (Case history 14.3).

Patients should be advised to quit smoking and blood pressure should be tightly controlled. There is some evidence that the use of ACE inhibitors or angiotensin receptor blockers may confer an additional benefit. Patients with diabetes should be treated with lipid-lowering therapy, including statins, although the use of fibrates or other drugs that target HDL-

---

BOX 14.11 Mechanisms leading to accelerated atherosclerosis in people with diabetes

- Hyperglycaemia
  - advanced glycaemic end-products
- Higher prevalence of traditional risk factors
  - hypertension
  - dyslipidaemia
  - obesity

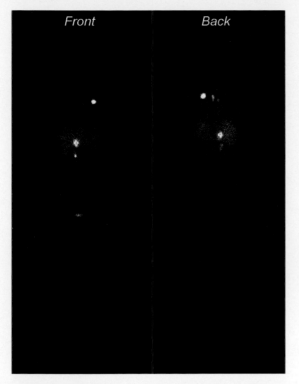

Front   Back

Plate 4.1 mIBG uptake by a phaeochromocytoma. A whole body I¹²³ mIBG scan with imaging from the front and back shows a right phaeochromocytoma with pulmonary and bony metastases. This type of imaging is helpful to investigate the potential for multisite disease prior to adrenalectomy. Image kindly provided by Dr Val Lewington, Royal Marsden Hospital.

1 month pre-op : 6 months post-op

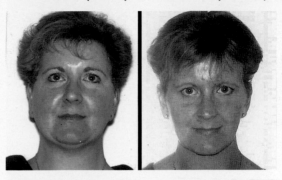

Plate 6.1 Cushing syndrome due to an adrenocortical adenoma secreting cortisol and sex steroid precursors. The face is shown immediately prior to operation and 6 months after right adrenalectomy (also see Fig. 4.7). The striking difference required the patient to renew her passport.

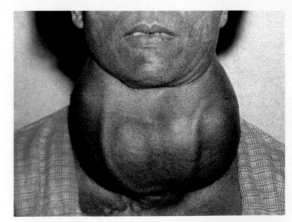

Plate 8.1 A large goitre due to iodine deficiency. Note the engorged veins overlying the gland, implying an obstruction by the goitre to venous drainage. The photograph was kindly provided by Professor David Phillips, University of Southampton.

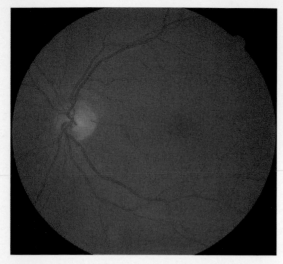

Plate 14.1 Normal fundus. Reproduced with the kind permission of the Southampton Mobile Retinal Screening Programme.

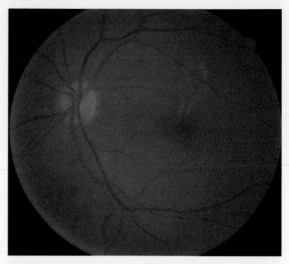

Plate 14.3 Diabetic maculopathy. The appearance is similar to Plate 14.2 but there are lesions within one disc diameter of the macula. Note how the hard exudates appear as an ellipse where fat has leaked from a single vessel. Reproduced with the kind permission of the Southampton Mobile Retinal Screening Programme.

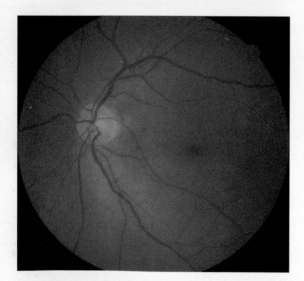

Plate 14.2 Mild background diabetic retinopathy. There are scattered 'dots and blots' and occasional hard exudates in the upper part of the fundus. Reproduced with the kind permission of the Southampton Mobile Retinal Screening Programme.

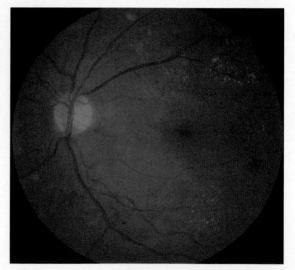

Plate 14.4 Preproliferative diabetic retinopathy. The changes are much more extensive and we start to see cotton wool spots (areas of retinal ischaemia), venous abnormalities and intraretinal microvascular abnormalities. Reproduced with the kind permission of the Southampton Mobile Retinal Screening Programme.

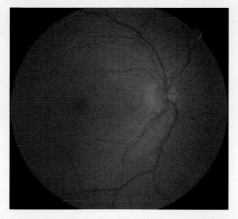

Plate 14.5 Proliferative diabetic retinopathy. There are new vessels growing at the disc (NVD). Reproduced with the kind permission of the Southampton Mobile Retinal Screening Programme.

Plate 14.7 High power view of new vessels seen in Plate 14.6. Reproduced with the kind permission of the Southampton Mobile Retinal Screening Programme.

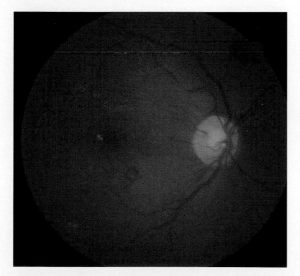

Plate 14.6 Proliferative diabetic retinopathy. There are new vessels growing close to the macula (new vessels elsewhere (NVE)). Reproduced with the kind permission of the Southampton Mobile Retinal Screening Programme.

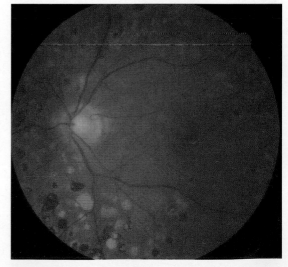

Plate 14.8 Fundal photograph showing extensive scarring of the retina following laser treatment of proliferative diabetic retinopathy.

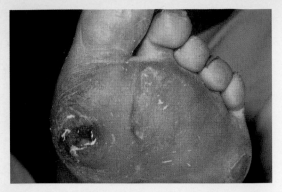

Plate 14.9 Plantar ulcer in a diabetic patient. Note how dry the skin appears and see how the callous has built up around the ulcer. Reproduced with the kind permission of Professor Cliff Shearman, University of Southampton.

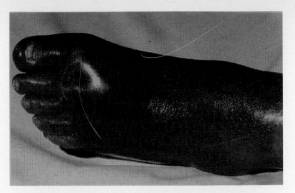

Plate 14.12 Moist gangrene. Not all necrosis appears as in Plate 14.10. Reproduced with the kind permission of Professor Cliff Shearman, University of Southampton.

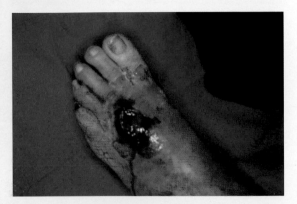

Plate 14.10 Infected diabetic ulcer on the dorsum of the foot. Reproduced with the kind permission of Professor Cliff Shearman, University of Southampton.

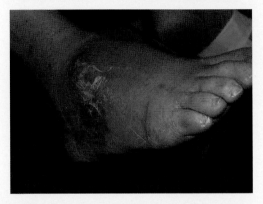

Plate 14.13 Active Charcot arthropathy. Reproduced with the kind permission of Mr Graham Bowen, Chief Podiatrist, Southampton University Hospitals NHS Trust.

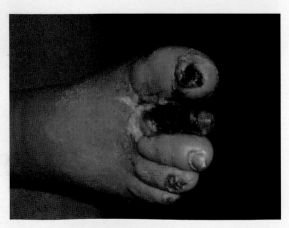

Plate 14.11 The combination of infection and vascular disease puts the diabetic foot at risk of necrosis as is seen in the toe of this patient. Reproduced with the kind permission of Mr Graham Bowen, Chief Podiatrist, Southampton University Hospitals NHS Trust.

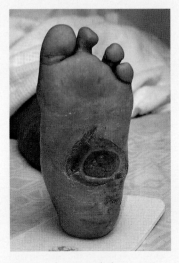

Plate 14.14 Plantar ulcer in a diabetic patient whose foot has become deformed by a Charcot arthropathy. Note also the amputation. Reproduced with the kind permission of Professor Cliff Shearman, University of Southampton.

CASE HISTORY 14.3

A 65-year-old man with diabetes for 20 years was treated with glibenclamide 15 mg daily and rosiglitazone 8 mg daily; HbA_{1c} 8.5%; past medical history of myocardial infarction; intolerant of metformin; microalbuminuria but no other microvascular complications; weighs 120 kg; blood pressure 150/100; serum total cholesterol 5.1 mmol/L; HDL cholesterol 0.7 mmol/L; and triglycerides 2.0 mmol/L.

What do you do now?

Answers, see p. 251

---

cholesterol, such as nicotinic acid, are appropriate in patients with low HDL concentration despite statin therapy. Although aspirin may not be as effective in patients with diabetes as in the general population because of the procoagulant state seen in diabetes, aspirin is also recommended in patients whose blood pressure is adequately controlled unless there is a specific contraindication. The benefits seen with thiazolidinediones may reflect their effect on multiple risk factors rather than blood glucose control alone.

Angina in patients with diabetes should be managed conventionally. Cardioselective β-blockers may be particularly useful. If symptoms worsen, early consideration should be given to coronary angiography and revascularization. Acute coronary syndrome and myocardial infarction have higher mortality rates among patients with diabetes than within the general population and therefore intensive therapy using thrombolysis, low molecular weight heparin, a β-blocker and either the platelet inhibitor clopidogrel or an inhibitor of platelet glycoprotein IIb/IIIa such as tirofiban or eptifibatide is required. It is also important to control blood glucose tightly at the time of the acute coronary event is this has been shown to improve survival (Case history 14.4).

Coronary revascularization is technically more difficult in patients with diabetes because of the diffuse and distal pattern of coronary atheroma. Coronary angioplasty with stenting is the preferred procedure for accessible large-vessel disease, with coronary artery bypass grafting being reserved for difficult or multiple occlusions and for restenosis after angioplasty.

BOX 14.12 International Diabetes Federation criteria for the metabolic syndrome

- Ethnic specific waist circumference
  - White European (≥94 cm for men, ≥80 cm for women)
  - Chinese and South Asian (≥90 cm for men, ≥80 cm for women)

Plus two of the following or treatment of the following:

- Hypertriglyceridaemia (≥150 mg/dl or 1.69 mmol/L)
- HDL cholesterol
  - men <40 mg/dL (1.04 mmol/L)
  - women <50 mg/dL (1.29 mmol/L)
- Hypertension ≥130/85
- High fasting glucose ≥100 mg/dL (≥5.6 mmol/L)

CASE HISTORY 14.4

A 60-year-old nondiabetic man presents with an uncomplicated acute myocardial infarction. His blood glucose on admission is 11.0 mmol/L. His blood pressure is 150/100. Serum total cholesterol 6.0 mmol/L, HDL cholesterol 1.0 mmol/L and triglycerides 2.0 mmol/L.

What are you immediate plans?

Answers, see p. 251

Psychological complications of diabetes

Patients with diabetes are at increased risk of several psychological problems, including anxiety and depression. Children may also have difficulties with cognitive functioning and academic achievement, particularly if they have repeated hypoglycaemia or hospitalization. Cognitive dysfunction also occurs more frequently in the elderly. Although most children and adolescents cope well during the course of diabetes, some individuals find it hard to adjust to their diagnosis. This may result in social withdrawal, sleeping difficulties and somatic complaints. The diabetes may be used by adolescents as a means of rebelling against their parents.

These psychological factors affect diabetes management and health outcomes. The patient, and not the healthcare professional, is responsible for nearly all of diabetes care, and psychological distress can lead to poor adherence to self-care behaviours such as taking medicine, complying with diet and monitoring. Support from family members and good communication can improve diabetic control. Interventions to reduce psychological distress include individual psychotherapy or counselling as well as group therapy. Depression may require pharmacological treatment.

Social aspects of diabetes

Diabetes affects the lifestyle of patients in the number of ways. There are limitations to driving and employment opportunities.

Driving

The main problems for drivers with diabetes are hypoglycaemia and visual impairment from either retinopathy or cataract. Diabetic drivers must actively avoid hypoglycaemia as this may impair motor skills and judgement (Box 14.13). Impaired awareness of hypoglycaemia is therefore a relative contraindication to driving. Diabetic drivers are required to inform the relevant authorities in most countries. Several tips can reduce the chance of accidents and it is important to ensure that all diabetic drivers are aware of their responsibilities to themselves and other road users.

> **BOX 14.13 Advice to reduce the risk of a road traffic accident**
>
> - Check blood glucose before driving and regularly on long journeys
>   - testing strips should be available within the vehicle
> - Take frequent rests with snacks and meals
> - Ensure that there is fast and longer-acting carbohydrate in the vehicle in case of hypoglycaemia
> - Do not drive if hypoglycaemia occurs; switch off the engine and leave the driver's seat
> - Do not drive within 45–60 min of an episode of hypoglycaemia

Employment

Certain employment opportunities are restricted where hypoglycaemia may pose a risk to the diabetic worker or their colleagues. This includes work in the Armed Forces, civil aviation or emergency services. Commercial driving or work in dangerous areas such as offshore or overhead working is restricted

Diabetes and pregnancy

Epidemiology

Diabetes is the commonest medical problem seen in pregnant women. It affects 2 to 5% of all pregnancies within the UK. Among pregnancies complicated by diabetes, 25% of cases involve pre-existing type 1 diabetes, 10% involve pre-existing type 2 diabetes and the remaining 65% involve gestational diabetes, which may or may not resolve after the pregnancy.

Effect of diabetes on pregnancy

Women with diabetes are at increased risk of losing a baby during pregnancy, having a baby with a congenital malformation or the infant dying within the first year of life. The perinatal mortality rate is approximately three to fivefold higher than the general population and the congenital malformation rate is six to 10-times higher.

In the first trimester, hyperglycaemia is terato-genic and all major malformations are increased in diabetic pregnancies. The miscarriage rate is increased. During the second half of the pregnancy, maternal hyperglycaemia leads to accelerated fetal growth and so macrosomia (defined as a baby whose weight is above the 95th centile for gestational age) is common. This increases the risk of an operative or traumatic birth. Despite its size, the baby born to a diabetic mother behaves like a premature baby in many ways: the risk of respiratory distress, jaundice and hypoglycaemia are all increased. Still birth rates are increased, particularly post-term. Tight control of blood glucose will reduce all pregnancy-related complications of diabetes but even in the best centres, the outcomes in diabetic mothers remain worse than the general population.

Effect of pregnancy on diabetes

Pregnancy induces a state of insulin resistance which is maximal in the second and third trimesters. This encourages nutrient transfer to the growing fetus and is largely caused by placental hormones. The change in insulin resistance affects the management of diabetes as insulin requirements change dramatically during pregnancy. Insulin requirement usually goes up by 50 to 100% in the latter half of pregnancy. In contrast, the insulin requirement may fall in the first trimester and this can be associated with increased hypoglycaemia and hypoglycaemia unawareness rates at this time.

The pregnancy may accelerate diabetic retinopathy and nephropathy. This may be caused by the rapid tightening of glycaemic control but a specific but unknown aspect of pregnancy may also have a role.

Management of diabetic pregnancy

Pre-existing diabetes
The outcome of a diabetic pregnancy is heavily dependent on the optimization of glycaemic control from the outset of pregnancy and so the management of a diabetic pregnancy begins well before the woman considers pregnancy. It is important that once a woman reaches childbearing age, she is educated about the risks of diabetes in pregnancy and the need for a planned pregnancy.

Preconception care
Many centres now run preconception clinics to allow these issues to be discussed more fully. It is important to check for microvascular complications of diabetes in the preconception period. Potentially harmful drugs should be discontinued and other medical therapy reviewed. The insulin regimen should be adjusted to bring blood glucose concentrations into the nondiabetic range. In women with pre-existing diabetes there is a higher risk of spina bifida and anencephaly and so a higher dose of folic acid (5 mg) is recommended.

Antenatal care
Once the pregnancy is confirmed, women should attend a specialized joint antenatal diabetes clinic. Regular contact with the diabetes team is important to ensure that suitable adjustment to the insulin regimen is made. Patients should be supplied with glucagon and instructed how to treat hypoglycaemia. It is important to screen for microvascular complications regularly during the pregnancy. The obstetrician is responsible for screening for malformations. Growth scans and other tests of fetal well-being should also be performed during the third trimester.

Birth
Most babies born to diabetic mothers are delivered before term because of the higher risk of still birth. For many women this will involve the induction of labour or caesarean section. During labour it is important that glycaemic control is maintained by an intravenous insulin glucose infusion.

Postnatal care
Following birth, the insulin requirement will drop dramatically and most women will return to their preconception doses immediately. Where possible the neonatal baby should remain with the mother although increased monitoring for hypoglycaemia will be required. Breast-feeding should be encouraged.

Gestational diabetes
Gestational diabetes is defined as diabetes occurring for the first time in pregnancy and occurs in at-risk women because of the insulin resistance of

pregnancy (Box 14.14). The risk factors for gestational diabetes are the same as for type 2 diabetes and so gestational diabetes can be regarded as the early unmasking of a metabolic abnormality brought on by the demands of pregnancy.

The management of gestational diabetes begins with lifestyle modification. This is similar to the advice given to patients with type 2 diabetes. Although the diet should provide sufficient calories and nutrients to meet the needs of the pregnancy, micronutrient-rich foods, such fruit, vegetables and low-fat dairy products rather than energy-dense, high-fat foods, will help control maternal blood glucose levels. The mother should be encouraged to include at least 30 min per day of physical activity in her daily routine.

When this is insufficient to control the glucose, pharmacotherapy is required. Although insulin is the most commonly used means of maintaining glucose control, there is research suggesting that certain oral hypoglycaemic agents can be used safely in pregnancy.

Women with gestational diabetes are at increased risk of developing type 1 and type 2 diabetes in the future. Approximately 50% of women will develop diabetes within 10 years of the index pregnancy. They should be targeted for lifestyle intervention to reduce their risk and should be screened regularly for diabetes.

The annual review

The provision of high-quality diabetes care is essential for all people with diabetes in order to achieve the best possible health outcomes. The growing numbers of people with diabetes has meant that traditional specialist care services are being swamped and new models of care are being developed. No single person or setting can provide all that is required in diabetes care. Consequently, both primary and secondary sectors are needed to ensure the delivery of appropriate structured care that is the hallmark of a good diabetes service.

The diabetes team is truly multidisciplinary, involving dieticians, podiatrist, pharmacists and psychologists as well as doctors and nurses. Diabetes specialist nurses play a crucial role in diabetes care, with important duties in clinical care and advice, education of patients and healthcare professionals as well as providing counselling and help to patients with diabetes. It is important that care is structured to ensure that patients receive all appropriate aspects. One way of doing this is to perform an annual review, during which the different aspects of care are systematically considered (Box 14.15)

BOX 14.15 The annual review

- Lifestyle
  - smoking
  - driving/DVLA (website www.dvla.gov.uk)
  - weight and diet (including alcohol)
  - physical activity
  - review social situation (e.g. carers)
  - pregnancy and prepregnancy advice
- Macrovascular screening
  - medication review
  - lipids
  - blood pressure
  - aspirin
  - angina
  - claudication—consider referral for intervention if deterioration of symptoms
  - cerebrovascular disease
- Glycaemia
  - HbA_{1c}
  - hypoglycaemia
  - insulin—injection sites, technical problems
- Microvascular screening
  - eyes
  - microalbuminuria
  - feet
  - erectile dysfunction
- Education
  - assess need for formal education
  - promote Diabetes UK

BOX 14.14 Diagnosis of gestational diabetes

There is a lot of controversy about the diagnosis of gestational diabetes. The World Health Organization recommends a 75-g oral glucose tolerance test at ~26 to 28 weeks gestation with the following cut-off values:
- Fasting glucose ≥ 7.0 mmol/L or
- 2-h 75 g oral glucose tolerance ≥ 7.8 mmol/L
This is similar to impaired glucose tolerance and diabetes outside pregnancy

KEY POINTS

- Diabetes is associated with a number of long-term complications

- These can be divided into microvascular and macrovascular

- Microvascular complications include:
  — retinopathy
  — nephropathy
  — neuropathy

- The aetiology of the microvascular complication is not fully understood but improved glycaemic control and blood pressure can slow the progression

- The burden of myocardial infarction, stroke and peripheral vascular disease increases in patients with diabetes

- The cause is multifactorial and so a systematic review of all cardiovascular risk factors is needed

- Diabetes is associated with psychosocial problems

- Pregnancy outcomes in diabetes are worse than the general population but may be improved by assiduous glycaemic control

- A systematic approach to the management of diabetes is needed, with a multidisciplinary team

Answers to case histories

Case history 14.1

An infected foot ulcer in a patient with diabetes is a medical emergency. Left untreated it can develop into a limb-threatening condition within a few days. Treatment will include debridement of the ulcer, culture of swabs and broad-spectrum antibiotics. Pressure must be taken off the foot and so bedrest should be advised. It is important to obtain good glycaemic control to improve healing and resolution of the infection. It is likely that insulin will be needed acutely. Her presentation will provide a good opportunity to assess her feet for neuropathy and peripheral vascular disease. Advice and education about foot care and appropriate shoes should be given.

Case history 14.2

There are a number of reasons why this man may have developed erectile dysfunction. It is likely that the cause is organic because of the lack of early morning erections. Furthermore, he has a good relationship with his wife. Diabetes, through autonomic neuropathy and endothelial dysfunction, are likely to be major contributors and his antihypertensive medication and simvastatin may also worsen the erectile dysfunction. He is drinking too much alcohol and this may also worsen his erectile dysfunction.

It is important to institute simple measures such as advice to reduce his alcohol consumption. It may be possible to switch some of the antihypertensives to drugs that are less associated with erectile dysfunction. However, this must be balanced against the cardioprotective effect of the drugs. The drug of choice for this man would be sildenafil.

Case history 14.3

This man is at high risk of further cardiovascular events and all risk factors should be targeted. His total cholesterol is above ideal and so a statin is indicated. His HDL cholesterol is low and a fibrate or nicotinic acid may be indicated if the HDL is not corrected by the statin. His blood pressure is above ideal and aggressive treatment of this is needed. Although the blood pressure target is more important than the agent used, it is likely that an ACE inhibitor or angiotensin receptor blocker should be included as he has microalbuminuria. He is overweight and efforts should be made to help bring down his weight through lifestyle modification but using drugs if necessary. Aspirin is indicated.

Case history 14.4

His myocardial infarction should be managed in the usual way with thrombolysis, analgesia, low molecular weight heparin, β-blockers, aspirin, clopidogrel and oxygen. Although we cannot make a formal diagnosis of diabetes at this stage, it is important to manage his blood glucose aggressively. This is most easily achieved with intravenous insulin.

CHAPTER 15

15 Obesity

LEARNING OBJECTIVES

- To understand the importance of obesity, including its links with diabetes
- To understand the hormonal and social determinants of eating behaviours
- To understand the pathogenesis of obesity and the

public health measures needed to reduce the prevalence of obesity
- To know the treatment options for the patient with obesity

In this chapter we will examine the epidemic of obesity

Introduction

The prevalence of obesity has increased dramatically over the last two decades throughout the world and is associated with a range of medical and psychological complications. It is now recognized that obesity is one of the most important public health problems of our time. Despite this, the trend of increasing obesity continues, indicating that current public health measures to prevent obesity are failing.

Although there is a high degree of heritability for obesity, the rapid rise in the prevalence of obesity suggests that environmental factors, such as altered diets and decreased energy expenditure, are more important in the change in obesity patterns within countries. Body weight is tightly regulated such that even small mismatches of less than 100 kcal/day in energy intake and expenditure may result in massive obesity. Despite this, the management of the individual with obesity is challenging. There is much pes-

simism regarding weight reducing programmes and it has been said that 'most obese people do not enter treatment, most who do fail to lose weight and most who lose weight regain it'.

If we are to implement changes to reduce the health burden of obesity, it is important to understand the causes of obesity and realistic aims of weight-management programmes. The purpose of this chapter is to examine the latest evidence around obesity to help prepare doctors to reduce the obesity burden among their patients.

What is obesity?

Normal weight and degrees of either overweight or underweight are defined by the World Health Organization using the body mass index (Box 15.1).

The definition of obesity and overweight, as well as underweight, are based on the actuarial observation that mortality has a J-shaped relation to body mass index with mortality being lowest within the BMI range of 20 to 25 kg/m² and increasing at BMIs above and below this range (Box 15.2). The effect of low BMI on mortality may have been overestimated because of the effect of smoking and consequent illness and clinical disorders causing weight loss (Fig. 15.1). These data are based on white European subjects and for individuals of South Asian ethnicity, the upper limit of normal BMI may need to be reduced.

Why worry about weight excess?

'Thou seest that I have more flesh than another man and therefore more frailty . . .' King Henry IV Part 1 Act III, Scene III

It is estimated that obesity reduces life expectancy by around 9 years and accounts for 30000 deaths in the UK per annum. It costs the UK National Health Service £480 million or 1.5% of total expenditure. In addition, indirect costs are probably £2 billion. Overweight and obesity are also associated with a number of metabolic and cardiovascular complications, musculoskeletal disease and several cancers (Table 15.1), accounting for 18 million days sickness absence per annum.

Obesity increases the risk of diabetes, dyslipidaemia and insulin resistance by more than threefold while increasing coronary heart disease and hypertension two to threefold. It is estimated that up to 80% of all new cases of diabetes can be attributed to obesity. The risk of developing type 2 diabetes increases across the normal range, such that the risk of

---

BOX 15.1 How to calculate body mass index

Body mass index is calculated according to the following formula:
   Weight in kilograms/(height in metres)²

BOX 15.2 The WHO definitions of underweight, overweight and obesity

- Underweight BMI <18.5 kg/m²
- Normal weight BMI 18.5–25 kg/m²
- Overweight >25 kg/m²
- Obesity BMI >30 kg/m²
- Morbid obesity BMI >40 kg/m².

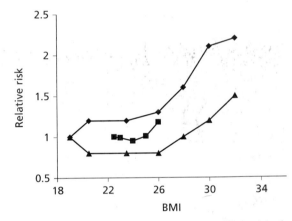

Figure 15.1 Relationship between BMI and relative risk of all cause mortality in US men and women. ■ Men ▲ All women ◆ Nonsmoking women with stable weight. Note how the J-shaped relationship disappears in women when only nonsmoking women with stable weight are considered. Note also that absolute risk is lower in non-smokers (date not shown).

Table 15.1 Health risks of obesity

Relative risk >3	Relative risk 2–3	Relative risk 1–2
Diabetes	Cardiovascular disease	Cancers—postmenopausal breast, endometrial, colon
Gallbladder disease	Hypertension	Reproductive hormone abnormalities—polycystic ovary syndrome, impaired fertility, fetal defects
Dyslipidaemia	Osteoathritis	Back pain
Insulin resistance	Hyperuricaemia	↑Anaesthetic risk
Breathlessness	Gout	
Sleep apnoea		

diabetes in a middle-aged woman whose BMI is greater than $35\,kg/m^2$ is 93.2 times greater than woman whose BMI is below $22.5\,kg/m^2$.

There is compelling evidence that our society discriminates against 'fat people' and this is damaging to the psychological well-being of obese individuals. Obese women are likely to leave school earlier, are less likely to be married and have higher rates of household poverty than women who are not overweight. These findings are independent of baseline socioeconomic status and are not seen in people with other chronic conditions such as asthma or musculoskeletal abnormalities.

The limitations of body mass index

As the health risks associated with obesity relate to an excess storage of body fat, and in particular visceral fat, certain individuals will be misclassified with body mass index. For any given BMI, women have a higher percentage of body fat than men (Box 15.3). This can lead to the anomalous situation where a lean young male bodybuilder may have an identical body mass index to a middle-aged obese woman. Nevertheless, across populations, body mass index correlates well with percentage body fat making this an easy measure of obesity.

Body fat may be preferentially located in the abdomen (central obesity) or surrounding the hips and thighs (peripheral obesity). Central obesity is associated with the metabolic syndrome and is a better predictor of health risk; at the same level of obesity, the more visceral fat, the greater the risk of developing cardiovascular and metabolic complications of obesity. Differences in the distribution of body fat explain why individuals from Asian backgrounds are at higher risk of the complications of obesity for any given BMI than white Europeans, as Asians tend to have greater central fat distribution. There are also gender differences in body fat distribution with most

> **BOX 15.3 Percentage body fat in men and women**
>
> In adult men of average weight, the percentage body fat is around 15 to 20%, while in women this percentage is higher at 25 to 30%.

women developing peripheral obesity while men develop central adiposity.

The use of the waist measurement can be used to identify those at high risk of developing the metabolic complications of obesity, particularly if combined with a fasting triglyceride concentration. Waist measurements of 100 to 102 cm in men and 88 to 90 cm in women alone provide useful reference values to identify obese patients who may be at high risk for chronic metabolic diseases. If hypertriglyceridaemia (>2.0 mmol/L) is also present, over 80% of men with waist measurements greater than 90 cm will be at risk of the metabolic syndrome.

Obesity trends

The WHO MONICA project has been following obesity trends in 21 countries among randomly selected middle-aged participants from the early 1980s to the mid-1990s. Mean BMI as well as the prevalence of overweight has increased in virtually every Western European country, Australia, USA and China.

Within the UK, the prevalence of obesity in adults has almost trebled since 1980, such that in 2002, 23% of men and 25% of women were obese. The prevalence of obesity among children is lower but the increase in the prevalence of overweight is similar to the rise in obesity in adults. Obesity rates are higher in low social classes and in some ethnic minority groups, particularly from South Asia.

The Centers for Disease Control's Behavioral Risk Factor Surveillance System (BRFSS) provides dramatic evidence to demonstrate the continuing rise in the prevalence of obesity within the United States. Each year, state health departments use standard procedures to collect data through a series of monthly telephone interviews with US adults. In 1991, four states had obesity prevalence rates of 15 to 19% and no states had rates at or above 20%. In 2003, 15 states had obesity prevalence rates of 15 to 19%; 31 states had rates of 20 to 24%; and four states had rates greater than 25%. As these data rely on self-reported height and weight, it is likely that these represent underestimates of the true prevalence of obesity.

The cause of obesity

The causes of obesity are multifactorial, and range

from purely genetic conditions, such as leptin deficiency, to entirely environmental conditions as seen in sumo wrestlers. It is, however, certain that obesity can only occur when energy intake remains greater than energy expenditure for a long period of time. Thus, if either energy intakes increases, or energy expenditure decreases or both, the individual will gain weight. Both energy intake and expenditure are affected by internal homeostatic mechanisms as well as external environmental factors.

Given the diversity of factors affecting energy balance, it is remarkable how well body weight can be regulated. Most adults are able to maintain their body weight to within a few kilograms over 40 or more years in spite of having eaten in excess of 20 tonnes of food. Even in individuals who become obese the mismatch between energy intake and energy expenditure is extremely small. Daniel Lamberts lived in Leicestershire, UK during the 18th century and earned a living by exhibiting himself as a natural curiosity, having reached the weight of 700 pounds (320 kg). It is estimated that when he died at the age of 39, he weighed 52 stone 11 pounds (336 kg), of which

approximately 230 kg would have been fat, containing approximately 2 million kcal. Assuming that there was progressive weight gain throughout his life, the excess consumption would have been only around 140 kcal/day, equivalent to an apple a day!

Control of appetite

Appetite is largely regulated by the ventromedial and lateral hypothalamus, with the ventromedial hypothalamus being a satiety centre and the lateral hypothalamus being thought of as a hunger centre. Lesions in the lateral hypothalamus cause complete cessation of feeding while stimulation of this area leads to overeating. The reciprocal is seen in the ventromedial hypothalamus. The neurobiology of appetite control is only now being unravelled (Fig. 15.2). The discovery of adipose tissue hormone, leptin, provided a new paradigm for our understanding of the control of body weight. Under normal circumstances, circulating leptin concentrations increase as fat mass increases and decrease as fat mass decreases.

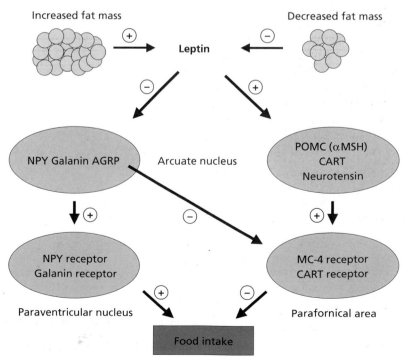

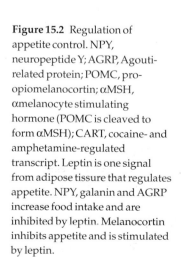

Figure 15.2 Regulation of appetite control. NPY, neuropeptide Y; AGRP, Agouti-related protein; POMC, pro-opiomelanocortin; αMSH, αmelanocyte stimulating hormone (POMC is cleaved to form αMSH); CART, cocaine- and amphetamine-regulated transcript. Leptin is one signal from adipose tissure that regulates appetite. NPY, galanin and AGRP increase food intake and are inhibited by leptin. Melanocortin inhibits appetite and is stimulated by leptin.

Leptin is secreted from adipocytes and signals to the brain to regulate fat mass. Leptin is actively transported across the blood–brain barrier and reaches the hypothalamus, where it binds to specific leptin receptors located on the surface of neuropeptide Y (NPY) containing cells. NPY has a powerful stimulating effect on appetite and leptin suppresses the secretion of NPY, leading to suppression of appetite. Thus as fat mass increases, the increased leptin suppresses NPY and appetite decreases. This provides a classical endocrine negative feedback mechanism by which appetite and basal metabolic expenditure is regulated in response to changing levels of adiposity. Leptin also acts to alter the secretion of several other hypothalamic neuropeptide hormones that are shown in Fig. 15.2.

The central action of leptin was first demonstrated by studies carried out in mice that had defective leptin secretion and who developed severe obesity. Abnormalities in the leptin receptor also led to severe obesity. This led to the hope that abnormalities in leptin action may be responsible for human obesity. While rare genetic abnormalities in humans in leptin and its receptor have been identified in cases of severe, early-onset obesity, in most situations leptin is increased in obesity and treatment with leptin does not lead to a fall in body weight. This is in contrast to the rare individuals with leptin deficiency whose body mass index falls dramatically with leptin therapy.

Genetic factors

The contribution of genetic factors has been shown from twin, family and adoption studies, which suggest that up to 70% of the variance of body mass index is accounted for by genetic variance. Over the last decade, in addition to genetic mutations in leptin and its receptor, a number of other human genes have been identified in which major missense or nonsense mutations have caused severe, early-onset obesity, usually through the disruption of normal appetite control mechanisms (Box 15.4). Although these cases only represent a minority of all obesity, these studies will begin to identify the critical molecular components of the human energy balance regulatory systems, which should allow the targeting of more effective therapies in the future.

BOX 15.4 Genetic syndromes and monogenic causes of obesity

- Conditions where obesity is the major feature
  - Leptin deficiency
  - Leptin receptor deficiency
  - Pro-opiomelanocortin deficiency
  - Melanocortin 4 receptor deficiency
  - Prohormone convertase 1 deficiency
- Genetic Syndromes in which obesity occurs
  - Prader–Willi syndrome
  - Laurence–Moon–Biedl syndrome
  - Biemond syndrome II
  - Alstrom syndrome
  - Carbohydrate-deficient glycoprotein syndrome type 1
  - Short stature obesity
  - Albright hereditary osteodystrophy
  - Borjeson–Forssman–Lehmann syndrome
  - Fragile X syndrome
  - Germinal cell aplasia Sertoli cell only syndrome
  - Simpson dysmorphia

Environmental changes

Despite the strong contribution of genetics to the development of obesity, the current obesity epidemic cannot be explained by genetics alone. The change in obesity patterns has arisen as the result of an adverse environment interacting with a susceptible genotype.

Dietary intake

The National Food Survey in United Kingdom provides the longest running continuous survey of household consumption in the world. This has shown that, over the last 50 years, food consumption within the home has decreased. At first sight these data appear to be paradoxical until it is remembered that as much as 50% of all food is consumed outside the home. Since the Second World War, within Europe more food is produced than is required. This has led to intense competition and incentives to bulk buy; there can be few people who have never taken advantage of 'two for the price of one' offers or the better value 'jumbo' pack.

The National Food Survey has also indicated that there are changes in the types of food that we are eating. There has been a shift from carbohydrate to fat consumption. This is important because most individuals regulate their meals size according to weight or volume rather than caloric intake. Fat contains approximately 9 kcal/g while carbohydrate and protein contain 4 kcal/g. Short-term metabolic studies show that when the fat content of the diet is increased, individuals continue to eat the same quantity of food and consequently move into positive energy balance.

There is some evidence from cross-sectional and longitudinal studies that the proportion of energy consumed as fat is linked with an increase in the prevalence of obesity. More recently, however, particularly in the UK and US, there has been a decline in the proportion of energy consumed as fat, while the prevalence of obesity continues to rise. This may reflect the relatively long lag phase in the development of obesity and so it may be many years before this dietary change affects the prevalence of obesity.

Physical activity

We have evolved to undertake vigorous physical activity and therefore it should be unsurprising that inactivity is associated with ill health. Total energy expenditure is the sum of our basal metabolic rate, dietary-induced thermogenesis, adaptive thermogenesis, such as shivering, and physical activity. Of these, physical activity offers the greatest scope for an individual to increase their energy expenditure. Physical activity can be defined as any bodily movement produced by skeletal muscle which results in energy expenditure and can be subdivided into different components, such as exercise or sport. Activity can be also divided according to its intensity and duration (Table 15.2). Low-intensity activities may include walking or household work while more intense activities may include running or cycling faster than 10 miles an hour or up hills. Sedentary behaviour, such as television viewing, is also significant when considering weight gain as it constrains the opportunity to be active and therefore reduces energy expenditure.

Physical inactivity is a major determinant of the current obesity epidemic. Several studies have shown that physically active people have lower levels of body fat and weight than inactive people. There are also strong relationships between indicators of inactivity, such as television viewing and car ownership, and secular trends in obesity. Unfortunately, epidemiological studies have shown that we are becoming progressively less active. The Allied Dunbar National Fitness Survey, undertaken in 1995, indicated that 29% of men and 28% of women were classed as sedentary while only 16% of men and 5% of women participated in regular vigorous activity. Inactivity increases with age but social class differences are not strong because occupational activity is often balanced with leisure time activity. In the US, 60% of adults were not regularly active and 25% reported no significant activity at all.

Table 15.2 Examples of light, moderate and vigorous physical activity

Activity	Light EE < 3.0 × BMR	Moderate EE: 3.0–6.0 × BMR	Vigorous EE: > 6.0 × BMR
Walking	Slowly	Briskly	Fast or jogging
Cycling	Slowly	Steadily or up slopes	>10 mph or up hills
Swimming	Slowly	Moderate exertion	Fast or treading water
Gym work	Stretching exercises	Sit-ups	Stair ergometer, ski machine
House work	Vacuum cleaning	Heavier cleaning	Moving furniture
Gardening	Weeding	Mowing the lawn with a power mower, sweeping, raking	Hand mowing or digging

EE, energy expenditure; BMR, basal metabolic rate.

Similarly, children are also becoming increasingly inactive.

Technological advances have reduced our physical activity in many spheres. The increasing number of cars has reduced the amount of physical activity we undertake travelling to and from work. It is estimated that household appliances have reduced our energy expenditure by around 500 kcal/day within the home. These trends have meant that we have endeavoured to compartmentalize our exercise into 30 to 40 min in the gym two or three times a week rather than focusing on increasing our energy expenditure throughout the day.

Psychological factors

As well as eating because we need to eat, many of us also eat for pleasure. Much of the research into obesity has been concerned with the former homeostatic control of eating rather than focusing on the latter hedonistic reasons why we eat. Yet these two aspects of eating are complementary and have two different CNS systems controlling them.

There is much to be learnt from studying the eating behaviours of people who gain weight. It is known that overweight individuals select more energy-dense food, display enhanced hunger traits with less satiety and eat larger and more frequent meals. Their eating behaviour is also less inhibited. Individuals who tend to gain weight have a greater readiness to eat and will eat opportunistically. There are differences in the timing of eating; obese individuals tend to eat more in the afternoon and less in the morning. In contrast, enjoyment from food is seen as being less important in those who do not gain weight and health rather than taste becomes a more important factor when choosing food (Case history 15.1).

Prevention of obesity

Despite the apparent simplicity of the solution for the prevention of obesity, there is little evidence of the efficacy of health education programmes within the general population. Education alone is probably insufficient and behaviour modification is also needed. Healthcare professionals need to take obesity seriously and must collectively support obesity prevention strategies to prevent the undermining of healthy lifestyle advice.

A public health and governmental response is also needed to reduce the obesity epidemic. This could include legislation or a more 'ecological' approach in which there is a co-ordinated strategy to influence the individual by education and behaviour change and the toxic environment through economic, physical and sociocultural pressures.

Management of the individual with obesity

The major aim of a weight-management programme is to improve health by reducing morbidity and mortality associated with obesity rather than simply lowering weight and adiposity. A 10% weight loss is associated with a major reduction in death and metabolic complications of obesity (Table 15.3).

Patient selection
The scale of the problem means that we are unable to treat all patients with obesity and therefore it is important to select patients that we are most likely to help. Characteristics of patients likely to lose weight during a weight-management programme are:
- High initial body mass
- High central obesity

CASE HISTORY 15.1

A 25-year-old female secretary attends to ask for help with her weight (BMI 27.4 kg/m²). She has read many magazines about slimmer of the year and has tried weightwatchers. She buys most of her food as ready prepared meals at the supermarket. She eats her lunch sitting at her desk with her work colleagues and eats her supper at home in front of the TV. She snacks on biscuits while at work.

What advice can you offer her?

Answers, see p. 263

Table 15.3 Benefits associated with 10% weight loss

Death	↓20–25% in premature mortality
Diabetes	↓50% in type 2 diabetes ↓30–50% in blood glucose
Lipids	↓10% in total cholesterol ↓30% in triglycerides
Blood pressure	↓10 mmHg in systolic BP ↓20 mmHg in diastolic BP

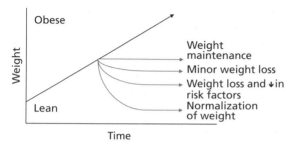

Figure 15.3 What is a successful outcome?

- High energy intake
- Initial weight loss

Early weight loss probably reflects the patient's ability to comply with the weight-management programme. Patients need to be well motivated to undertake the lifestyle changes. High self-esteem and the acceptance of the need to change also predict weight loss. This is particularly challenging in the arena of mental illness where obesity may well complicate the mental state of the patient.

It is important to set appropriate goals to prevent disappointment and frustration during the programme. A 10% weight loss is an appropriate goal because it is achievable, results in significant health benefits and can be maintained. However, in one study when most patients were asked how much weight they would like to lose, only 1% reported they would be happy with a weight loss of less than 10% while 63% expected to lose more than 20% of weight. The natural history of body weight throughout a lifetime is a gradual increase, and therefore the first aim of a weight-management programme is to prevent further weight gain before moving on to weight loss (Fig. 15.3). Congratulating patients on maintaining

weight can improve self-esteem and therefore lead on to a long-term adherence to the programme.

Patient should also be aware of the long-term challenge of weight loss. In the same way that weight gain occurred over many years, a lifelong change to their lifestyle is needed to reduce weight. Patient should be encouraged not to think of 'short-term fixes'. A significant portion of our total energy intake is made up from the basal metabolic rate. If energy intake falls below basal metabolic rates, strong protective adaptations occur to try to maintain weight. The patient feels lethargic, tired and listless and will be unable to maintain this situation for any length of time. Too great a calorie deficit will therefore lead to failure! On the other hand if a deficit of around 500 kcal is advocated, the patient can lose around 1 kg of weight per week and this is sustainable over the long term (Fig. 15.4).

Dietary strategies

There is a huge popular literature about diets that will aid weight loss. Most of these diets fail to appreciate that nutrition is a demand led process and therefore any diet should meet the requirements of the body. There is a need to include both fats and carbohydrates as energy supplies and any diet that excludes one or other of these components will create a mismatch between supply and demand. Diets need to be sustainable over the long-term and most diets that exclude many different food types, such as the Atkins or Ornish diet, cannot be maintained for more than several months (Box 15.5).

The first aim of dietary advice therefore must be to ensure that the individuals eat sufficient food to meet their metabolic needs (Fig. 15.4). Patient should be advised to avoid extreme eating restraints and dieting. In order to reduce calorie consumption, two dietary changes should be considered: the types of food should be changed and portion sizes reduced. A systematic review of all dietary interventions lasting greater than 1 year found that there is little evidence to support the use of diets apart from low fat diets for weight reduction. Low fat diets for up to 36 months resulted in modest weight losses of around 3.5 kg. The consumption of low-energy-dense foods and sweeteners may also reduce meal energy intake.

Portion size is also extremely important. There is good evidence that energy intake is proportional to

BOX 15.5 Eating and activity objectives in weight-management programme

Eating objectives
- Regain control (rehabilitation)
  - avoid extreme eating restraint/dieting
  - eat sufficient food to ensure metabolic control and adequate intake of nutrients
  - re-establish 'normal' eating behaviour and attitudes towards food
  - appreciate scale of challenge
- Modest reduction in energy intake (−500 kcal/d)
  - eat well but with lower fat, sugar and alcohol intake
  - maintain sufficient energy (>BMR) and nutrients to satisfy minimal requirements

Activity objectives
- Decrease amount of time sitting and supine
- Low intensity activity—not exercise!
- Total time spent active does not have to be a single bout of 'continuous activity sufficiently vigorous to make you out of breath or sweaty', i.e. 10 times 3 min as good as 1 times 30 min
- Activity must fit in with daily life and functional capabilities of individual
- Activity should be pleasurable

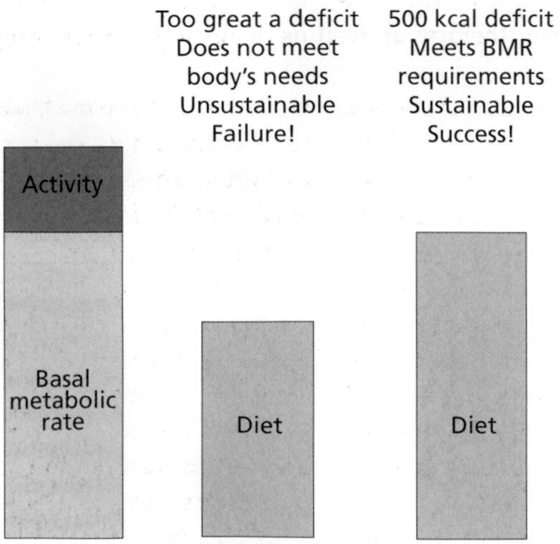

Figure 15.4 Rationale of 500 kcal deficit diet.

the amount of food available at mealtimes and by reducing portion size energy consumption falls. Over the last decade the average size of dinner plate in the United States restaurant has gone up from 9 inches to 12 inches! The same volume of food on a larger plate appears smaller and therefore this will lead to overconsumption while the use of a small plate is a useful means by which patients can reduce portion size.

It is important to re-establish 'normal' eating behaviour and attitudes towards food. Many people eat for reasons that have nothing to do with hunger. For example, people might eat from boredom, to cope with sadness or to be sociable. Encouraging healthy eating patterns can lead to a reduction in energy intake. It is important that while food is consumed, the individual's attention is focused on the food. If the attention is divided, such as by working at a computer, the reward gained from eating is reduced and therefore people eat more. It is important that food does not become associated with other activities, such as watching television, because this will lead to less healthy eating behaviours. Patients should be advised to eat only at a dining-room or kitchen table at mealtimes. Cravings for food are often short lived and therefore a useful strategy can be to distract the patient with an alternative activity such as a 5-min walk when a craving occurs. The value of commercial weight loss programmes has not been fully established but they may lead to greater weight loss than an individual's own attempts to lose weight.

Exercise

Exercise can play an important part in a weight-management programme (Box 15.5). While high energy expenditure can outstrip energy intake and therefore promotes weight loss in its own right, exercise also has a role in the prevention of weight regain when combined with dietary interventions. It is important that patients decrease the amount of time that they spend sitting or occupied in sedentary activities. Low intensity activity is also of great importance; for example an 80-year-old patient with agitated Alzheimer's disease will expand more calories per day than an Olympic athlete because the patient with Alzheimer's is walking for nearly 24 h every day. The total time spent active is important and exercise does not need to be undertaken in a single period. Patients need to think about ways of including physical activity in their everyday lives. This can be achieved in many areas; for example patients can be encouraged to use the stairs rather than lifts, to get off the bus one stop early, or to park at the far end of the car park rather than right next to the door. Physical activity needs to fit in with daily life and the functional capabilities of individual and ideally should be pleasurable. The most appropriate type of exercise that patients can undertake is the one that will still be pursued a decade later.

Drugs

Pharmacological treatment of obesity has a chequered history and many physicians still regard these drugs with suspicion and scepticism. Whilst it is true that the currently available drugs are relatively ineffective when used alone, when used in combination with lifestyle and behavioural modification programs, they are a useful adjunct in the management of obesity (Fig. 15.5). The drugs that are currently available can be divided into two main categories, those acting on the gastrointestinal system and centrally acting drugs which affect appetite. The three drugs that are currently available for the management of obesity are:

- orlistat, which is a pancreatic lipase inhibitor
- sibutramine, which is a serotonin and noradrenaline reuptake inhibitor.
- rimonabant, which is an endocannabinoid receptor antagonist

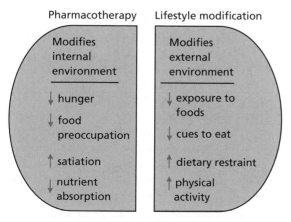

Figure 15.5 Additive effects of diet and drugs.

Orlistat inhibits pancreatic and gastric lipases, thereby reducing ingested triglyceride hydrolysis. It produces a dose-dependent reduction in dietary fat absorption that is near maximal at the currently available dose of 120 mg three times a day. In clinical trials lasting up to 4 years it leads to modest weight loss of up to 10%. This weight loss is associated with a reduction in other cardiovascular risk factors including waist circumference, blood pressure, dyslipidaemia and hyperglycaemia. In patients with impaired glucose tolerance, it reduces the risk of incident diabetes by 37% over and above the effect of lifestyle intervention alone. In patients with pre-existing diabetes, many may be able to reduce or discontinue their oral hypoglycaemic medication.

The main limiting factor for the use of orlistat is the development of gastrointestinal side-effects secondary to fat malabsorption. These include loose or liquid stools, faecal urgency and anal discharge and can be associated with fat soluble vitamins malabsorption. As the consumption of a high fat diet will inevitably lead to severe gastrointestinal side-effects, it is important that the prescription of orlistat is accompanied by behavioural and dietary advice. Prior to the use of orlistat, it is important to educate the patient about the drug's mode of action and the dietary changes needed to reduce the side-effects. As facilities may not always be available locally, Roche, who manufacture the drug, have established a free telephone and online patient support programme that has been shown to improve the compliance with drug therapy as well as achieving greater weight loss.

When orlistat was first introduced into the United Kingdom, its license limited its usage to 2 years. However, as longer studies have been reported and there is a greater appreciation of the chronic relapsing nature of obesity, this restriction has now been removed and patients can continue to use the drug as long as it remains effective. It is important to note that the drug should not be considered ineffective because weight loss has stopped, provided the new lowered weight is maintained. Discontinuation of the drug at this stage may well lead to weight regain. There is no published literature to suggest that the use of orlistat is associated with dependency on the drug.

Sibutramine is a centrally acting serotonin and noradrenaline reuptake inhibitor which leads to diminished appetite and decreased food intake through activation of the β_1 and $5HT_{2a/2c}$ receptors. Clinical studies have shown that patients lose up to around 10% of body weight before reaching a plateau. If the drug is discontinued, weight is then regained. The weight loss is associated with a reduction in waist circumference, improved lipid profile and decreased insulin resistance. The noradrenergic effects of sibutramine can cause an increase in heart rate and blood pressure. However, this may be offset by the reduction in blood pressure that occurs with weight loss. Other side-effects include:

- dry mouth
- constipation
- insomnia
- irritability
- unusual impatience or excitation
- headache
- rhinitis and nausea

Within the UK, weight reducing drugs are recommended for use in patients whose BMI is greater than $30 kg/m^2$ or in patients with comorbidity whose BMI is greater than $28 kg/m^2$. Initially, the drug should be used for a 3-month trial period and should only be continued if the patient loses more than 5% of body weight. Furthermore, it should be reconsidered if the patient has not lost more than 10% of body weight within the first 6 months.

Rimonabant is an endocannabinoid 1 receptor antagonist, which has been shown to be effective in reducing body weight and in weight maintenance with up to 2 years of therapy in several phase III studies. It has recently entered clinical practice. Endocannabinoids increase food intake through endocannabinoid 1 receptor activation and animal experiments show that antagonism of this receptor reduces sucrose and food intake. Endocannabinoid 1 receptors are also found in peripheral tissues where activation of this receptor leads to increased insulin resistance, possibly through alteration in adipocytokine production, such as decreased adiponectin secretion. Antagonism of this receptor leads to weight loss and a reduction in features of the metabolic syndrome, with only around half of the improvements in meta-bolic profile being explained by changes in weight. The main side-effects of rimonabant are depressed mood, anxiety and nausea and therefore caution may be needed if this drug is to be used in patients with psychiatric illness. There have been small trials of CB1 antagonists in the treatment of schizophrenia and while inconclusive have not shown any worsening of psychiatric symptoms.

Several other drugs have been considered for the use in the management of obesity including pseudophedrine, ephedra, sertraline, yohimbine, amphetamine or its derivatives, bupropion, benzocaine, threachlorocitric acid, sertraline and bromocriptine. There is currently a paucity of data about their effectiveness and these were not recommended in a recent Cochrane systematic database review.

Bariatric surgery

Bariatric surgery is currently the only long-term cure for obesity. There are two main types of operation to treat obesity. Malabsorption techniques bypass part of the stomach or small intestine while restrictive surgery lead to reduced dietary intake by reducing the size of the stomach and therefore improves satiety. The best evidence for the long-term effects of gastric surgery for obesity comes from the Swedish Obese Subjects Study where the weight loss after 2 years was typically between 30 and 40 kg. Quality-of-life improves dramatically following surgery and this is associated with major improvements in meta-bolic side-effects of obesity. A review of bariatric surgery has also suggested that gastric bypass surgery is associated with a 99 to 100% prevention of diabetes in patients with impaired glucose tolerance and an 80 to 90% clinical resolution of diagnosed early type 2 diabetes.

At present, obesity surgery is only recommended for those with morbid obesity. Each patient requires an extensive preoperative assessment which includes a psychological assessment as surgery will not treat an eating disorder and may lead to worsening of the mental state if patients are dependent on food.

Conclusions

Obesity has become a major health problem throughout the world. While genetics can explain much of the variability of body mass index within a given population, it is environmental changes over the last 50 years that have precipitated the obesity epidemic. A public health and governmental response is needed to reduce the toxic environment in which we live. The management of the individual with obesity is challenging but successful results can be obtained through lifestyle modification when combined with realistic goals and patient selection. Drug therapy is currently in its infancy but the use of orlistat or sibutramine is a useful adjunct to weight loss. Bariatric surgery is the only long-term solution for patients with morbid obesity. There can no longer be a place for therapeutic nihilism and therefore we need to develop strategies within health settings to promote lifestyles that will both prevent and treat overweight and obesity.

Answer to case history

Case history 15.1

It is important to take a full dietary and exercise history although she has given you clues that she has unhealthy eating behaviours. Her expectations may be unrealistic if she wants to win the slimmer of the year and she needs to know what is achievable. It would be better for her to eat away from her desk at lunch—partly to increase her activity levels and partly because eating at her desk may become associated with feelings of relaxation. We see she is snacking on biscuits—is this a coping behaviour for a stressful job? Lower calorie snacks could be suggested but snacking should be discouraged. Cravings do not last long and so it might be worth suggesting she gets up and does something else for a few minutes when she has the urge to eat. It is likely that eating by the TV will increase her calorie intake and will lead to eating outside meal times. Encourage her to eat at a table where she can devote all her attention to the food. She has a sedentary job and should be encouraged to become more physically active.

Index

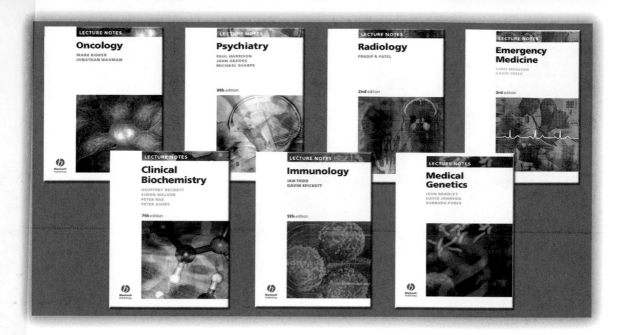

at a Glance

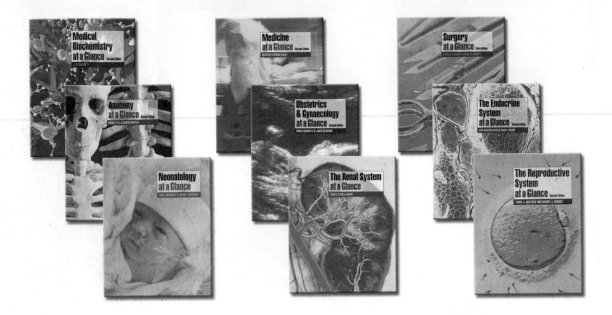

- The most simple and concise approach to all your subjects
  - Each bite-sized chapter covered in a double-page spread with key facts and fundamentals and a summary diagram
    - Perfect for exam preparation and use on clinical rotations

Titles in the at a Glance series

www.blackwellmedstudent.com

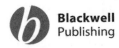

Blackwell Publishing